Handbook of Sepsis

W. Joost Wiersinga
Christopher W. Seymour
Editors

Handbook of Sepsis

Springer

ESGBIS
ESCMID STUDY GROUP FOR BLOODSTREAM INFECTIONS AND SEPSIS
European Society of Clinical Microbiology and Infectious Diseases

EUROPEAN SEPSIS ACADEMY

Editors
W. Joost Wiersinga
University of Amsterdam
Amsterdam
The Netherlands

Christopher W. Seymour
University of Pittsburgh
Pittsburgh
Pennsylvania
USA

ISBN 978-3-319-73505-4 ISBN 978-3-319-73506-1 (eBook)
https://doi.org/10.1007/978-3-319-73506-1

Library of Congress Control Number: 2018935395

Printed on acid-free paper

This Springer imprint is published by the registered company Springer International Publishing AG part of Springer Nature
The registered company address is: Gewerbestrasse 11, 6330 Cham, Switzerland

Preface

Sepsis is one of the most common deadly diseases. Despite its remarkable incidence, and despite the progress which has been made in understanding this complex syndrome, for both clinicians at the bedside and scientists at the bench many key questions remain unanswered.

In order to address this unmet need, we now present the first edition of the *Handbook of Sepsis*. This practically oriented book provides an up-to-date overview of all significant aspects of the pathogenesis of sepsis and its management. Readers will find information on the involvement of the coagulation and endocrine systems during sepsis and on the use of biomarkers to diagnose sepsis and allow early intervention. International clinical practice guidelines for the management of sepsis are presented, and individual chapters focus on aspects such as fluid resuscitation, vasopressor therapy, response to multiple organ failure, antimicrobial therapy, and adjunctive immunotherapy. The closing section looks forward to the coming decade, discussing novel trial designs, sepsis in low- and middle-income countries, and emerging management approaches. The book is international in scope, with contributions from leading experts across the world. It will be of value to professionals/practitioners that take care of patients with severe infections in all fields of medicine in addition to those who are in training or study sepsis in depth.

We would like to thank all our colleagues who all worked hard and full of enthusiasm on each and every chapter of this book. In this respect, the continued support of members of the European Sepsis Academy, the Surviving Sepsis Campaign guidelines committee, the European Society of Clinical Microbiology and Infectious Diseases, and the International Sepsis Forum has been truly inspiring. In addition, we gratefully acknowledge the continued and wonderful support of the editorial staff at Springer Nature. At the end, we do hope that this handbook can make a small contribution to the further improvement of care for patients with sepsis who present with this devastating syndrome on emergency departments, wards, and intensive care units in all corners of the world.

Amsterdam, The Netherlands — W. Joost Wiersinga
Pittsburgh, PA, USA — Christopher W. Seymour
March 2018

Contents

Part I

Sepsis: An Overview

What Is Sepsis?

1

Luuk Giesen and Mervyn Singer

1.1 Introduction

Sepsis is an enigmatic clinical syndrome that arises when a patient reacts adversely to an infection and develops organ dysfunction as a consequence. It can affect practically all organ systems, though the organs involved and the degree of dysfunction will vary markedly between patients. It can lead to death in a high proportion of cases.

Sepsis is now officially defined as a dysregulated host response to an infection, causing life-threatening organ dysfunction [1]. This new definition, and accompanying clinical criteria, will hopefully provide a stronger, more consistent base to better inform incidence, outcomes and research. The nature of sepsis is extremely complex, and the disease course can differ markedly between patients. As yet, sepsis cannot be determined with certainty in many cases. Diagnosis often relies upon clinician gestalt as definitive microbiological evidence of a precipitating infection is often absent. Moreover, attempts to find a magic cure for sepsis have been fruitless [2]. This is, in large part, due to a highly variable biological phenotype, even in patients presenting with similar clinical features. Management is mainly supportive at present with resuscitation, organ support and eradication of the underlying infection with antibiotics ± source control [2]. On a more positive note, our understanding of sepsis has profoundly increased, and better diagnostics are being developed to aid identification and target the dosing and timing of therapeutic interventions.

In the developed world, sepsis has an incidence of 2.5 million patients per year and a mortality rate of approximately 650,000 patients per year (when corrected for the new definition using only recent data) [3]. This would translate to roughly 19 million cases of sepsis a year globally, with approximately 5 million deaths [3]. This estimation is probably wildly inaccurate, as there is a general lack of

L. Giesen, M.D. · M. Singer, M.D., F.R.C.P.(Lon) (✉)
Bloomsbury Institute of Intensive Care Medicine, University College London, London, UK
e-mail: m.singer@ucl.ac.uk

W. J. Wiersinga, C. W. Seymour (eds.), *Handbook of Sepsis*,
https://doi.org/10.1007/978-3-319-73506-1_1

comprehensive epidemiological data in low- and middle-income countries. The lack of good primary care, adequate infection prevention, timely antibiotic treatment, poor staffing levels and adequate critical care provision account for a completely different situation in these countries. The World Health Organization provides additional insights into this conundrum. While the WHO does not yet monitor sepsis, it does track communicable diseases. According to WHO data, three infectious diseases were in the top ten causes of death worldwide in 2015: lower respiratory disease, diarrheal disease and tuberculosis with a combined mortality of 7.3 million people [4]. The majority of these fatalities occur in developing countries. It is likely that most die from sepsis as infection without organ dysfunction cannot be life-threatening. Chapter 15 will address sepsis in low- and middle-income countries in more detail.

The mortality rate of sepsis is declining in the developing world, in part because of earlier recognition and clinical management but also because increased recognition has considerably enlarged the denominator [5]. In some healthcare structures, there is also a financial reimbursement incentive to code patients as 'sepsis' rather than, for example, pneumonia [6]. Current cited mortality rates range from 15 to 25% in industrialized countries; however many uncertainties remain [3]. For example, sepsis may not always be recorded as the cause of death in the presence of other comorbidities such as cancer or heart failure. Second, death in a septic patient may relate to secondary or unrelated complications. Furthermore, to paraphrase Osler [7], sepsis may be the 'old man's friend', being the final event of a terminal and/or debilitating illness such as severe dementia, stroke and chronic heart failure. In such cases, it may be inappropriate and not in the patient's best interests to offer aggressive, life-prolonging, medical intervention. In the next chapter, the epidemiology of sepsis will be discussed in more depth.

1.2 The Origins of Sepsis

The riveting tale of sepsis is one of controversy and paradox, of huge success amidst grand failure and of the long-running debate on the relative importance of pathogen versus host response. Sepsis must be preceded by infection. Both histories start out intertwined, since sepsis was long viewed as a systemic infection with terms such as 'septicaemia' applied to a critically ill patient. Sepsis finally got its own narrative once it was appreciated that the consequent organ dysfunction is what defines the condition. Arguably, this matters most to patient outcomes.

The meaning of the term sepsis has undergone remarkable changes over the course of thousands of years (Fig. 1.1). Hippocrates (460–370 BC) first wrote of *sepsis* and *pepsis* [8]. He considered that both occurred simultaneously in the body in a balanced way; sepsis was associated with putrefaction (decay) and bad odour and pepsis with odourless fermentation. Aristotle (384–322 BC) hypothesized that the process of sepsis (as decay) also occurred outside the body, generating a conception of small creatures in smelly, muddy places. The Romans improved upon Aristotle's theory. As proximity to swamps induced sickness and fever in humans,

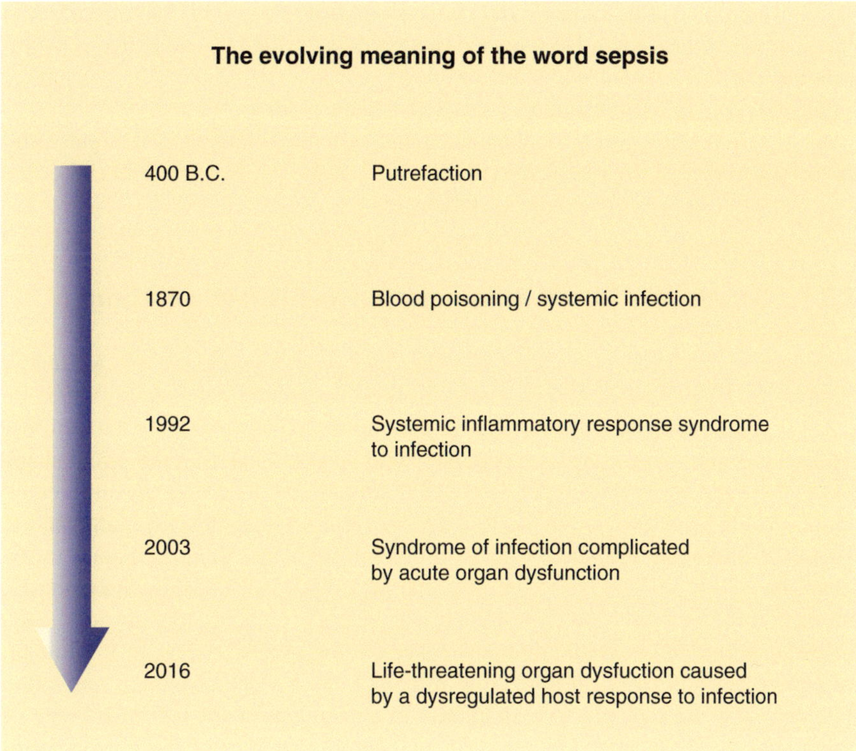

Fig. 1.1 The evolving meaning of sepsis

they believed Aristotle's small, invisible creatures were the actual cause of disease. They promptly created a novel goddess, *Febris*, and drained their swamps [8].

After the fall of the Roman Empire, efforts related to discovery and treatment of infection and sepsis either diminished or went unreported. In the following centuries, infectious epidemics wiped out large swathes of populations. This caused enormous terror as people could not understand how these diseases spread nor how they could be treated. The most infamous epidemic, the plague or the Black Death, was caused by the bacterium *Yersinia pestis* [9]. This bacterium generated a severe infection complicated by organ failure (thus, sepsis) and eradicated a third of all Europeans in the thirteenth century [10].

It was not until the scientific revolution in the seventeenth century that the understanding of infection and sepsis progressed further, and Aristotle's ideas were challenged. Two advances were important. The first was the development of the microscope, which allowed visualization of those invisible creatures. The second was the discovery that microbes could indeed cause human disease, and this was called germ theory [8].

Davaine (1812–1882), a French physician, shifted the perception from sepsis as decay to sepsis as infection [8]. He injected rotten blood subcutaneously into a rabbit, which died after 40 h. He then took blood from this rabbit and injected it in the next, which also died. He repeated this process 25 times. Hence, and notwithstanding the lack of bad odour of the blood, Davaine introduced the concept of septicaemia or 'blood poisoning' [11]. Sepsis then became synonymous with systemic infection [8]. It was widely believed that systemic infection, and in particular the pathogenicity of the bug, led to the patient's death [2]. Not until the end of the twentieth century was this concept challenged.

1.3 Sepsis Was About Inflammation and Not the Pathogen

Advances in infection prevention and the discovery of penicillin by Alexander Fleming in 1928 marked crucial events in both preventing and treating infection [12, 13]. The establishment of intensive care units (ICUs) from the 1950s further reduced mortality from sepsis as patients could be resuscitated in the initial shock state, and organ support could be provided to prop up the failed organs until recovery occurred [14]. However, in the 1970s, it was realized that, despite eradication of the initial pathogen and successful resuscitation, patients often continued to die from sepsis [2, 15]. This led to the idea that the culprit was not only the pathogen but also, and perhaps more importantly, the patient's inflammatory response [15, 16]. Attenuating the host inflammatory response was considered as, or even more, important as eliminating the infecting microorganism. Animal models supported this idea. The use of high-dose endotoxin (a constituent of the cell membrane of Gram-negative bacteria) led to a massive and abrupt rise in pro-inflammatory cytokines—a 'cytokine storm'—and other mediators of inflammation, which caused certain death [17]. Efforts to block these cytokines in young, previously healthy animals significantly improved survival, though administration of these agents at, or even before, the initiation of sepsis was far removed from real-life patient management. Nonetheless, these studies reinforced the notion that patients with sepsis had a systemic hyperinflammatory response to an infection, which could lead to organ dysfunction and death.

In 1992, a North American Consensus Committee officially defined sepsis as a systemic inflammatory response syndrome (SIRS) to infection [18]. This could lead to organ dysfunction (severe sepsis) and progress to a shock state (septic shock). This definition placed the systemic hyperinflammatory response at centre stage. SIRS was characterized by abnormalities in ≥2 of 4 clinical criteria: heart rate, respiratory rate (or $PaCO_2$), temperature and white cell count (Table 1.1).

Table 1.1 SIRS (systemic inflammatory response syndrome) criteria (from Bone et al. [18]) (two or more of the following)

Temperature	>38 or <36 °C
White blood cell count	>12,000 or <4000/mm^3
Heart rate	>90 beats/min
Respiratory rate	>20 breaths/min or $PaCO_2$ < 32 mmHg

While the use of SIRS criteria improved recognition of sepsis, these were far too general. A patient with a straightforward gastroenteritis or a bad cold would fulfil a sepsis definition despite having self-limiting illnesses. Thus, septic patients could not be distinguished in a uniform manner. The true incidence and mortality of sepsis became blurred as different criteria were applied.

In part driven by the repeated failure of various anti-inflammatory and immunosuppressive approaches, there was also a growing appreciation of an excess overfocus upon systemic inflammation as the predominant pathophysiological process to the detriment of other, perhaps equally relevant, pathways. In 2003 a North American-European Task Force published the second iteration of the sepsis definitions. They acknowledged the inadequacies of the existing definitions, but as there was insufficient evidence to support a change, they simply expanded the list of possible diagnostic criteria for sepsis [19].

1.4 Sepsis Is Now About Organ Dysfunction and Not Inflammation

In the last decade, the knowledge base regarding sepsis pathophysiology has increased significantly, and the relevance of noninflammatory pathways is increasingly appreciated [20]. Furthermore, most patients now survive the initial hyperinflammatory state but die of unresolved organ failure or new infection to which sepsis-associated immunosuppression increases susceptibility [21, 22]. Pharmacological agents attenuating the inflammatory response were very successful in preclinical studies but have all failed to show outcome benefit in large clinical trials [2, 23]. The relatively late administration of these drugs in a patient's disease course (as time to admission to hospital or intensive care may be days or even longer), as opposed to before, at or soon after the insult in a laboratory model, had likely missed the zenith of the inflammatory response; the figurative horse had already bolted [23, 24]. The pre-existing model of sepsis as an infection-triggered inflammatory disorder failed to embrace these developments. In addition, no clear guidance had been offered as to what precisely constitutes 'organ dysfunction' or 'shock'; this too impacted considerably on the variable incidence and mortality of sepsis and septic shock discussed earlier. A new paradigm and clear operationalization were needed.

In 2016, the latest sepsis definitions—'Sepsis-3'—were introduced [1]. Sepsis is now defined as 'life-threatening organ dysfunction caused by a dysregulated host response to infection' [1]. Under this new terminology, the old term *severe sepsis* becomes obsolete as organ dysfunction is now necessary for the diagnosis of sepsis. Sepsis and septic shock (defined as a subset of sepsis in which profound circulatory, cellular and metabolic abnormalities are associated with a greater risk of mortality than with sepsis alone) are now identified. Specific clinical criteria are used to identify sepsis (i.e. a change in Sequential (sepsis-related) Organ Failure Assessment (SOFA) score ≥2 above baseline values) (Table 1.2) and septic shock (i.e. vasopressor requirement to maintain a mean arterial pressure ≥ 65 mmHg and a serum lactate >2 mmol/L in the absence of hypovolaemia) [1]. Importantly, these criteria were

Table 1.2 Sequential (sepsis-related) Organ Failure Assessment (SOFA) score

	SOFA score				
System	0	1	2	3	4
Respiration *PaO_2/FiO_2 mmHg (kPa)*	≥400 (53.3)	<400 (53.3)	<300 (40)	<200 (26.7) with respiratory support	<100 (13.3) with respiratory support
Coagulation *platelets*	≥150	<150	<100	<50	<20
Liver *bilirubin, mg/dL (μmol/L)*	<1.2 (20)	1.2–1.9 (20–32)	2.0–5.9 (33–101)	6.0–11.9 (102–204)	>12.0 (204)
Cardiovascular (doses in *μg*/ kg/min)	MAP >70 mmHg	MAP <70 mmHg	Dopamine <5 or dobutamine (any dose)	Dopamine 5.1–15 or epinephrine <0.1 or norepinephrine <0.1	Dopamine >15 or epinephrine >0.1 or norepinephrine >0.1
Central nervous system *Glasgow Coma Scale*	15	13–14	10–12	6–9	<6
Renal *creatinine, mg/ dL (μmol/L), or urine output, mL/day*	<1.2 (110)	1.2–1.9 (110–170)	2.0–3.4 (171–299)	3.5–4.9 (300–440) <500	>5.0 (440) <200

MAP mean arterial pressure, *FiO_2* fraction of inspired oxygen, *PaO_2* partial pressure of oxygen
Catecholamine doses are given as μg/kg/min for at least 1 h
The Glasgow Coma Scale range from 3 to 15, with a higher score indicating better neurological function
Adapted from Vincent et al. [26]

developed from big data amassed from databases containing 850,000 hospital patient encounters that were cultured and treated for infection. A rise in SOFA ≥2 equates to a ≥ 10% risk of hospital mortality, while fulfilling the septic shock criteria was associated with a 42% risk of dying. While the overall reception to Sepsis-3 has been positive, there are detractors who feel that the removal of SIRS is a backward step [25]. The Sepsis-3 Task Force however did encourage prospective validation of these criteria in multiple healthcare settings; early studies support their findings.

1.5 Multiple Organ Dysfunction

With Sepsis-3, organ dysfunction has been pushed to the forefront of diagnosis and treatment. Many patients develop infection, often with a SIRS response, that does not require antibiotic treatment, let alone hospitalization. The key is to identify organ dysfunction at an early stage and intervene accordingly. The degree and type of organ dysfunction differ from patient to patient. Both the initial site of infection and the organism and host traits (genetic, epigenetic, comorbidities and medication) can influence the degree of organ dysfunction [2]. As a general rule, more pronounced organ failure is associated with worse outcome [26, 27].

All major organ systems may be impacted by the septic process [2, 28]. Patients often have impaired myocardial function which can lead to a low cardiac output and hypotension [29]. This may compound both a loss of vascular smooth muscle tone that is poorly responsive to catecholamines and activation of the vascular endothelium leading to increased extravasation of fluid as well as increased production of both pro- and anti-inflammatory mediators. Patients may suffer from respiratory distress as a direct consequence of lung involvement and/or progressive metabolic acidosis or respiratory muscle fatigue. This may be apparent as tachypnoea or progressive obtundation related to hypoxaemia and/or hypercapnoea. The nervous system can be affected, leading to altered mental status ('septic encephalopathy') and peripheral issues such as neuropathy and disturbed autonomic function. Acute kidney injury leads to elevated creatinine levels and decreased urine output. Liver dysfunction is noted as an increase in hepatic markers such as bilirubin and coagulopathy recognized by consumptive thrombocytopenia, hypercoagulability and, rarely, full-blown diffuse intravascular coagulation (DIC). Many other organ systems can be affected including the skeletal muscle (leading to a generalized myopathy), alimentary system (e.g. ileus, pancreatitis, cholecystitis) and hormonal system (including relative adrenal insufficiency, the low T3 syndrome and marked decreases in circulating vasopressin and sex hormone levels) [28, 30].

Intriguingly, despite severe clinical organ failure, remarkably little cell death is found, even in septic non-survivors [31, 32]. In those surviving an episode of sepsis, long-term organ support (e.g. dialysis) is usually not required if the affected organs were normal beforehand. These findings suggest that organ failure is more of a functional phenomenon rather than being due to a loss of structural integrity [33]. This has led to the hypothesis that organ dysfunction may represent a protective mechanism, akin to hibernation, that is designed to save the body from further damage. There may be a regulated shutdown of body metabolism, triggered in part by decreases in energy availability and altered hormone levels, that enables the affected organs to switch off during the acute illness phase but to regain functionality once the illness subsides. Many other features of sepsis support this notion. For example, the transcriptome, proteome and metabolome show generally similar changes in both septic survivors and non-survivors, but the magnitude of change (either down- or upregulated) is more extreme in eventual non-survivors [34]. Adaptation may thus spill over into maladaptation.

1.6 Clinical Recognition of Sepsis

Correctly recognizing a septic patient can be difficult, even for the experienced doctor. Presentation may be protean and, in the early stages, often vague and non-specific. For example, a rash is only seen in ~50% of cases of meningococcal sepsis on presentation [35]. Features of sepsis may be confounded by pre-existing comorbidities, and organ dysfunction may not be immediately apparent. Deterioration may be gradual over days or abrupt and severe over just a few hours. Patients are initially treated empirically for sepsis, but in 20–25% of cases, a sepsis mimic is belatedly identified [36]. Many mimics exist, ranging from pulmonary embolus and heart failure to beriberi, phaeochromocytoma, haemophagocytotic syndrome and various autoimmune diseases such as SLE.

A number of 'early warning scores' are proposed to identify patients at risk of having sepsis and poor outcomes. Examples include the quick SOFA (qSOFA) score consisting of respiratory rate $\geq$ 22 breaths/min, altered mentation (GCS <15) and systolic BP $\leq$100 mmHg which can be performed in minutes at the bedside and the National Early Warning Score (NEWS) which provides a score (of 0–4 depending on the degree of abnormality) to each of seven criteria (the three used in qSOFA plus PaO_2:FiO_2 ratio, serum creatinine or urine output, platelets and bilirubin) [1]. Such scores can offer prognostication and enable the trajectory of illness to be determined; however they should complement rather than replace sound clinical judgment.

To improve recognition and treatment, scientists have long sought biomarkers that can accurately identify the type of infection (either 'rule in' or 'rule out') and the early onset of organ dysfunction and offer some prognostic capability [37]. Multiple choices are available, increasingly as point-of-care tests and increasingly utilizing panels of biomarkers rather than a single variable [38]. However, the majority are still research tools and require large-scale prospective validation in multiple different populations (e.g. young/old, different ethnicities, post-surgery) [37]. Chapter 6 will address biomarkers in sepsis more in depth.

1.7 Risk Factors and Disease Course

The risk of sepsis depends on multiple factors including age, health status, genetic predisposition and comorbidity. Impaired immunity is an important risk factor, whether because of immunosuppressive drugs, cancer, malnutrition or stressors such as surgery, trauma or burns [39]. The very young and the elderly are more susceptible as their immune system functions less well. Many comorbid illnesses increase the chances of developing sepsis, though not all increase the eventual risk of mortality [39, 40]. Certain types of medication, e.g. statins, beta-blockers and calcium channel blockers, are associated with reduced mortality [41–43]. Intriguingly, body weight appears to impact upon outcome—the 'obesity paradox' [44]; this may offer general protection against critical illness through increased energy reserves and/or the endocrine and paracrine properties of adipose tissue.

The course of disease differs in each patient, and this, in part, reflects patient predisposition.

A subset of patients will recover remarkably quickly and will need little time in intensive care. Such patients are often young and resilient with no comorbidity. Others have a very protracted disease course with failure to thrive and delayed recovery. Such patients have ongoing activation of their inflammatory system marked, for example, by a persisting high C-reactive protein, yet often without a clear aetiology such as an undrained abscess. This condition has recently been coined the persistent immunosuppression, inflammation and catabolism syndrome (PICS) [45]. How to optimally manage PICS, either preventing, attenuating or hastening recovery, remains unclear. Although affected patients may eventually be discharged from intensive care, many have an ongoing poor quality of life, and subsequent hospital readmission and mortality are high. They often have long-term cognitive impairment and physical disability and a higher prevalence of mood disorders [46]. Attention is being increasingly directed towards this problematic subset with different strategies to be explored to improve outcomes such as immunostimulation and personalized rehabilitation regimens [47, 48].

Patients who die from sepsis can also be roughly divided in two groups. In a study that included only patients suffering from septic shock, approximately 30% of deaths occurred quickly, within 72 h of presentation [49]. These patients already had severe organ dysfunction on presentation and died from fulminant multiple organ failure. The remainder died much later, most after a protracted stay in intensive care [49]. In clinical practice, these late deaths often occur from a secondary complication (notably nosocomial infection) or an elective withdrawal due to failure to recover, usually on a background of underlying significant comorbidity.

1.8 Finding a Cure for Sepsis

The quest for novel therapies for sepsis has been highly disappointing. Most large multicentre trials have failed to show any benefit, and some have even been discontinued early because of harm [20, 23, 24]. This underlies how our incomplete grasp of sepsis pathophysiology and a poor appreciation of the biological phenotype of the individual patient fail to select an appropriate treatment given at appropriate dose and duration. Apart from clinical heterogeneity, the biological phenotype is variable in terms of magnitude of response and duration, as exemplified by a widely varying disease course between patients. So, for instance, administering an anti-inflammatory agent, the once-believed holy grail of sepsis treatment, will not prove beneficial if the pro-inflammatory phase has largely abated.

In addition, animal models often fail to simulate the clinical situation. Young, healthy rodents without comorbidity are predominantly used, and they often receive the septic insult that is non-representative of a clinical situation such as a bolus injection of endotoxin. The animals subsequently receive no or minimal or minimal standard sepsis management such as fluid [50]. Furthermore, the treatment is often given before, concurrent with or soon after the septic insult, and the model duration is relatively short and thus does not account for late deaths.

1.9 Clinical and Public Misunderstandings

To this day, many members of the public are still unaware of sepsis, despite campaigns such as the Surviving Sepsis Campaign. Those with some awareness often use outdated and fundamentally incorrect terminology such as blood poisoning and septicaemia. These terms were intended to reflect the presence of microorganisms in blood, yet this finding is infrequently made in most patients, especially if they have received prior antibiotics [2]. Likewise, patients with bacteraemia, viraemia or parasitaemia do not necessarily have sepsis. Indeed, transient bacteraemia is well recognized after toothbrushing [51].

1.10 Challenges and the Way Forward

While significant strides have been made in our understanding of sepsis, there is still a long way to go. Better education of healthcare workers regarding the nature of sepsis, including earlier identification and optimal treatment, should improve outcomes. This is particularly relevant in view of the rising incidence of sepsis as the population ages and more aggressive medical interventions are given. Better technologies to accurately identify infection and the causative agent and the early onset of organ dysfunction are needed, as are theranostics to guide choice and dosing of treatment. New treatments will be developed, but it is also worth reinvestigating discarded therapies as many may have a role in selected patients. It is also important to use a common language to describe incidence and epidemiology more precisely than at present. As more people survive sepsis, attention must also be paid to long-term outcomes, including morbidity, which can significantly impair quality of life and increase long-term healthcare costs.

References

1. Singer M, Deutschmann CS, Seymour CW, et al. The Third International Consensus Definitions for Sepsis and Septic Shock (Sepsis-3). JAMA. 2016;315:801–10.
2. Angus DC, van der Poll T. Severe sepsis and septic shock. N Engl J Med. 2013;369:840–51.
3. Fleischmann C, Scherag A, Adhikari NKJ, et al. Assessment of global incidence and mortality of hospital-treated sepsis. Current estimates and limitations. Am J Respir Crit Care Med. 2016;193:259–72.
4. World Health Organization. The top 10 causes of death (Fact sheet updated January 2017). http://www.who.int/mediacentre/factsheets/fs310/en/. Accessed 9 Feb 2018.
5. Kaukonen K-M, Bailey M, Suzuki S, et al. Mortality related to severe sepsis and septic shock among critically ill patients in Australia and New Zealand, 2000–2012. JAMA. 2014;311:1308–16.
6. Rhee C, Gohil S, Klompas M. Regulatory mandates for sepsis care--reasons for caution. N Engl J Med. 2014;370:1673–6.
7. Osler W. Principles and practice of medicine designed for the use of practitioners and students of medicine. 3rd ed. Edinburgh: Pentland; 1898.
8. Majno G. The ancient riddle of sigma eta psi iota sigma (sepsis). J Infect Dis. 1991;163:937–45.
9. Haensch S, Bianucci R, Signoli M, et al. Distinct clones of Yersinia pestis caused the black death. PLoS Pathog. 2010;6:e1001134.
10. Benedictow OJ. The black death 1346–1353: the complete history. Woodbridge: Boydell Press; 2004.
11. Davaine MC. Recherches sur quelques questions relatives a la septicemie. Paris: G. Masson; 1872.

12. Lister J. On the antiseptic principle in the practice of surgery. Lancet. 1867;90:353–6.
13. Fleming A. On the antibacterial action of cultures of a Penicillium, with special reference to their use in the isolation of B. influenzæ. Br J Exp Pathol. 1929;10:226–36.
14. Kelly FE, Fong K, Hirsch N, et al. Intensive care medicine is 60 years old: the history and future of the intensive care unit. Clin Med. 2014;14:376–9.
15. Thomas L. Germs. N Engl J Med. 1972;287:553–5.
16. Cerra FB. The systemic septic response: multiple systems organ failure. Crit Care Clin. 1985;1:591–607.
17. Fink MP, Heard SO. Laboratory models of sepsis and septic shock. J Surg Res. 1990;49:186–96.
18. Bone RC, Balk RA, Cerra FB, et al. Definitions for sepsis and organ failure and guidelines for the use of innovative therapies in sepsis. The ACCP/SCCM Consensus Conference Committee. American College of Chest Physicians/Society of Critical Care Medicine. Chest. 1992;101:1644–55.
19. Levy MM, Fink MP, Marshall JC, et al. 2001 SCCM/ESICM/ACCP/ATS/SIS International Sepsis Definitions Conference. Crit Care Med. 2003;31:1250–6.
20. Hotchkiss R, Karl I. The pathophysiology and treatment of sepsis. N Engl J Med. 2003;348(2):138–50.
21. Mira JC, Gentile LF, Mathias BJ, et al. Sepsis pathophysiology, chronic critical illness, and persistent inflammation-immunosuppression and catabolism syndrome. Crit Care Med. 2017;XX:1–10.
22. van Vught LA, Klein Klouwenberg PMC, Spitoni C, et al. Incidence, risk factors, and attributable mortality of secondary infections in the intensive care unit after admission for sepsis. JAMA. 2016;315:1469.
23. Zeni F, Freeman B, Natanson C. Anti-inflammatory therapies to treat sepsis and septic shock: a reassessment. Crit Care Med. 1997;25:1095–100.
24. Angus DC. The search for effective therapy for sepsis: back to the drawing board? JAMA. 2011;306:2614–5.
25. Sprung CL, Schein RMH, Balk RA. The new sepsis consensus definitions: the good, the bad and the ugly. Intensive Care Med. 2016;42:2024–6.
26. Vincent JL, Moreno R, Takala J, et al. The SOFA (Sepsis-related Organ Failure Assessment) score to describe organ dysfunction/failure. On behalf of the working group on sepsis-related problems of the European Society of Intensive Care Medicine. Intensive Care Med. 1996;22:707–10.
27. de Grooth H-J, Geenen IL, Girbes AR, et al. SOFA and mortality endpoints in randomized controlled trials: a systematic review and meta-regression analysis. Crit Care. 2017;21:38.
28. Hotchkiss RS, Moldawer LL, Opal SM, et al. Sepsis and septic shock. Nat Rev Dis Prim. 2016;2:16045.
29. Rudiger A, Singer M. Mechanisms of sepsis-induced cardiac dysfunction. Crit Care Med. 2007;35:1599–608.
30. Haak BW, Wiersinga WJ. The role of the gut microbiota in sepsis. Lancet Gastroenterol Hepatol. 2017;2:135–43.
31. Hotchkiss RS, Swanson PE, Freeman BD, et al. Apoptotic cell death in patients with sepsis, shock, and multiple organ dysfunction. Crit Care Med. 1999;27:1230–51.
32. Takasu O, Gaut JP, Watanabe E, et al. Mechanisms of cardiac and renal dysfunction in patients dying of sepsis. Am J Respir Crit Care Med. 2013;187:509–17.
33. Singer M, De Santis V, Vitale D, et al. Multiorgan failure is an adaptive, endocrine-mediated, metabolic response to overwhelming systemic inflammation. Lancet (London, England). 2004;364:545–8.
34. Langley RJ, Tsalik EL, van Velkinburgh JC, et al. An integrated clinico-metabolomic model improves prediction of death in sepsis. Sci Transl Med. 2013;5:195ra95.
35. Stephens DS, Greenwood B, Brandtzaeg P. Epidemic meningitis, meningococcaemia, and Neisseria meningitidis. Lancet. 2007;369:2196–210.
36. Heffner AC, Horton JM, Marchick MR, et al. Etiology of illness in patients with severe sepsis admitted to the hospital from the emergency department. Clin Infect Dis. 2010;50:814–20.

37. Pierrakos C, Vincent J-L. Sepsis biomarkers: a review. Crit Care. 2010;14:R15.
38. Davenport EE, Burnham KL, Radhakrishnan J, et al. Genomic landscape of the individual host response and outcomes in sepsis: a prospective cohort study. Lancet Respir Med. 2016;4:259–71.
39. Angus DC, Linde-Zwirble WT, Lidicker J, et al. Epidemiology of severe sepsis in the United States: analysis of incidence, outcome, and associated costs of care. Crit Care Med. 2001;29:1303–10.
40. van Vught LA, Holman R, de Jonge E, et al. Diabetes is not associated with increased 90-day mortality risk in critically ill patients with sepsis. Crit Care Med. 2017;45(10):e1026–35. https://doi.org/10.1097/CCM.0000000000002590.
41. Wan Y-D, Sun T-W, Kan Q-C, et al. Effect of statin therapy on mortality from infection and sepsis: a meta-analysis of randomized and observational studies. Crit Care. 2014;18:R71.
42. Morelli A, Ertmer C, Westphal M, et al. Effect of heart rate control with esmolol on hemodynamic and clinical outcomes in patients with septic shock. JAMA. 2013;310:1683.
43. Wiewel MA, van Vught LA, Scicluna BP, et al. Prior use of calcium channel blockers is associated with decreased mortality in critically ill patients with sepsis: a prospective observational study. Crit Care Med. 2017;45:454–63.
44. Arabi YM, Dara SI, Tamim HM, et al. Clinical characteristics, sepsis interventions and outcomes in the obese patients with septic shock: an international multicenter cohort study. Crit Care. 2013;17:R72.
45. Gentile LF, Cuenca AG, Efron PA, et al. Persistent inflammation and immunosuppression: a common syndrome and new horizon for surgical intensive care. J Trauma Acute Care Surg. 2012;72:1491–501.
46. Angus DC, Carlet J. Surviving intensive care: a report from the 2002 Brussels Roundtable. Intensive Care Med. 2003;29:368–77.
47. Mehlhorn J, Freytag A, Schmidt K, et al. Rehabilitation interventions for postintensive care syndrome: a systematic review. Crit Care Med. 2014;42:1263–71.
48. Hutchins NA, Unsinger J, Hotchkiss RS, et al. The new normal: immunomodulatory agents against sepsis immune suppression. Trends Mol Med. 2014;20:224–33.
49. Daviaud F, Grimaldi D, Dechartres A, et al. Timing and causes of death in septic shock. Ann Intensive Care. 2015;5:16.
50. Zolfaghari PS, Pinto BB, Dyson A, et al. The metabolic phenotype of rodent sepsis: cause for concern? Intensive Care Med Exp. 2013;1:6.
51. Lockhart PB, Brennan MT, Sasser HC, et al. Bacteremia associated with tooth brushing and dental extraction. Circulation. 2008;117:3118–25.

The Epidemiology of Sepsis

2

Hallie C. Prescott

Key Points

- The global burden of sepsis is estimated at 19.4 million cases each year and 5.3 million sepsis-related deaths annually. However, this estimate is based on the incidence of hospital-treated sepsis in the developed world and may underestimate the true global burden of sepsis.
- The incidence of sepsis is rising over time, and there are disparities in incidence by age, gender, comorbidity burden, and socioeconomic status.
- The most common sites of infection are the lung, abdomen, urinary tract, bloodstream, and skin/soft tissue.
- About 35–45% of sepsis cases have gram-negative organisms identified, 30–40% have gram-positive organisms identified, and 12–16% have fungal organisms identified. Thirty to forty percent of cases are culture negative, and 20% have multiple pathogens identified.
- The case-fatality rate is falling, but sepsis survivors are at increased risk for morbidity, recurrent sepsis, and late death.
- Thirty to forty percent of sepsis survivors are rehospitalized within 90 days, most commonly for recurrent sepsis.

2.1 Introduction

Sepsis, a life-threatening organ dysfunction resulting from the host response to infection [1], is a worldwide public health threat. This chapter will review the epidemiology of sepsis, including incidence, etiology, long-term outcomes, and risk

H. C. Prescott, M.D., M.Sc.
Department of Internal Medicine, University of Michigan, Ann Arbor, MI, USA

VA Center for Clinical Management Research, HSR&D Center of Innovation, Ann Arbor, MI, USA
e-mail: hprescot@med.umich.edu

W. J. Wiersinga, C. W. Seymour (eds.), *Handbook of Sepsis*,
https://doi.org/10.1007/978-3-319-73506-1_2

for recurrent sepsis in children and adults. Throughout this chapter, sepsis refers to infection complicated by acute organ dysfunction, consistent with updated Sepsis-3 terminology, or what was previously termed “severe sepsis” in the 1992 and 2001 consensus definitions [2, 3].

2.2 Incidence and Acute Mortality

There is incomplete data on the global incidence and mortality from sepsis. The Global Burden of Diseases Study—a worldwide observational epidemiological study that quantifies the burden death and disability due to specific diseases—does not include sepsis as its own category, except in infants. However, lower respiratory infections, the most common cause of sepsis, were the second leading cause of disability-adjusted life years (DALY) and the fourth leading cause of mortality worldwide in the 1990–2010 Global Burden of Diseases analysis [4, 5]. Meanwhile, diarrheal diseases were the fourth most common cause of DALY and seventh most common cause of mortality [4, 5]. From this, we can conclude that sepsis is a leading cause of death and disability, although the exact magnitude of burden is unknown.

In a 2016 meta-analysis by Fleischmann et al., the average population incidence rate of sepsis hospitalization in developed countries (the USA, Germany, Australia, New Zealand, Taiwan, Norway, Spain, and Sweden) was estimated at 270 per 100,000 person-years, with an in-hospital mortality rate of 26% [6]. However, the incidence varied widely across studies, from 90 to more than 1000 cases per 100,000 person-years, depending on the time-period of the study, country of origin, and method used to identify sepsis [6]. (To put these incidence rates into perspective, there are estimated 125 new breast cancer diagnoses per 100,000 women and 60 new lung cancer diagnoses per 100,000 adults in the USA each year [7].)

In the developed world, hospitalization for sepsis is more common than hospitalizations for myocardial infarction and stroke combined—and accounts for about 6% of all inpatient hospitalization costs among elderly US patients [8]. Approximately 2–3% of adults admitted to a hospital ward [9], 25–40% of patients admitted to an ICU [10–12], and 8% of children admitted to a pediatric ICU [13] have sepsis. Sepsis contributes to an estimated one-third to one-half of hospital deaths [14].

At the time of the 2016 meta-analysis by Fleischmann et al., there were no population-level studies of sepsis incidence in lower-income countries, which contain 87% of the world’s population [6]. However, by extrapolating from the available studies from developed countries, the authors estimated that—among 7.2 billion people worldwide—there are 19.4 million cases of sepsis each year and 5.3 million sepsis-related deaths annually [6]. This estimate assumes that the incidence of sepsis in lower-income countries is the same as the incidence of hospital-treated sepsis in developed countries. However, the incidence of infection is higher in lower-income countries, so the 19.4 million cases are likely an underestimate [15].

Nonetheless, while the precise impact of sepsis has been difficult to quantify, there is growing awareness that sepsis is a leading cause of death and disability and that it has not received sufficient attention. In May 2017, in recognition of the global burden of sepsis, the World Health Organization adopted a resolution on improving the prevention, recognition, and management of sepsis [15]. The resolution recognizes sepsis as a global health priority and urges member states to develop national policies and process to address sepsis [15].

2.2.1 Sepsis Incidence and Outcomes by Age

The incidence of sepsis follows a bimodal distribution, with higher rates at the extremes of age. Rates of sepsis are moderate in infants (5 per 1000 people), are lowest in children and young adults (<5 per 1000 people), and then rise exponentially from ages 50 to 85 years and beyond [16]. The incidence of sepsis in octogenarians is more than 15 per 1000 people [16]. In developed countries, most (58%) sepsis hospitalizations and most sepsis-related hospital deaths (71%) are in patients aged 65 years or older [17]. The greater incidence of sepsis in older patients is likely explained by both a greater prevalence of chronic medical conditions that may predispose patients to sepsis (e.g., cancer, chronic kidney disease) and changes in age-related deterioration in immune function, known as immunosenescence.

In studies using administrative data, the case-fatality rate of sepsis appears to increase steadily with age, from less than 10% in infants to more than 35% in patients 85 years and older [16]. However, a recent study with prospective data collection from 128 pediatric ICUs in 26 countries reported a case-fatality rate of 25% in children in both developed and resource-limited countries, suggesting that sepsis in pediatric patients may be more lethal than was previously believed [13].

2.2.2 Changes in Incidence and Outcomes Over Time

The incidence of sepsis appears to be rising steadily over the past few decades, while the case-fatality rates have fallen [18–20]. Some of this change is explained by temporal trends in the recognition and coding of sepsis, with increased labeling of less severely ill patients as septic over time [21]—a condition known as stage migration, or "Will Rogers" phenomenon [22]. However, even studies with stable sepsis definitions find that the incidence of sepsis is rising over time, albeit more modestly [23]. For example, in one study that identified sepsis based on clinical evidence of infection and organ dysfunction in electronic medical records, septic shock cases rose from 12.8 cases per 1000 hospitalizations in 2005 to 18.6 cases per 1000 hospitalizations in 2014, while the case-fatality rate fell from 55 to 51% [24]. In another study of ICU patients in Australia and New Zealand over a 13-year time frame, in which the presence of acute organ dysfunction was collected by bedside nurse abstractors, the incidence of sepsis in ICU patients rose from 7.2% (2708 of 35,012 ICU admissions) in 2000 to 11.1% (12,512 of 100,286 ICU admissions) in 2012, while the case-fatality rate fell from 35.0 to 18.4%.

The rising incidence of sepsis is likely multifactorial, related to both better survival from other medical conditions such as cancer and increasing use of immunosuppressive therapies and invasive medical procedures, which together result in a greater number of patients who are at heightened risk for developing sepsis.

Beyond those gradual changes in sepsis incidence and mortality from year to year, the incidence and lethality of sepsis also vary by season. Both incidence and case-fatality rates are about 17% higher in the winter months and show greater fluctuations in cold climates [25]. This difference is largely explained by differences in pulmonary infection, as respiratory causes of sepsis increase about 40% during winter months [25].

2.2.3 Sepsis Incidence by Chronic Medical Conditions

The incidence of sepsis is higher in patients with chronic medical conditions that impair immune function, particularly in patients with cancer, acquired immunodeficiency syndrome (AIDS), diabetes, and chronic obstructive pulmonary disease (COPD), in patients taking immunosuppressive medications, and in patients on hemodialysis. For example, the incidence of sepsis is approximately 40-fold higher in patients on maintenance hemodialysis compared to patients not on hemodialysis [26]. Sepsis incidence is also four- to tenfold higher in cancer patients than non-cancer patients and higher still in patients with certain malignancies (e.g., 65-fold increased risk with myeloid leukemia) [27, 28]. A study examining a nationally representative sample of US hospital discharge records estimated incidence rates of 1075, 1051, and 755 per 100,000 patients with cancer, AIDS, and COPD, respectively [28]. The risk for sepsis hospitalization is 2.5-fold higher in patients with versus without diabetes [29]. In addition to higher incidence rate, the case fatality of sepsis also varies by the presence of comorbid conditions and is 55% greater in patients with cancer [28].

More than half of patients who develop sepsis have at least one chronic medical condition, commonly cancer (15–16%), COPD (10–12%), congestive heart failure (15%), chronic kidney disease (5–12%), diabetes (3–20%), or alcohol abuse (2–5%) [16, 30–33], with varying frequencies depending on the population studied. Among children with sepsis, three in four have at least one chronic condition, most commonly a respiratory (30%), gastrointestinal (25%), or cardiovascular condition (24%) [13].

2.2.4 Maternal Sepsis

Sepsis is a rare but devastating complication of childbirth, accounting for about 11% of all maternal deaths [34]. Puerperal sepsis—infection of the reproductive tract following childbirth or miscarriage—is estimated to result in at least 75,000 maternal deaths each year, mostly in low-income countries [35]. In a national UK cohort study, 14% of maternal critical care admissions were for sepsis [36]. The incidence of ICU admission for sepsis was 4.1/10,000 maternities, while the risk of sepsis-associated mortality was 1.8/100,000 maternities [36]. The most common sources of infection are pneumonia and polymicrobial genital tract infections, accounting for 40 and 24% of maternal sepsis cases, respectively [36].

2.2.5 Sepsis Incidence by Demographics and Socioeconomic Status

The incidence of sepsis varies by patient demographics and socioeconomic status. Across the age spectrum, both incidence and case-fatality rates of sepsis are higher in males than females [16]. Sepsis is more also common in black patients than white patients [37, 38]. In a study of the 2002 New Jersey State Inpatient Database, risk of sepsis hospitalization was higher in black versus white patients, with the greatest discrepancy in rates seen among patients aged 35–44 years (relative risk for sepsis hospitalization 4.4, $p < 0.001$). The racial discrepancy in sepsis incidence is explained by both higher rates of infection and higher rates of acute organ dysfunction during infection among black patients [37]. The case-fatality rate for sepsis hospitalizations is similar between black and white patients, suggesting similar quality of inpatient care [38]. However, rates of comorbid conditions are higher, and rates of insurance are lower—suggesting that disparities in preventative care and chronic disease management may explain some of the differences [38].

Sepsis is also more common in patients with lower socioeconomic status [31]. For example, in the USA, patients living in ZIP codes with higher poverty rates have a higher incidence of sepsis [39]. Risk of sepsis and sepsis-related death also differ by insurance type in the USA, with higher rates in patients with government-provided insurance, relative to patients with private insurance [40].

2.3 Etiology and Characteristics of Sepsis

2.3.1 Context

In the developed world, about 11% of sepsis is acquired during hospitalization, 26% is healthcare associated (acquired outside of a hospital by patients with recent exposure to healthcare facilities, such as nursing home residents, hemodialysis recipients, or patients hospitalized within the prior 30 days), and 63% of sepsis is acquired de novo in the community [41].

2.3.2 Site of Infection

Pneumonia is the most common inciting infection in adults and children [10, 13, 16, 42]. It accounts for about 40% adult hospitalized sepsis cases in studies using administrative data, which examine both ward and ICU patients [16]. In prospective studies of ICU patients, pneumonia accounts for over 60% of adult sepsis cases [10, 42] and 40% of pediatric sepsis cases [13]. After pneumonia, the next most common sites of infection are

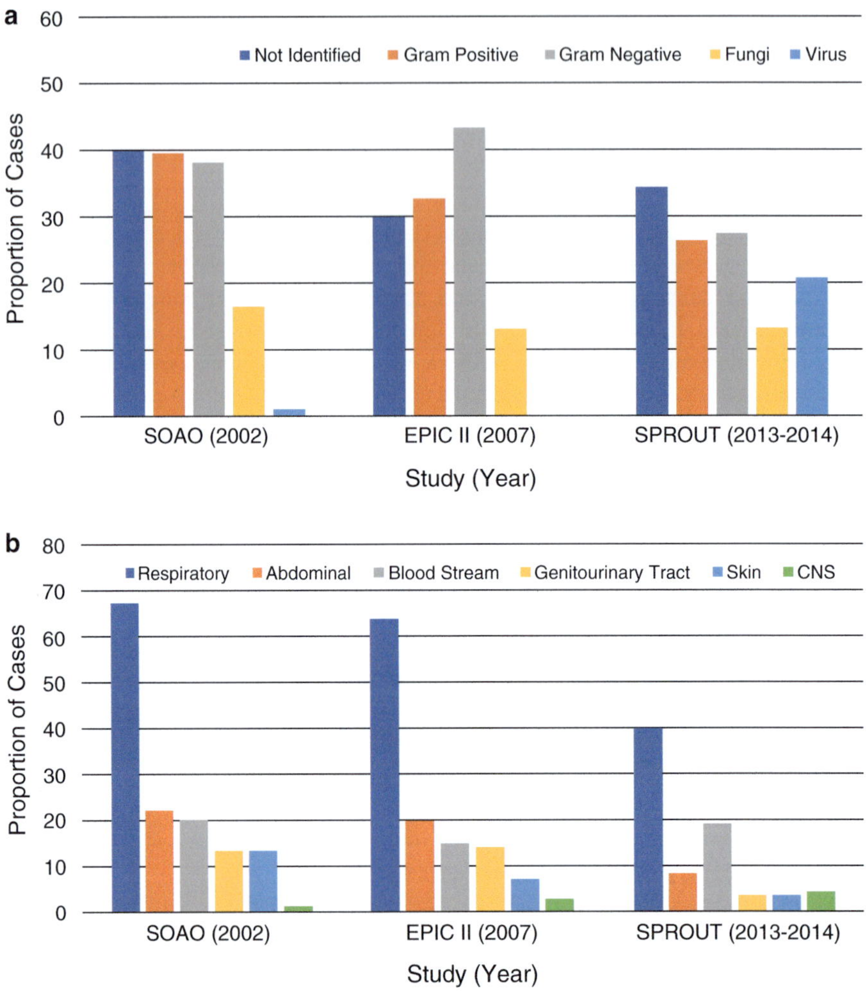

Fig. 2.1 Characteristics of sepsis, from selected multicenter studies with prospective data collection. (**a**) Infectious organism isolated (**b**) site of infection. The proportion of cases is determined by the number of cases with a specific etiologic agent (**a**) or specific site of infection (**b**) divided by all cases with sepsis (SOAP and SPROUT) or infection (EPIC II). The proportions for an individual study do not add up to 100 because patients may have more than one infectious agent identified or more than one site of infection. *SOAP*, Sepsis in European Intensive Care Units, was a 2-week, prospective period-prevalence study involving 198 adult ICUs in 24 European countries; *SPROUT*, Sepsis Prevalence, Outcomes, and Treatment, was a 5-day point-prevalence study of sepsis involving 128 pediatric ICUs in 26 countries; EPIC II, European Prevalence of Infection in Intensive Care, was a 1-day prospective point-prevalence study involving adult 1265 ICUs from 75 countries

abdominal, genitourinary, primary bacteremia, and skin/soft tissue infections (Fig. 2.1a) [16, 43, 44]. These top sites account for over 85% of all adult sepsis cases [16, 43, 44]. In children, pneumonia is the most common site of infection (40%), followed by primary bacteremia (19%), abdominal (8%), and central nervous system infections (4%) [13].

Common sites of infection differ depending on patients' comorbid medical conditions, with infection commonly occurring in diseased organs or in sites of instrumentations. For example, patients on chronic dialysis have higher rates of abdominal and catheter-related infection [45]. Meanwhile, patients with COPD or who are taking inhaled steroids have higher rates of lower respiratory tract infection [46, 47].

2.3.3 Pathogen

An infectious organism is identified in about 60–65% of patients with sepsis [10, 13, 32, 33, 44] and 75% of patients with ICU-acquired sepsis [10]. In adult sepsis patients treated in an ICU, about 35–45% have gram-negative organisms identified, 30–40% have gram-positive organisms identified, 12–16% have fungal organisms, and 1% have viruses identified (Fig. 2.1b) [10, 32, 42]. Eighteen percentage of patients have multiple organisms identified [10]. Among pediatric ICU patients with sepsis, rates of identification of gram-positive bacteria, gram-negative bacteria, and viruses are 28%, 27%, and 21%, respectively [13]. The higher rates of viral infection in pediatric patients likely reflect both differences in the epidemiology of infection between children and adults and the increasing use of polymerase chain reaction testing to identify viruses in the more recent pediatric study.

Common organisms isolated in children and adults include methicillin-sensitive *Staphylococcus aureus*, methicillin-resistant *Staphylococcus aureus*, *Pseudomonas* species, *Klebsiella* species, *Streptococcus pneumococcus*, *Escherichia coli*, and *Candida* species [10, 13, 32]. In children, the most common viral pathogens detected are rhinovirus, respiratory syncytial virus, and adenovirus [13]. Group B *Streptococcus* and *Escherichia coli* have dominated as the causes of early neonatal sepsis, accounting for about 35% and 20% of cases, respectively [48].

Site of infection, organism, and the interaction between site and organism are strongly associated with survival from sepsis [49]. For example, gram-negative bacteremia is more lethal than gram-positive bacteremia, while urinary tract infection is rarely fatal regardless of the infectious organism [49]. Mortality from pulmonary sepsis varies widely by pathogen, from 13% for *Streptococcus pneumoniae* to 77% for *Pseudomonas aeruginosa* [49]. However, this is likely a reflection of the context by which infection occurs, rather than the pathogenicity of the particular organisms. *Pseudomonas* species are not particularly pathogenic (they rarely cause infection in normal hosts) [50], but can cause serious infection in vulnerable hosts, and are a much more common cause of ICU-acquired versus non-ICU-acquired sepsis, 21 versus 12%, $p < 0.01$ [10].

2.3.4 Acute Organ Dysfunction and Failure

About half of patients with sepsis are treated in an ICU, while half are managed exclusively in a hospital ward [16, 19, 51]. Three-quarters of adult patients have single-organ dysfunction, one in five has two organ dysfunctions, and one in 20 has three or more acute organ dysfunctions [16]. The most common types of acute organ dysfunction are respiratory (46%), followed by cardiovascular (24%), renal (22%), and hematologic (20%) [16].

Among ICU patients with sepsis treated in European ICUs, about 75–80% of patients have at least two acute organ failures, and 36–50% have three or more acute organ failures [10, 32]. The most common acute organ failures requiring life support in ICU-treated sepsis patients are respiratory failure (50–75%), shock or cardiovascular failure (50–63%), and renal failure (20–50%) [10, 32, 33].

In the multinational point-prevalence study of pediatric sepsis, 83% of patients had respiratory dysfunction, 70% had cardiovascular dysfunction, and 30% had hematological dysfunction. Seventy-four percentage of ICU-treated pediatric sepsis patients received mechanical ventilation, 55% received vasoactive medications, 41% received blood product transfusion, 14% received renal replacement therapy, and 5% received extracorporeal membrane oxygenation (ECMO) [13].

Each additional organ dysfunction or failure is associated with increased risk for in-hospital mortality [33, 52]. In a multinational point-prevalence study, adult septic patients with single-organ failure had an 18% in-hospital mortality, while patients with two, three, or four failing organs had in-hospital mortality rates of 30%, 50%, and 65%, respectively [10].

2.4 Long-Term Outcomes

2.4.1 Late Mortality

Over the past decade, there has been greater recognition of the long-term consequences of surviving sepsis. While in-hospital mortality has fallen steadily over the past two decades [18–20], patients surviving hospital treatment for sepsis remain at increased risk for death [53–55]. The highest risk period is the first 90 days after sepsis hospitalization, but risk for death remains increased relative to carefully matched controls for years after the acute septic episode has resolved [53–55]. Approximately one in five older patients who survives a sepsis hospitalization died within 2 years due to the lasting effects of sepsis [53]. Risk for death is not elevated in only older or more frail patients who survive a sepsis hospitalization. In a large retrospective study of pediatric sepsis patients treated in the state of Washington, 6.5% of children who survived hospitalization had a late death, most commonly in the 2 years following hospital discharge [56].

2.4.2 Physical, Cognitive, and Mental Health Impairment

Patients who survive a hospitalization for sepsis frequently develop new functional disability and/or cognitive impairment [57]. Elderly acquire an average of 1–2 new functional limitations (e.g., inability to manage medications, inability to manage money, inability to toilet independently, inability to bathe independently) after sepsis hospitalization, and the prevalence of moderate-to-severe cognitive impairment rises from about 6% in the year prior to sepsis hospitalization to 16% in the year following sepsis hospitalization [57]. The incidence of new mild cognitive impairment is unknown, but likely even more common. The risk for new cognitive impairment is similar among older and younger patients who survive a critical medical illness [58]. Risk is also similar among patients who survive more and less severe sepsis hospitalizations [59].

Anxiety, depression, and post-traumatic stress disorder all affect about 30–40% of patients who survive an ICU stay for any cause [60–62]. However, it is not clear that the prevalence of these conditions is actually increased after sepsis. In one of the few prospective studies with baseline measurement prior to sepsis hospitalization, the rate of clinically important depressive symptoms was 28% before sepsis hospitalization and 28% after sepsis hospitalization [63]—suggesting that mental health impairments are more common in patients who are hospitalized with sepsis than the general population, but not that depression is triggered or exacerbated by sepsis.

Beyond the relatively well-described impairments in physical function, cognitive function, and mental health after sepsis, patients surviving sepsis hospitalization also report a range of other symptoms are worse after sepsis, such as numbness, fatigue, pain, visual disturbance, hair loss, and problems with dentition and nails [64]. While the extent to which these symptoms, and mental health impairments, are due to sepsis is unclear, they are important to be addressed as they herald a more complicated post-sepsis course.

2.4.3 Healthcare Utilization and Hospital Readmission

As a result of new functional disability, sepsis survivors are frequently discharged to post-acute care facilities after hospital discharge, such as skilled nursing facilities or long-term acute care facilities [51]. Thirty to forty percent of adult sepsis survivors are rehospitalized in the next 90 days, most commonly for another episode of sepsis [65]. Other common and potentially preventable causes of hospital readmission include congestive heart failure, acute renal failure, exacerbation of chronic obstructive pulmonary disease, and aspiration pneumonitis [65]. Approximately 40% of all hospital readmissions in the 90 days after sepsis are for "potentially preventable" or "ambulatory care-sensitive" diagnoses, suggesting an opportunity for improvement [65].

Children surviving sepsis are also frequently discharged to rehabilitation or long-term care facilities for additional medical care [56]. In a retrospective study of pediatric sepsis patients in Washington state, almost half (47%) of the survivors were rehospitalized during the study period. The median patients were rehospitalized three times, with the first readmission occurring a median of 95 days after initial hospital discharge [56]. Similar to adults, the most common reason for readmission was respiratory infection [56].

2.4.4 Recurrent Sepsis

Patients' risk for further health deterioration is increased after surviving a hospitalization for sepsis. In population-based study in Taiwan, 35% of sepsis survivors were again hospitalized with sepsis in the following 8 years, compared to just 4% of carefully matched observational controls [66]. The adjusted risk for subsequent sepsis in patient surviving a sepsis hospitalization was nearly ninefold higher than the matched controls [66]. Among elderly US Medicare beneficiaries who survive a sepsis hospitalization, 6.4% are rehospitalized with another episode of sepsis within 90 days of hospital discharge. This rate of readmission for sepsis is markedly higher than is experienced by matched patients hospitalized for other acute medical conditions [65]. 6.4% of patients who survive hospitalizations for sepsis versus 2.8% of matched controls are readmitted for sepsis within 90 days, $p < 0.001$ [65].

At least half of recurrent sepsis hospitalizations are for new infections (different site and/or different pathogen), as opposed to relapse or recrudescence of the initial infection (Fig. 2.2) [67]. Only 20% of recurrent sepsis hospitalizations are due to infections with both the same site and same pathogen as the initial septic episode. In 30% of recurrent sepsis cases, cultures are negative in one or both hospitalizations, so it is unclear whether the recurrent sepsis is due to a new or relapsed infection [67]. The high rate of sepsis due to new infection suggests that there are multiple mechanisms by which patients develop recurrent sepsis—not merely treatment failure—and that longer or stronger initiation antibiotic courses alone are unlikely to solve the problem [68].

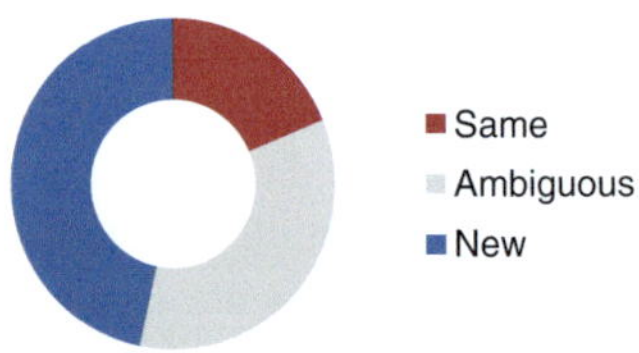

Organism Concordance	Site Concordance		
	Different Site	Same Site	Unknown
Different Organism	14 (10%)	30 (22%)	3 (2%)
Same Organism	0 (0%)	26 (19%)	1 (1%)
Culture Negative	17 (12%)	38 (28%)	8 (6%)

Fig. 2.2 Etiology of recurrent sepsis. This figure, which is adapted from DeMerle et al. [67], depicts the relationship between initial sepsis and recurrent sepsis in 139 patients with recurrent sepsis hospitalization. Nineteen percentage of patients with recurrent sepsis had an infection with the same organism and same site at the initial septic episode, while 47 had a definitively new infection (new site and/or new organism)

2.4.5 Cardiovascular Events

Two matched cohort studies indicate that risk for subsequent cardiovascular events is elevated in patients who survive sepsis. First, Yende et al. found that sepsis survivors have a 1.9-fold higher risk for subsequent cardiovascular events relative to population controls [69]. However, risk for subsequent events was only 1.1-fold higher relative to matched hospitalized controls and equivalent to other ICU survivors—suggesting that risk for subsequent cardiovascular events may be mediated by critical illness in general, rather than sepsis specifically [69]. In a population-based observational study in Taiwan, Ou et al. similarly found that patients who survived a sepsis hospitalization had a 1.4-fold increased risk for cardiovascular events relative to matched population controls and a 1.3-fold increased risk relative to matched hospitalized controls [55].

Conclusions

Sepsis is a leading cause of disability and death around the world. There are estimated 19.4 million cases of sepsis each year and 5.3 million sepsis-related deaths annually. However, as these estimates are extrapolated from high-income countries, they likely underestimate the true burden of disease. The most common sites of infection are respiratory, abdominal, bloodstream, genitourinary, and skin/soft tissue. The most common infectious agents isolated are gram-negative bacteria (35–45%), gram-positive bacteria (30–40%), and fungi (12–16%), although 30–40% of septic patients have no infectious organism identified. Three out of four patients who are hospitalized with sepsis survive to hospital discharge, but often in a weakened state. Sepsis survivors are at increased risk for new physical disability, cognitive impairment, recurrent infection, hospital readmission, and death. These poor long-term outcomes add to the total burden of sepsis-related death and disability.

References

1. Singer M, Deutschman CS, Seymour CW, et al. The third international consensus definitions for Sepsis and Septic Shock (Sepsis-3). JAMA. 2016;315:801–10.
2. Levy MM, Fink MP, Marshall JC, et al. 2001 SCCM/ESICM/ACCP/ATS/SIS International Sepsis Definitions Conference. Intensive Care Med. 2003;29:530–8.
3. Bone RC, Sibbald WJ, Sprung CL. The ACCP-SCCM consensus conference on sepsis and organ failure. Chest. 1992;101:1481–3.
4. Murray CJL, Vos T, Lozano R, et al. Disability-adjusted life years (DALYs) for 291 diseases and injuries in 21 regions, 1990–2010: a systematic analysis for the Global Burden of Disease Study 2010. Lancet Lond Engl. 2012;380:2197–223.
5. Lozano R, Naghavi M, Foreman K, et al. Global and regional mortality from 235 causes of death for 20 age groups in 1990 and 2010: a systematic analysis for the Global Burden of Disease Study 2010. Lancet Lond Engl. 2012;380:2095–128.
6. Fleischmann C, Scherag A, Adhikari NKJ, Hartog CS, Tsaganos T, Schlattmann P, Angus DC, Reinhart K, International Forum of Acute Care Trialists. Assessment of global incidence and

mortality of hospital-treated sepsis. Current estimates and limitations. Am J Respir Crit Care Med. 2016;193:259–72.
7. SEER cancer stat facts. https://seer.cancer.gov/statfacts/. Accessed 13 Jul 2017.
8. Torio C, Moore BJ. National Inpatient Hospital Costs: the most expensive hospital conditions by payer, 2013. HCUP statistical brief #204. Rockville, MD: Agency for Healthcare Research and Quality; 2016. https://hcup-us.ahrq.gov/reports/statbriefs/sb204-Most-Expensive-Hospital-Conditions.pdf. Accessed 14 Feb 2017
9. Szakmany T, Lundin RM, Sharif B, et al. Sepsis prevalence and outcome on the general wards and emergency departments in Wales: results of a Multi-Centre, Observational, Point Prevalence Study. PLoS One. 2016;11:e0167230.
10. Vincent JL, Sakr Y, Sprung CL, et al. Sepsis in European intensive care units: results of the SOAP study. Crit Care Med. 2006;34:344–53.
11. Zhou J, Qian C, Zhao M, et al. Epidemiology and outcome of severe sepsis and septic shock in intensive care units in mainland China. PLoS One. 2014;9:e107181.
12. Harrison DA, Welch CA, Eddleston JM. The epidemiology of severe sepsis in England, Wales and Northern Ireland, 1996 to 2004: secondary analysis of a high quality clinical database, the ICNARC Case Mix Programme Database. Crit Care Lond Engl. 2006;10:R42.
13. Weiss SL, Fitzgerald JC, Pappachan J, et al. Global epidemiology of pediatric severe sepsis: the sepsis prevalence, outcomes, and therapies study. Am J Respir Crit Care Med. 2015;191:1147–57.
14. Liu V, Escobar GJ, Greene JD, Soule J, Whippy A, Angus DC, Iwashyna TJ. Hospital deaths in patients with sepsis from 2 independent cohorts. JAMA. 2014;312:90–2.
15. Reinhart K, Daniels R, Kissoon N, Machado FR, Schachter RD, Finfer S. Recognizing sepsis as a global health priority – a WHO resolution. N Engl J Med. 2017;377:414–7. https://doi.org/10.1056/NEJMp1707170.
16. Angus DC, Linde-Zwirble WT, Lidicker J, Clermont G, Carcillo J, Pinsky MR. Epidemiology of severe sepsis in the United States: analysis of incidence, outcome, and associated costs of care. Crit Care Med. 2001;29:1303–10.
17. HCUPnet, Healthcare Cost and Utilization Project. Agency for healthcare research and quality. Rockville, MD. http://hcupnet.ahrq.gov/. Accessed 23 Nov 2016.
18. Kaukonen KM, Bailey M, Suzuki S, Pilcher D, Bellomo R. Mortality related to severe sepsis and septic shock among critically ill patients in Australia and New Zealand, 2000–2012. JAMA. 2014;311:1308–16.
19. Prescott HC, Kepreos KM, Wiitala WL, Iwashyna TJ. Temporal changes in the influence of hospitals and regional healthcare networks on severe sepsis mortality. Crit Care Med. 2015;43:1368–74.
20. Stevenson EK, Rubenstein AR, Radin GT, Wiener RS, Walkey AJ. Two decades of mortality trends among patients with severe sepsis: a comparative meta-analysis*. Crit Care Med. 2014;42:625–31.
21. Lindenauer PK, Lagu T, Shieh MS, Pekow PS, Rothberg MB. Association of diagnostic coding with trends in hospitalizations and mortality of patients with pneumonia, 2003–2009. JAMA. 2012;307:1405–13.
22. Will Rogers phenomenon. Wikipedia; 2017.
23. Iwashyna TJ, Angus DC. Declining case fatality rates for severe sepsis: good data bring good news with ambiguous implications. JAMA. 2014;311:1295–7.
24. Kadri SS, Rhee C, Strich JR, Morales MK, Hohmann S, Menchaca J, Suffredini AF, Danner RL, Klompas M. Estimating ten-year trends in septic shock incidence and mortality in United States academic medical centers using clinical data. Chest. 2017;151:278–85.
25. Danai PA, Sinha S, Moss M, Haber MJ, Martin GS. Seasonal variation in the epidemiology of sepsis. Crit Care Med. 2007;35:410–5.
26. Sakhuja A, Nanchal RS, Gupta S, Amer H, Kumar G, Albright RC, Kashani KB. Trends and outcomes of severe sepsis in patients on maintenance dialysis. Am J Nephrol. 2016;43:97–103.

27. Williams MD, Braun LA, Cooper LM, Johnston J, Weiss RV, Qualy RL, Linde-Zwirble W. Hospitalized cancer patients with severe sepsis: analysis of incidence, mortality, and associated costs of care. Crit Care Lond Engl. 2004;8:R291–8.
28. Danai PA, Moss M, Mannino DM, Martin GS. The epidemiology of sepsis in patients with malignancy. Chest. 2006;129:1432–40.
29. Shah BR, Hux JE. Quantifying the risk of infectious diseases for people with diabetes. Diabetes Care. 2003;26:510–3.
30. Martin GS, Mannino DM, Eaton S, Moss M. The epidemiology of sepsis in the United States from 1979 through 2000. N Engl J Med. 2003;348:1546–54.
31. Esper AM, Moss M, Lewis CA, Nisbet R, Mannino DM, Martin GS. The role of infection and comorbidity: factors that influence disparities in sepsis. Crit Care Med. 2006;34:2576–82.
32. Blanco J, Muriel-Bombín A, Sagredo V, et al. Incidence, organ dysfunction and mortality in severe sepsis: a Spanish multicentre study. Crit Care. 2008;12:R158.
33. Brun-Buisson C, Meshaka P, Pinton P, Vallet B, EPISEPSIS Study Group. EPISEPSIS: a reappraisal of the epidemiology and outcome of severe sepsis in French intensive care units. Intensive Care Med. 2004;30:580–8.
34. Say L, Chou D, Gemmill A, Tunçalp Ö, Moller A-B, Daniels J, Gülmezoglu AM, Temmerman M, Alkema L. Global causes of maternal death: a WHO systematic analysis. Lancet Glob Health. 2014;2:e323–33.
35. van Dillen J, Zwart J, Schutte J, van Roosmalen J. Maternal sepsis: epidemiology, etiology and outcome. Curr Opin Infect Dis. 2010;23:249–54.
36. Acosta CD, Harrison DA, Rowan K, Lucas DN, Kurinczuk JJ, Knight M. Maternal morbidity and mortality from severe sepsis: a national cohort study. BMJ Open. 2016;6:e012323.
37. Mayr FB, Yende S, Linde-Zwirble WT, Peck-Palmer OM, Barnato AE, Weissfeld LA, Angus DC. Infection rate and acute organ dysfunction risk as explanations for racial differences in severe sepsis. JAMA. 2010;303:2495–503.
38. Dombrovskiy VY, Martin AA, Sunderram J, Paz HL. Occurrence and outcomes of sepsis: influence of race. Crit Care Med. 2007;35:763–8.
39. Barnato AE, Alexander SL, Linde-Zwirble WT, Angus DC. Racial variation in the incidence, care, and outcomes of severe sepsis: analysis of population, patient, and hospital characteristics. Am J Respir Crit Care Med. 2008;177:279–84.
40. O'Brien JM, Lu B, Ali NA, Levine DA, Aberegg SK, Lemeshow S. Insurance type and sepsis-associated hospitalizations and sepsis-associated mortality among US adults: a retrospective cohort study. Crit Care Lond Engl. 2011;15:R130.
41. Page DB, Donnelly JP, Wang HE. Community-, healthcare-, and hospital-acquired severe sepsis hospitalizations in the University HealthSystem Consortium. Crit Care Med. 2015;43:1945–51.
42. Vincent J-L, Rello J, Marshall J, et al. International study of the prevalence and outcomes of infection in intensive care units. JAMA. 2009;302:2323–9.
43. Leligdowicz A, Dodek PM, Norena M, Wong H, Kumar A, Kumar A. Association between source of infection and hospital mortality in patients who have septic shock. Am J Respir Crit Care Med. 2014;189:1204–13.
44. Finfer S, Bellomo R, Lipman J, French C, Dobb G, Myburgh J. Adult-population incidence of severe sepsis in Australian and New Zealand intensive care units. Intensive Care Med. 2004;30:589–96.
45. Clark E, Kumar A, Langote A, et al. Septic shock in chronic dialysis patients: clinical characteristics, antimicrobial therapy and mortality. Intensive Care Med. 2016;42:222–32.
46. Almirall J, Bolíbar I, Serra-Prat M, et al. Inhaled drugs as risk factors for community-acquired pneumonia. Eur Respir J. 2010;36:1080–7.
47. Sethi S. Infection as a comorbidity of COPD. Eur Respir J. 2010;35:1209–15.
48. Schrag SJ, Farley MM, Petit S, Reingold A, Weston EJ, Pondo T, Hudson Jain J, Lynfield R. Epidemiology of invasive early-onset neonatal sepsis, 2005 to 2014. Pediatrics. 2016;138(6):e20162013. https://doi.org/10.1542/peds.2016-2013.

49. Cohen J, Cristofaro P, Carlet J, Opal S. New method of classifying infections in critically ill patients. Crit Care Med. 2004;32:1510–26.
50. Sadikot RT, Blackwell TS, Christman JW, Prince AS. Pathogen–host interactions in Pseudomonas aeruginosa pneumonia. Am J Respir Crit Care Med. 2005;171:1209–23.
51. Prescott HC, Langa KM, Liu V, Escobar GJ, Iwashyna TJ. Increased 1-year healthcare use in survivors of severe sepsis. Am J Respir Crit Care Med. 2014;190:62–9.
52. Shankar-Hari M, Harrison DA, Rowan KM. Differences in impact of definitional elements on mortality precludes international comparisons of sepsis epidemiology-a cohort study illustrating the need for standardized reporting. Crit Care Med. 2016;44:2223–30.
53. Prescott HC, Osterholzer JJ, Langa KM, Angus DC, Iwashyna TJ. Late mortality after sepsis: propensity matched cohort study. BMJ. 2016;353:i2375.
54. Quartin AA, Schein RM, Kett DH, Peduzzi PN. Magnitude and duration of the effect of sepsis on survival. Department of Veterans Affairs Systemic Sepsis Cooperative Studies Group. JAMA. 1997;277:1058–63.
55. Ou S-M, Chu H, Chao P-W, Lee Y-J, Kuo S-C, Chen T-J, Tseng C-M, Shih C-J, Chen Y-T. Long-term mortality and major adverse cardiovascular events in sepsis survivors. A Nationwide population-based study. Am J Respir Crit Care Med. 2016;194:209–17.
56. Czaja AS, Zimmerman JJ, Nathens AB. Readmission and late mortality after pediatric severe sepsis. Pediatrics. 2009;123:849–57.
57. Iwashyna TJ, Ely EW, Smith DM, Langa KM. Long-term cognitive impairment and functional disability among survivors of severe sepsis. JAMA. 2010;304:1787–94.
58. Pandharipande PP, Girard TD, Jackson JC, et al. Long-term cognitive impairment after critical illness. N Engl J Med. 2013;369:1306–16.
59. Shah FA, Pike F, Alvarez K, et al. Bidirectional relationship between cognitive function and pneumonia. Am J Respir Crit Care Med. 2013;188:586–92.
60. Nikayin S, Rabiee A, Hashem MD, Huang M, Bienvenu OJ, Turnbull AE, Needham DM. Anxiety symptoms in survivors of critical illness: a systematic review and meta-analysis. Gen Hosp Psychiatry. 2016;43:23–9.
61. Rabiee A, Nikayin S, Hashem MD, Huang M, Dinglas VD, Bienvenu OJ, Turnbull AE, Needham DM. Depressive symptoms after critical illness: a systematic review and meta-analysis. Crit Care Med. 2016;44:1744–53.
62. Parker AM, Sricharoenchai T, Raparla S, Schneck KW, Bienvenu OJ, Needham DM. Posttraumatic stress disorder in critical illness survivors: a metaanalysis. Crit Care Med. 2015;43:1121–9.
63. Davydow DS, Hough CL, Langa KM, Iwashyna TJ. Symptoms of depression in survivors of severe sepsis: a prospective cohort study of older Americans. Am J Geriatr Psychiatry. 2013;21:887–97.
64. Huang C, Daniels R, Lembo A, Heymann T, O'Brien J, Hartog C, Reinhart K, Nguyen HB. Mental, physiologic, and functional disabilities in post-sepsis syndrome: an international survey. Crit Care Med. 2016;44:429.
65. Prescott HC, Langa KM, Iwashyna TJ. Readmission diagnoses after hospitalization for severe sepsis and other acute medical conditions. JAMA. 2015;313:1055–7.
66. Shen H-N, Lu C-L, Yang H-H. Risk of recurrence after surviving severe sepsis. Crit Care Med. 2016;44:1833–41.
67. DeMerle K, Royer S, Mikkelsen M, Prescott H. Readmissions for recurrent sepsis: new or relapsed infection? Crit Care Med. 2017;45(10):1702–8.
68. Prescott HC. Toward a nuanced understanding of the role of infection in readmissions after sepsis. Crit Care Med. 2016;44:634–5.
69. Yende S, Linde-Zwirble W, Mayr F, Weissfeld LA, Reis S, Angus DC. Risk of cardiovascular events in survivors of severe sepsis. Am J Respir Crit Care Med. 2014;189:1065–74.

Part II

The Pathogenesis of Sepsis

Pathogenesis of Sepsis

3

Tjitske S. R. van Engelen, W. Joost Wiersinga, and Tom van der Poll

3.1 Introduction

Before the turn of the century, the pathogenesis of sepsis was considered to be driven by an abundant inflammatory response following the invasion of pathogens [1]. Current consensus acknowledges the occurrence of two opposite host reactions to severe infection with proinflammatory and anti-inflammatory features [2]. In sepsis, the normally careful inflammatory balance is disturbed, and hyperinflammation together with immune suppression ensue. This dysregulated immune response to infection is associated with a failure to return to homeostasis and harms the host, resulting in the life-threatening condition called sepsis [3]. While insights in the pathogenesis of sepsis have rapidly grown, this complex syndrome is not yet fully understood, and our increased understanding of pathophysiological mechanisms underlying sepsis has thus far failed to improve health outcome. This chapter provides a brief overview of the pathogenesis of sepsis (Fig. 3.1).

T. S. R. van Engelen, M.D. (✉)
Center for Experimental Molecular Medicine, Academic Medical Center, University of Amsterdam, Amsterdam, The Netherlands
e-mail: t.s.vanengelen@amc.uva.nl

W. Joost Wiersinga, M.D. · T. van der Poll, M.D.
Center for Experimental Molecular Medicine, Academic Medical Center, University of Amsterdam, Amsterdam, The Netherlands

Division of Infectious Diseases, Academic Medical Center, University of Amsterdam, Amsterdam, The Netherlands
e-mail: w.j.wiersinga@amc.uva.nl; t.vanderpoll@amc.uva.nl

W. J. Wiersinga, C. W. Seymour (eds.), *Handbook of Sepsis*,
https://doi.org/10.1007/978-3-319-73506-1_3

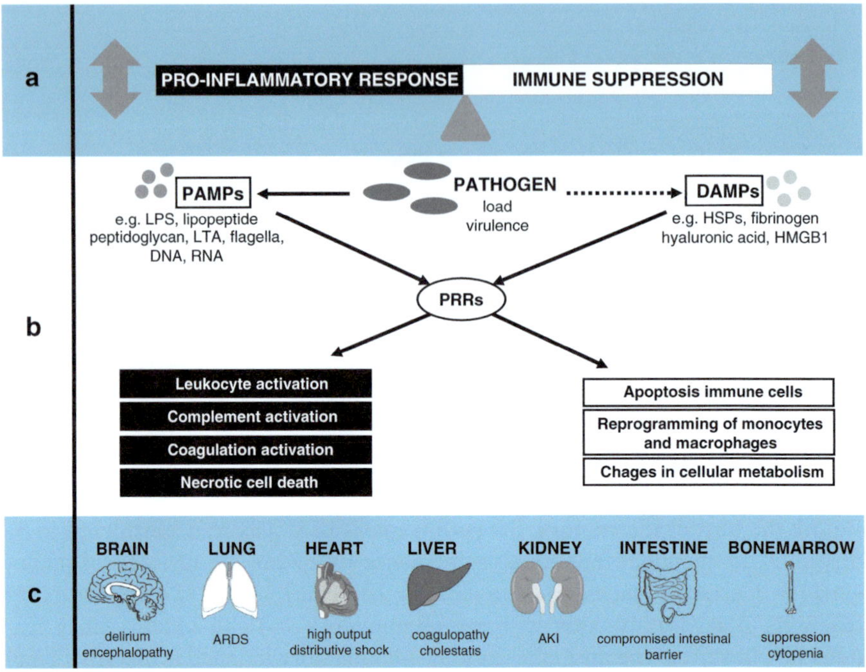

Fig. 3.1 Pathogenesis of sepsis. (**a**) Sepsis is defined as a dysregulated host response to infection, leading to life-threatening organ dysfunction. The normally careful inflammatory balance is disturbed, and this dysregulation is associated with a failure to return to homeostasis. Hyperinflammation and immune suppression ensue, to an extent that is detrimental to the host. (**b**) Once a pathogen has succeeded to cross the mucosal barrier of the host, it can cause sepsis depending on its load and virulence. The host defense system can recognize molecular components of invading pathogens (PAMPs) with specialized receptors (PRRs). Stimulation of PRRs has proinflammatory and immune suppressive consequences. It leads to activation of target genes coding for proinflammatory cytokines (leukocyte activation), inefficient use of the complement system, activation of the coagulation system, and concurrent downregulation of anticoagulant mechanisms and necrotic cell death. This starts a vicious cycle with further progression to sepsis, due to the release of endogenous molecules by injured cells (DAMPs or alarmins), which can further stimulate PRRs. Immune suppression is characterized by massive apoptosis and thereby depletion of immune cells, reprogramming of monocytes and macrophages to a state of a decreased capacity to release proinflammatory cytokines and a disturbed balance in cellular metabolic processes. (**c**) Sepsis is by definition a disease with organ failure. The clinical manifestation can be heterogeneous. Clinicians use physical examination, laboratory testing, and imaging techniques to determine the severity and origin of organ failure. Antimicrobial treatment is aimed to eliminate the causative pathogen, where supportive care is aimed to restore organ function. *ARDS* acute respiratory distress syndrome, *AKI* acute kidney injury, *DAMPs* danger-associated molecular patterns, *DNA* deoxyribonucleic acid, *HMGB1* high-mobility group box-1 protein, *HSPs* heat shock proteins, *LPS* lipopolysaccharide, *LTA* lipoteichoic acid, *PAMPs* pathogen-associated molecular patterns, *PPRs* pattern recognition receptors, *RNA* ribonucleic acid

3.2 Pathogens and Infection Sites

A successful pathogen must attach to and cross the mucosal barrier, escape the host defense system, and multiply to ensure its own survival. All invading microorganisms with a sufficient load and virulence can cause sepsis. However, several pathogens are well known for their impressive arsenal to attack the host. In a point-prevalence study entailing 14,000 intensive care unit (ICU) patients in 75 countries, 62% of positive isolates were gram-negative bacteria, versus 47% gram-positive and 19% fungal [4]. The most common gram-negative isolates in sepsis patients are *Escherichia coli*, *Klebsiella* sp., and *Pseudomonas aeruginosa*; the most frequent gram-positive organisms are *Staphylococcus aureus* and *Streptococcus pneumoniae* [5, 6]. The incidence of fungal infections as the cause of sepsis is rising, which is problematic due to the associated increased mortality. The most common site of infection is the respiratory tract with 63.5% of the culture-positive infections in the ICU, followed by abdominal infections (19.6%), bloodstream infections (15.1%), renal or urinary tract infections (14.3%), skin infections (6.6%), catheter-related infections (4.7%), infections of the central nervous system (2.9%), and others [4].

3.3 Host Recognition of Pathogens

The host can recognize molecular components of invading pathogens, called pathogen-associated molecular patterns (PAMPs), with specific receptors. Examples of key bacterial PAMPs are lipopolysaccharide (LPS, also known as endotoxin, a cell wall component of gram-negative bacteria), peptidoglycan, lipopeptides (constituents of many pathogens), lipoteichoic acid (a cell wall component of gram-positive bacteria), flagellin (factor in the mobility of bacteria), and bacterial DNA [7]. In the early response to infection, pathogens or more specifically PAMPs are recognized by a limited number of specialized host receptors, known as pattern recognition receptors (PRRs). PRR-mediated pathogen recognition is an important defense mechanism of the host against invading pathogens and results in upregulation of inflammatory gene transcription and initiation of innate immunity [2, 7, 8]. However, if the innate immune system fails to eradicate the pathogen, overstimulation of PRRs by a growing bacterial load can result in dysregulation of the host response, which then no longer benefits the host but causes tissue injury, organ dysfunction, and progression to sepsis. A contributing factor herein is that PRRs can also be stimulated by endogenous molecules released by injured cells, so-called danger-associated molecular patterns (DAMPs or alarmins) [9]. Examples of DAMPs are heat shock proteins, fibrinogen, hyaluronic acid, and high-mobility group box-1 protein (HMGB-1) [9]. Thus, PRRs recognize molecular components of both the pathogen (PAMPs) and the host (DAMPs), resulting in a vicious cycle and perpetuation of inflammation. Four main PRR families have been identified: Toll-like receptors (TLRs), C-type lectin receptors (CLRs), retinoic acid-inducible gene (RIG)-I-like receptors (RLRs), and NOD-like receptors (NLRs) [7, 8].

TLRs comprise the most well-known family of PRRs [7]. They are expressed both extracellularly (TLR1, 2, 4, 5, 6) and intracellularly (TLR3, 7, 8, 9, 10, 11, 12, 13) in endosomes and lysosomes. Ten different TLRs have so far been identified in humans (TLR1–10); 12 are found in mice (TRL1–9, TLR11, TLR12, TLR13) [10]. TLRs are activated by a broad range of ligands presented by bacteria, viruses, parasites, fungi, and the host itself. The signaling pathways of TLRs run via four adaptor proteins, namely, myeloid differentiation primary response protein 88 (MyD88), TIR domain-containing adaptor protein (TIRAP), TIR domain-containing adaptor protein-inducing IFN-β (TRIF), and TRIF-related adaptor molecule (TRAM). This signaling eventually leads to the translocation of nuclear factor (NF-κB) into the nucleus which starts the transcoding of genes and is crucial for early activation of the immune system [8]. As an example of TLR signaling, TLR4 is stimulated through its ligand LPS, the virulence factor of gram-negative bacteria. It activates both the MyD88- and the TIRAP-dependent pathways for early-phase activation of NF-κB and results in late-phase activation of NF-κB via the TRIF-dependent pathway [7]. TLR3 is stimulated by dsRNA derived from viruses or virus-infected cells and activates the TRIF-dependent pathway [8].

NLRs are cytoplasmic proteins composed of a central nucleotide-binding domain and C-terminal leucine-rich repeats [11]. NLRs are an important factor in the initial immune response through their formation of multiprotein complexes called "inflammasomes." These complexes activate caspase-1 leading to the maturation of proinflammatory cytokines interleukin 1β (IL-1β) and IL-18 [12]. RLRs are cytoplasmic proteins that can recognize the genomic RNA of RNA viruses [13, 14]. CLRs are transmembrane receptors with a carbohydrate-binding domain. CLR-mediated microbial recognition occurs through their ability to recognize carbohydrates on viruses, bacteria, and fungi (Table 3.1).

Table 3.1 Pattern recognition receptors and their ligands in humans

Pattern recognition receptor	Ligand	Origin of ligand
Toll-like receptors (TLRs)		
TLR1	Triacyl lipoprotein (forms heterodimer with TLR2), soluble factors	Bacteria
TLR2	Lipoprotein (forms heterodimer with TLR1 and TLR6)	Bacteria, viruses, fungi, self
TLR3	Double-stranded RNA	Viruses
TLR4	Lipopolysaccharide, envelop proteins (syncytial viruses), glycoinositol phospholipids, HSPs 60 and 70, S100a8 (ligand from dying cells)	Bacteria, viruses, self
TLR5	Flagellin	Bacteria
TLR6	Diacyl lipoprotein (forms heterodimer with TLR2)	Bacteria, viruses
TLR7	Single-stranded RNA, synthetic compounds (e.g., imidazoquinolines)	Bacteria, viruses, self
TLR8	Single-stranded RNA, small purine analog compounds (imidazoquinolines)	Viruses
TLR9	CpG-DNA, insoluble crystal hemozoin (*Plasmodium falciparum*)	Bacteria, viruses, parasites, self
TLR10	Unknown	
NOD-like receptors (NLRs)		
NOD1	Peptidoglycan (iE-DAP)	Bacteria
NOD2	Peptidoglycan (MDP)	Bacteria

Table 3.1 (continued)

Pattern recognition receptor	Ligand	Origin of ligand
C-type lectins (CLRs)		
Dectin-1	β-Glucan	Fungi
Dectin-2	β-Glucan	Fungi
MINCLE	SAP130	Fungi, self
Retinoic acid-inducible gene (RIG)-I-like receptors (RLRs)		
RIG-I	Short double-stranded RNA, 5′triphosphate dsRNA	Viruses
MDA5	Long double-stranded RNA	Viruses
LGP2	Double-stranded RNA	Viruses
DDX3	Viral RNA	Viruses

The innate immune system recognizes pathogens by four main classes of pattern recognition receptors. The table shows the main receptors, their main ligands, and the origin of these ligands. Note that some receptors also recognize "self" antigens, primarily in the context of injury, wherein self-antigens function as alarmins to the host

CpG-DNA cytosine-phosphate-guanosine-DNA, *DDX3* DEAD/H Box 3, *iE-DAP* g-D-glutamyl-meso-diaminopimelic acid, *LGP2* laboratory of genetics and physiology-2, *MDA5* melanoma differentiation-associated gene 5, *MDP* muramyl dipeptide, *MINCLE* macrophage-inducible C-type lectin, *SAP130* Sin3A-associated protein of 130 kDa

Table adapted from Refs. [8, 10, 59]

3.4 Hyperinflammation

Sepsis is associated with a strong activation of the immune system, by stimulation of PRRs by PAMPs and DAMPs, leading to the activation of target genes coding for proinflammatory cytokines such as tumor necrosis factor (TNF), IL-1β, IL-12, and IL-18 [2]. Cytokines are small proteins that can regulate the host response both locally and systemically, after their release from various cell types such as monocytes and neutrophils. These cells can further attribute to activation of the immune system by expression of the triggering receptor expressed on myeloid cells-1 (TREM-1) that amplifies TLR- and NLR-mediated inflammatory response [15]. Several mechanisms regulate the activation of PRRs to avoid overstimulation, including the negative regulators MyD88 short (MyD88s), ST2, single-immunoglobulin interleukin (IL)-1 receptor-related molecule (SIGIRR), toll-interacting protein (TOLLIP), suppressor of cytokine signaling (SOCS), A20, and IRAK-M [16]. If the delicate balance between activation and inhibition of the inflammatory response is disturbed, the pleiotropic hyperinflammatory response in sepsis ensues. This includes activation of the complement and coagulation systems and disturbance of vascular permeability [2], which have been considered important factors in sepsis mortality.

3.4.1 Complement System

The complement system comprises over 40 components that, when activated, work as a cascade and contribute to the innate immune surveillance system [17, 18]. A close collaboration between the complement system and other proinflammatory stimuli such as cytokines is necessary: the complement system tags dangerous cells or pathogens, and phagocytic cells can respond more properly after activation by proinflammatory mediators. This teamwork is dysregulated in sepsis resulting in inefficient use of the complement system. The complement system contributes directly to the activation of the immune system by the release of anaphylatoxins C3a and C5a. Anaphylatoxins are proinflammatory molecules that activate surrounding cells when they reach a threshold concentration, can lead to the recruitment of other immune cells (macrophages, basophils, neutrophils, eosinophils, and mast cells), and can activate endothelial and epithelial cells and platelets [17, 18]. The harmful role of C5a in sepsis has been linked to neutrophil dysfunction, apoptosis of lymphoid cells, exacerbation of systemic inflammation, cardiomyopathy, disseminated intravascular coagulation (DIC), and complications associated with multiple organ failure [19]. Several experimental sepsis studies have highlighted the beneficial effect of blockage of C5a signaling on outcome [20]. As such, C5a is considered a potential therapeutic target in sepsis.

3.4.2 Coagulation System and Vascular Endothelium

Activation of PRRs leads to upregulation of inflammatory mediators which results in a systemic inflammatory response, including activation of the coagulation system and concurrent downregulation of anticoagulant mechanisms [21]. Coagulation abnormalities can range from mild to clinically relevant fulminant coagulopathies. DIC is the most severe manifestation of disturbed hemostasis with microvascular thrombosis and, through consumption of clotting factors and platelets, simultaneous hemorrhage [22]. The most important initiator of coagulation in sepsis is tissue factor (TF). Indeed, inhibition of TF prevents DIC and improves survival in experimental sepsis [21]. TF is predominantly produced by macrophages and monocytes, and its expression is enhanced by proinflammatory cytokines, exemplifying the close interaction between inflammation and coagulation [23]. Furthermore, TF can reside in micro particles that are formed by hematopoietic and endothelial cells. These micro particles play a significant role in both coagulation and inflammation [24].

In healthy hosts, coagulation is controlled by three main anticoagulant pathways: the antithrombin system, tissue factor pathway inhibitor (TFPI), and the protein C system. In septic patients all these pathways are impaired in their function, partially due to endothelial dysfunction, resulting in low levels of these coagulation inhibitors [25, 26]. The physiological function of the protein C system has been supported by investigations in which interventions inhibiting this pathway resulted in severe coagulopathy and death in otherwise nonlethal infection models. During the early stages of inflammation, plasminogen activators are released to help break down fibrin. Sepsis is associated with high levels of plasminogen activator inhibitor type 1 (PAI-1), a main inhibitor of fibrinolysis, further facilitating microvascular thrombosis [27].

The interaction between inflammation and coagulation is not unilateral. Coagulation factors regulate inflammation in particular through proteolytic cleavage of protease-activated receptors (PARs) [28]. Activated protein C (APC) influences inflammation, by reducing the expression of receptors for cytokines and chemokines [29], by downregulating the production of inflammatory mediators [30, 31], and by blockage of cytokine release and leukocyte activation [32].

During sepsis the vascular endothelium is involved in the disturbance of anticoagulant mechanisms. Glycosaminoglycans on the endothelial surface support antithrombin-mediated inhibition of thrombin formation and platelet adhesion. Sepsis reduces the production of glycosaminoglycans averting not only antithrombin function but also that of TFPI with regard to inhibiting the main coagulation TF-factor VIIa complex. In healthy hosts endothelium generates APC from protein C through an interaction between thrombin and thrombomodulin (a receptor expressed by endothelial cells); formation of APC by the thrombomodulin-thrombin complex is accelerated by the endothelial protein C receptor (EPCR). APC inactivates coagulation cofactors Va and VIIIa by proteolysis, thereby inhibiting coagulation. In sepsis APC levels are reduced due to impaired production caused by downregulation of both thrombomodulin and EPCR on endothelial cells, as well as by increased consumption.

Adhesion of cells to the endothelium is increased in sepsis. Physiologically, injured endothelium activates von Willebrand factor which forms multimers at the site of injury as a primary step in protective coagulation [25]. Von Willebrand multimers are cleaved by a proteolytic enzyme ADAMTS13 to control adhesion and prevent formation of large obstructive von Willebrand multimers. In sepsis there is a relative deficiency of ADAMTS13 leading to ultra-large von Willebrand multimers at injured sites, contributing to overwhelming platelet adhesion and microvascular thrombosis and possibly eventually multiple organ dysfunction. Furthermore, activation of platelets because of vascular injury during sepsis starts a vicious cycle which leads to more activated endothelium and platelets which further increases coagulation [25].

Impaired vascular barrier function is a key pathogenic mechanism in sepsis, associated with protein leakage into the extravascular space, tissue edema, and diminished microvascular perfusion [25]. Important regulators of vascular barrier function are sphingosine-1-phosphate (S1P) and angiopoietin-1 [25, 33]. S1P activates the endothelial S1P receptor 1, thereby preserving vascular integrity [33]. Angiopoietin-1 activates TIE2, supporting barrier function. Angiopoietin-2 antagonizes angiopoietin-1, and a high angiopoietin-2/angiopoietin-1 ratio has been used as a marker for vascular barrier dysfunction in patients with sepsis [34].

3.4.3 Neutrophil Extracellular Traps

Activation of the coagulation system and vascular injury are amplified by the release of neutrophil extracellular traps (NETs) by neutrophils [35]. NETs are composed of DNA, histones, and neutrophil-derived proteinases and can protect the host by eliminating pathogens. However, NETs may also contribute to collateral damage and thrombosis in the dysregulated immune response in sepsis [35].

3.5 Immune Suppression

Much attention has been drawn to immune suppression in patients with sepsis, which in many patients can already be detected on admission to the ICU and is a prominent feature in those patients that remain in the ICU for extended periods of time [2, 36]. Targeted immune-enhancing therapy may be beneficial for selected patients with immune suppression [2, 36].

Transcriptomic analysis of peripheral blood leucocytes of septic patients recently resulted in the classifications of distinct sepsis endotypes with implications for main pathophysiological mechanisms and prognosis [37, 38]. These studies further confirmed the existence of subgroups of sepsis patients with a predominant immune suppressive phenotype [37, 38].

3.5.1 Apoptosis of Immune Cells

Sepsis-associated immune suppression involves several cell types. During sepsis massive apoptosis leads to depletion of immune cells, especially CD4+ and CD8+ T cells and B cells. This depletion is seen in lymphoid organs and body sites, such as the spleen, thymus, lymph nodes, and gut-associated lymphoid tissue [36, 39]. T regulatory (Treg) cells are more resistant to sepsis-induced apoptosis which, combined with the substantial apoptosis of CD4+ and CD8+ T cells and B cells, lead to a more immune suppressive phenotype. Furthermore, surviving CD4+ and CD8+ T cells shift from a Th1 proinflammatory phenotype to the more immune suppressive Th2 phenotype. Inhibition of lymphocyte apoptosis was associated with better outcomes in various experimental sepsis models, suggesting a causal relationship between lymphocyte apoptosis and sepsis mortality [2, 36]. A recently identified potential therapeutic target in sepsis is the programmed cell death 1 (PD1)–PD1 ligand (PDL1) pathway. Patients with sepsis showed enhanced expression of PD1 on CD4+ T cells together with increased expression of PDL1 on macrophages and endothelial cells [39]. Enhanced PD1–PDL1 interaction is expected to impair T-cell function, and in mice inhibition of this pathway conferred protection against lethality following experimentally induced sepsis [40]. Clinical trials seeking to inhibit PD1–PDL1 signaling in sepsis patients are under way.

Contrary to lymphocytes, apoptosis of neutrophils in sepsis is delayed [2, 36]. Furthermore, the bone marrow releases immature neutrophils which together result in high numbers of circulating neutrophils in different stages of maturation. The function of neutrophils is impaired in sepsis, with reduced chemotaxis and reactive oxygen production.

3.5.2 Reprogramming of Monocytes and Macrophages

Sepsis is further characterized by profound changes in the function of antigen presenting cells [2, 36]. Monocytes and macrophages demonstrate a strongly decreased capacity to release proinflammatory cytokines upon stimulation with bacterial agonists (a feature commonly referred to as "endotoxin tolerance") and reduced HLA-DR expression. Notably, monocytes/macrophages do not show a general unresponsiveness, but rather are reprogrammed: after stimulation with bacterial compounds, they produce equal or even increased amounts of anti-inflammatory cytokines. Correspondingly, mRNA expression levels of genes encoding proinflammatory mediators have been reported downregulated upon stimulation with concurrent upregulation of mRNAs of anti-inflammatory mediators [2, 36]. HLA-DR expression on monocytes has been suggested as a biomarker to select sepsis patients for immune stimulatory therapy.

Epigenetic regulation of gene function likely plays a significant role in the host response to infection through suppression of proinflammatory gene expression and/or activation of anti-inflammatory genes, thereby contributing to immune suppression [41]. Protein expression can be regulated both at the pre- and posttranscriptional level. Pretranscriptional regulation takes place on chromatin, the complex formed by the DNA double helix packaged by histones. The gene loci on chromatin can be organized in transcriptionally active "euchromatin" or transcriptionally silent "heterochromatin." The chromatin activation state is regulated by histone modifications due to acetylation, methylation, ubiquitination, and phosphorylation. For example, acetylation of lysine residues within histones usually facilitates transcription [41]. "Endotoxin tolerance" in monocytes has been linked to reduced expression of marks of open chromatin such as histone H3 lysine 4 trimethylation (H3K4me3) [42], and "endotoxin tolerant" macrophages showed enhanced levels of the repressive histone modification H3K9 dimethylation (H3K9m2) at the promoter sites of the genes encoding the proinflammatory cytokines TNF and IL-1β [43]. One mechanism by which microbial stimuli induce epigenetic gene regulation is through increased expression of the histone lysine demethylase KDM6B via NF-κB activation [44]. KDM6B primes genes for transcription, and it is postulated that this promotes IL-4 maturation. The latter is a potent cytokine to counteract various proinflammatory cytokines and contributes to immune suppression. This IL-4/KDM6B axis appears to be one of the important pathways in the epigenetic regulation of macrophage activation [41]. The immune suppressive effects of sepsis can remain for months, perhaps even longer. It is hypothesized that epigenetic imprints occur both on mature immune cells in the periphery and progenitor cells in the bone marrow, thereby contributing to this long-lasting immune suppression [41].

3.5.3 Cellular Metabolism

Changes in cellular metabolism may contribute to immune suppression [45]. A shift from oxidative phosphorylation to glycolysis (the so-called Warburg effect) is important for cells to generate an inflammatory response upon stimulation by LPS, and a failure to do so may render cells relatively unresponsive. As such, a disturbed balance in cellular metabolic processes has been implicated in the altered phenotype of monocytes in sepsis, although the underlying mechanisms seem to be more intricate than mere shifts between oxidative phosphorylation and glycolysis. In contrast to LPS (which induces a classical Warburg effect), other bacterial stimuli were found to induce a rise in both glycolysis and oxidative phosphorylation in monocytes [46]. Similarly, the deficits of monocyte metabolism in sepsis patients with immune suppression do not only involve glycolysis but include a broad inhibition of metabolic processes including glycolysis, fatty acid oxidation, and oxidative phosphorylation [47].

3.6 Microbiome

The microbiome consists of trillions of bacteria of which most are found in the gastrointestinal tract [48]. Dysbiosis of the microbiome (meaning a decreased microbial diversity) has been associated with altered immune responses (for instance, altered cytokine production capacity of immune cells). Sepsis affects the composition of the intestinal microbiome, characterized by a loss of diversity, lower abundances of key commensal genera (such as *Faecalibacterium*, *Blautia*, *Ruminococcus*), and overgrowth of opportunistic pathogens [49]. Small studies show that the gut is overrun by a single bacterial genus in patients with sepsis, most notably by *Clostridium difficile*, *Staphylococcus* spp., *Escherichia* spp., *Shigella* spp., *Salmonella* spp., and *Enterococcus* spp. [50]. This overgrowth by one genus occurs in roughly one third of the septic patients but increases with time spent on the ICU [51]. The underlying mechanism is not fully understood, but antibiotic treatment that is part of standard care in septic patients seems to have the most disruptive effect on the microbiome, possibly amplified by the use of (par)enteral feeding and gastric acid inhibitory drugs [52]. Murine studies support a role for the microbiome in regulation of granulocytosis, neutrophil homeostasis, and host resistance to sepsis [53]. In pneumonia-derived sepsis, disruption of the gut microbiome impaired host defense; underlying mechanisms likely include a reduced responsiveness to microbial stimulation and an impaired phagocytosis capacity of alveolar macrophages [54]. In addition, neutrophils from microbiota-depleted mice demonstrated a diminished capacity to migrate into inflamed tissues [55].

The immune response can further be compromised when translocation of pathological microbes through disintegrated epithelial barriers results in systemic and lymphatic spreading of pathogens. Theories of connections between the gut microbiome and distant organ function, the so-called gut-organ axis, are rapidly developing. For instance, a recent study showed evidence of gut bacteria present in the lung microbiome in mice with experimental sepsis and humans with acute respiratory distress syndrome, supporting the existence of the gut-lung axis [56]. Research concerning the pathophysiological mechanism underlying these phenomena is growing rapidly [52, 57], as are studies regarding the microbiome as a therapeutic target in critically ill patients [58].

Conclusion

Sepsis is defined as a life-threatening organ dysfunction caused by a dysregulated host response to infection characterized by sustained hyperinflammation and immune suppression. While much progress has been made in understanding the pathogenesis of sepsis, translation of this knowledge into effective novel sepsis therapies has been unsuccessful. The aim of future sepsis research should be just that.

References

1. van der Poll T, Opal SM. Host-pathogen interactions in sepsis. Lancet Infect Dis. 2008;8(1):32–43.
2. van der Poll T, van de Veerdonk FL, Scicluna BP, Netea MG. The immunopathology of sepsis and potential therapeutic targets. Nat Rev Immunol. 2017;17(7):407–20.
3. Singer M, Deutschman CS, Seymour CW, Shankar-Hari M, Annane D, Bauer M, et al. The third international consensus definitions for sepsis and septic shock (Sepsis-3). JAMA. 2016;315(8):801–10.
4. Vincent JL, Rello J, Marshall J, Silva E, Anzueto A, Martin CD, et al. International study of the prevalence and outcomes of infection in intensive care units. JAMA. 2009;302(21):2323–9.
5. Opal SM, Garber GE, LaRosa SP, Maki DG, Freebairn RC, Kinasewitz GT, et al. Systemic host responses in severe sepsis analyzed by causative microorganism and treatment effects of drotrecogin alfa (activated). Clin Infect Dis. 2003;37(1):50–8.
6. Ranieri VM, Thompson BT, Barie PS, Dhainaut JF, Douglas IS, Finfer S, et al. Drotrecogin alfa (activated) in adults with septic shock. N Engl J Med. 2012;366(22):2055–64.
7. Kawai T, Akira S. The role of pattern-recognition receptors in innate immunity: update on toll-like receptors. Nat Immunol. 2010;11(5):373–84.
8. Takeuchi O, Akira S. Pattern recognition receptors and inflammation. Cell. 2010;140(6):805–20.
9. Chan JK, Roth J, Oppenheim JJ, Tracey KJ, Vogl T, Feldmann M, et al. Alarmins: awaiting a clinical response. J Clin Invest. 2012;122(8):2711–9.
10. Satoh T, Akira S. Toll-like receptor signaling and its inducible proteins. Microbiol Spectr. 2016;4:6.
11. Inohara C, McDonald C, Nunez G. NOD-LRR proteins: role in host-microbial interactions and inflammatory disease. Annu Rev Biochem. 2005;74:355–83.
12. Franchi L, Munoz-Planillo R, Nunez G. Sensing and reacting to microbes through the inflammasomes. Nat Immunol. 2012;13(4):325–32.
13. Takeuchi O, Akira S. Innate immunity to virus infection. Immunol Rev. 2009;227(1):75–86.
14. Yoneyama M, Fujita T. Structural mechanism of RNA recognition by the RIG-I-like receptors. Immunity. 2008;29(2):178–81.
15. Klesney-Tait J, Turnbull IR, Colonna M. The TREM receptor family and signal integration. Nat Immunol. 2006;7(12):1266–73.
16. Liew FY, Xu D, Brint EK, O'Neill LA. Negative regulation of toll-like receptor-mediated immune responses. Nat Rev Immunol. 2005;5(6):446–58.
17. Merle NS, Noe R, Halbwachs-Mecarelli L, Fremeaux-Bacchi V, Roumenina LT. Complement system part II: role in immunity. Front Immunol. 2015;6:257.
18. Sarma JV, Ward PA. The complement system. Cell Tissue Res. 2011;343(1):227–35.
19. Ward PA. The harmful role of c5a on innate immunity in sepsis. J Innate Immun. 2010;2(5):439–45.
20. Guo RF, Ward PA. Role of C5a in inflammatory responses. Annu Rev Immunol. 2005;23:821–52.
21. Levi M, van der Poll T. Coagulation and sepsis. Thromb Res. 2017;149:38–44.
22. Gando S, Levi M, Toh CH. Disseminated intravascular coagulation. Nat Rev Dis Primers. 2016;2:16037.
23. Levi M, van der Poll T. Inflammation and coagulation. Crit Care Med. 2010;38(2 Suppl):S26–34.
24. Meziani F, Delabranche X, Asfar P, Toti F. Bench-to-bedside review: circulating microparticles--a new player in sepsis? Crit Care. 2010;14(5):236.

25. Opal SM, van der Poll T. Endothelial barrier dysfunction in septic shock. J Intern Med. 2015;277(3):277–93.
26. Levi M, Poll T. Coagulation in patients with severe sepsis. Semin Thromb Hemost. 2015;41(1):9–15.
27. Biemond BJ, Levi M, Ten Cate H, Van der Poll T, Buller HR, Hack CE, et al. Plasminogen activator and plasminogen activator inhibitor I release during experimental endotoxaemia in chimpanzees: effect of interventions in the cytokine and coagulation cascades. Clin Sci (Lond). 1995;88(5):587–94.
28. Coughlin SR. Thrombin signalling and protease-activated receptors. Nature. 2000;407(6801):258–64.
29. Kaneider NC, Forster E, Mosheimer B, Sturn DH, Wiedermann CJ. Syndecan-4-dependent signaling in the inhibition of endotoxin-induced endothelial adherence of neutrophils by antithrombin. Thromb Haemost. 2003;90(6):1150–7.
30. Esmon CT. New mechanisms for vascular control of inflammation mediated by natural anticoagulant proteins. J Exp Med. 2002;196(5):561–4.
31. Yuksel M, Okajima K, Uchiba M, Horiuchi S, Okabe H. Activated protein C inhibits lipopolysaccharide-induced tumor necrosis factor-alpha production by inhibiting activation of both nuclear factor-kappa B and activator protein-1 in human monocytes. Thromb Haemost. 2002;88(2):267–73.
32. Murakami K, Okajima K, Uchiba M, Johno M, Nakagaki T, Okabe H, et al. Activated protein C attenuates endotoxin-induced pulmonary vascular injury by inhibiting activated leukocytes in rats. Blood. 1996;87(2):642–7.
33. Sanchez T. Sphingosine-1-phosphate signaling in endothelial disorders. Curr Atheroscler Rep. 2016;18(6):31.
34. Mikacenic C, Hahn WO, Price BL, Harju-Baker S, Katz R, Kain KC, et al. Biomarkers of endothelial activation are associated with poor outcome in critical illness. PLoS One. 2015;10(10):e0141251.
35. Sorensen OE, Borregaard N. Neutrophil extracellular traps – the dark side of neutrophils. J Clin Invest. 2016;126(5):1612–20.
36. Hotchkiss RS, Monneret G, Payen D. Sepsis-induced immunosuppression: from cellular dysfunctions to immunotherapy. Nat Rev Immunol. 2013;13(12):862–74.
37. Davenport EE, Burnham KL, Radhakrishnan J, Humburg P, Hutton P, Mills TC, et al. Genomic landscape of the individual host response and outcomes in sepsis: a prospective cohort study. Lancet Respir Med. 2016;4(4):259–71.
38. Scicluna BP, van Vught LA, Zwinderman AH, Wiewel MA, Davenport EE, Burnham KL, et al. Classification of patients with sepsis according to blood genomic endotype: a prospective cohort study. Lancet Respir Med. 2017;5(10):816–26. Epub ahead of print
39. Boomer JS, To K, Chang KC, Takasu O, Osborne DF, Walton AH, et al. Immunosuppression in patients who die of sepsis and multiple organ failure. JAMA. 2011;306(23):2594–605.
40. Huang X, Venet F, Wang YL, Lepape A, Yuan Z, Chen Y, et al. PD-1 expression by macrophages plays a pathologic role in altering microbial clearance and the innate inflammatory response to sepsis. Proc Natl Acad Sci U S A. 2009;106(15):6303–8.
41. Carson WF, Cavassani KA, Dou Y, Kunkel SL. Epigenetic regulation of immune cell functions during post-septic immunosuppression. Epigenetics. 2011;6(3):273–83.
42. Foster SL, Hargreaves DC, Medzhitov R. Gene-specific control of inflammation by TLR-induced chromatin modifications. Nature. 2007;447(7147):972–8.
43. El Gazzar M, Yoza BK, Chen X, Garcia BA, Young NL, McCall CE. Chromatin-specific remodeling by HMGB1 and linker histone H1 silences proinflammatory genes during endotoxin tolerance. Mol Cell Biol. 2009;29(7):1959–71.
44. De Santa F, Narang V, Yap ZH, Tusi BK, Burgold T, Austenaa L, et al. Jmjd3 contributes to the control of gene expression in LPS-activated macrophages. EMBO J. 2009;28(21):3341–52.
45. O'Neill LA, Kishton RJ, Rathmell J. A guide to immunometabolism for immunologists. Nat Rev Immunol. 2016;16(9):553–65.

46. Lachmandas E, Boutens L, Ratter JM, Hijmans A, Hooiveld GJ, Joosten LA, et al. Microbial stimulation of different toll-like receptor signalling pathways induces diverse metabolic programmes in human monocytes. Nat Microbiol. 2016;2:16246.
47. Cheng SC, Scicluna BP, Arts RJ, Gresnigt MS, Lachmandas E, Giamarellos-Bourboulis EJ, et al. Broad defects in the energy metabolism of leukocytes underlie immunoparalysis in sepsis. Nat Immunol. 2016;17(4):406–13.
48. Jacobs MC, Haak BW, Hugenholtz F, Wiersinga WJ. Gut microbiota and host defense in critical illness. Curr Opin Crit Care. 2017;23(4):257–63.
49. McDonald D, Ackermann G, Khailova L, Baird C, Heyland D, Kozar R, et al. Extreme dysbiosis of the microbiome in critical illness. mSphere. 2016;1(4):e00199-16.
50. Lankelma JM, van Vught LA, Belzer C, Schultz MJ, van der Poll T, de Vos WM, et al. Critically ill patients demonstrate large interpersonal variation in intestinal microbiota dysregulation: a pilot study. Intensive Care Med. 2017;43(1):59–68.
51. Ojima M, Motooka D, Shimizu K, Gotoh K, Shintani A, Yoshiya K, et al. Metagenomic analysis reveals dynamic changes of whole gut microbiota in the acute phase of intensive care unit patients. Dig Dis Sci. 2016;61(6):1628–34.
52. Haak BW, Wiersinga WJ. The role of the gut microbiota in sepsis. Lancet Gastroenterol Hepatol. 2017;2(2):135–43.
53. Deshmukh HS, Liu Y, Menkiti OR, Mei J, Dai N, O'Leary CE, et al. The microbiota regulates neutrophil homeostasis and host resistance to Escherichia coli K1 sepsis in neonatal mice. Nat Med. 2014;20(5):524–30.
54. Schuijt TJ, Lankelma JM, Scicluna BP, de Sousa e Melo F, Roelofs JJ, de Boer JD, et al. The gut microbiota plays a protective role in the host defence against pneumococcal pneumonia. Gut. 2016;65(4):575–83.
55. Karmarkar D, Rock KL. Microbiota signalling through MyD88 is necessary for a systemic neutrophilic inflammatory response. Immunology. 2013;140(4):483–92.
56. Dickson RP, Singer BH, Newstead MW, Falkowski NR, Erb-Downward JR, Standiford TJ, et al. Enrichment of the lung microbiome with gut bacteria in sepsis and the acute respiratory distress syndrome. Nat Microbiol. 2016;1(10):16113.
57. Schirmer M, Smeekens SP, Vlamakis H, Jaeger M, Oosting M, Franzosa EA, et al. Linking the human gut microbiome to inflammatory cytokine production capacity. Cell. 2016;167(4):1125–36.e8.
58. Wischmeyer PE, McDonald D, Knight R. Role of the microbiome, probiotics, and 'dysbiosis therapy' in critical illness. Curr Opin Crit Care. 2016;22(4):347–53.
59. Tartey S, Takeuchi O. Pathogen recognition and toll-like receptor targeted therapeutics in innate immune cells. Int Rev Immunol. 2017;36(2):57–73.

4 The Coagulation System in Sepsis

Marcel Levi

4.1 Sepsis and Coagulation

Sepsis is a very serious and potentially life-threatening complication of infection. Sepsis occurs when host defense mediators released into the circulation to combat the infection elicit systemic inflammatory responses throughout the body [1]. Sepsis is a frequently occurring medical condition with an incidence of about 2.5 per 1000 in the Western world and an almost 10% annual rise over the last two decades [2]. About 20% of patients with sepsis die within the hospital, and severe sepsis leads to a mortality rate of approximately 40% [3, 4].

Sepsis is consistently associated with coagulation abnormalities [5]. These deviations range from delicate activation of coagulation that can only be identified by highly sensitive assays for hemostatic factor activation to somewhat more severe coagulation activation that may be noticeable by a subtle fall in platelet count and subclinical elongation of global clotting assays to fulminant disseminated intravascular coagulation (DIC), manifested by profuse microvascular thrombosis in small- and mid-size vessels and simultaneous widespread hemorrhage from various sites [5–7]. Patients with sepsis and extensive forms of DIC may develop overt thromboembolic complications or clinically less apparent microvascular clot formation that may contribute to multiple organ failures [7, 8]. In other cases, severe hemorrhage may be the dominant presentation [9], and frequently sepsis and DIC lead to simultaneous thrombosis and bleeding. Hemorrhage is due to consumption and subsequent depletion of coagulation factors and platelets, caused by ongoing activation of the hemostatic system [10]. In its most extreme manifestation, this combination may present as the

M. Levi, M.D., Ph.D., F.R.C.P.
University College London Hospitals, London, UK

Department of Vascular Medicine, Academic Medical Center, University of Amsterdam, Amsterdam, The Netherlands
e-mail: marcel.levi@uclh.nhs.uk

W. J. Wiersinga, C. W. Seymour (eds.), *Handbook of Sepsis*,
https://doi.org/10.1007/978-3-319-73506-1_4

Waterhouse-Friderichsen syndrome, typically observed during fulminant meningococcal septicemia, although many other microorganisms may cause this clinical situation as well [11].

4.2 Frequency of Clinically Relevant Coagulopathy in Sepsis

Clinically relevant hemostatic changes may occur in up to 70% of septic patients, and approximately 35% of patients with sepsis will meet the criteria for DIC [12, 13]. The majority of septic patients will develop thrombocytopenia (platelet count $<150 \times 10^9$/l) [14, 15]. Commonly, platelet count drops in the first 4 days following admission to the hospital [16]. The severity of sepsis correlates markedly with the decrease in platelet count [17]. Critical factors that cause thrombocytopenia in sepsis are decreased platelet production, enhanced consumption, obliteration, or sequestration in the spleen. Decreased production of megakaryocytes in the bone marrow may seem incongruous with the high levels of platelet production-stimulating pro-inflammatory mediators, such as tumor necrosis factor (TNF)-α and interleukin (IL)-6, and elevated levels of thrombopoietin in patients with sepsis, which theoretically should stimulate megakaryopoiesis [18]. However, in a substantial number of patients with sepsis, significant hemophagocytosis occurs, consisting of active phagocytosis of platelet precursors and other hematopoietic cells by mononuclear cells, presumably caused by elevated concentrations of macrophage colony-stimulating factor (M-CSF) in sepsis [19]. Platelet consumption is presumably also significant in sepsis, due to platelet activation secondary to continuous formation of thrombin. Platelet activation, consumption, and destruction take place at the endothelial surface as a result of the widespread endothelial cell-platelet interaction in sepsis, although the extent may differ between various vascular beds of different organs [20]. Prolonged global coagulation assays (such as the prothrombin time (PT) or the activated partial thromboplastin time (aPTT)) are detectable in 15–30% of septic patients [21]. Other coagulation assay changes include high fibrin degradation products (in more than 95% of patients with sepsis) [22, 23] and low levels of physiological anticoagulants, such as antithrombin and protein C (90% of sepsis patients) [23, 24].

4.3 Pathways Leading to Coagulation Abnormalities in Sepsis

In the last three decades, the pathways involved in the coagulopathy of sepsis have been elucidated for an important part [6]. It is clear that various mechanisms in the coagulation system act simultaneously toward a prohemostatic state. Apparently the most important factors that mediate this derangement of the coagulation system during sepsis are cytokines. Ample evidence indicates an extensive cross talk between inflammation and coagulation, where besides inflammation-induced coagulation activation, coagulation also markedly influences inflammatory activity (Fig. 4.1) [25]. Of note, systemic activation of coagulation and inflammation in

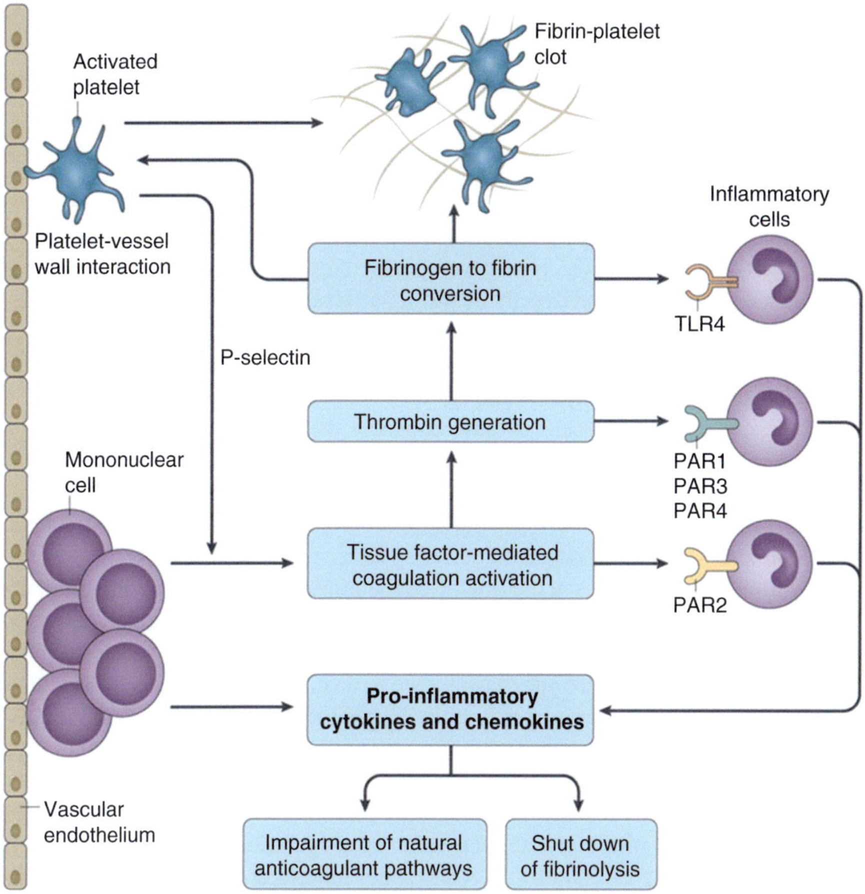

Fig. 4.1 Interaction between inflammation and coagulation in sepsis. Expression of tissue factor in mononuclear cells and subsequent exposure to blood results in thrombin generation followed by fibrinogen to fibrin conversion. Simultaneously, platelet vessel wall interaction and activation of platelets contribute to (micro)vascular clot formation. Platelet-derived P-selectin further enhances tissue factor expression. Binding of tissue factor, thrombin, and other activated coagulation proteases to specific protease-activated receptors (PARs) and binding of fibrin to Toll-like receptor (TLR) 4 on inflammatory cells affect inflammation through the consequent release of pro-inflammatory cytokines and chemokines, which further modulate coagulation and fibrinolysis [6]

sepsis may manifest with organ-specific presentations that are relevant for the specific organ failure resulting from severe sepsis [26].

The most important initiator of thrombin formation in sepsis is tissue factor. Studies of experimental or human endotoxemia or cytokinemia have demonstrated a central role of the tissue factor/factor VIIa system in the initiation of thrombin generation [27]. Abrogation of the tissue factor/factor VII(a) pathway by specific interventions aimed at tissue factor or factor VIIa activity resulted in a complete abrogation of thrombin generation in experimental settings [28, 29]. Also, in severe

Gram-negative sepsis, ex vivo tissue factor expression on monocytes of patients was demonstrated [30]. Experimental low-dose endotoxemia in healthy humans resulted in a 125-fold increase in tissue factor mRNA levels in blood monocytes [31]. An alternative source of tissue factor may be its localization on other blood cells [32], although it is not likely that these cells themselves produce tissue factor in substantial quantities [33]. Based on the assessment of transfer of tissue factor from mononuclear cells to activated platelets in an ex vivo perfusion setting, it was postulated that this "blood-borne" tissue factor is shuttled between cells through microparticles [34].

Platelets have a central role in the development of coagulation abnormalities in sepsis. Platelets can be triggered directly by pro-inflammatory mediators, such as platelet-activating factor [35]. Generated thrombin will further activate platelets. Activation of platelets may also stimulate fibrin formation by alternative mechanism. The expression of P-selectin on the platelet membrane not only mediates the adherence of platelets to leukocytes and endothelial cells but also enhances the expression of tissue factor on monocytes [36]. The underlying molecular pathway relies on nuclear factor kappa-B (NFκB) expression, induced by binding of activated platelets to neutrophils and monocytes. P-selectin can be shed from the surface of platelet membrane, and soluble P-selectin levels are indeed increased during systemic inflammation [36].

In normal circumstances activation of coagulation is controlled by three important physiological anticoagulant pathways: the antithrombin system, the activated protein C system, and the tissue factor pathway inhibitor (TFPI). In sepsis all three pathways are importantly deranged [37]. Due to a combination of impaired synthesis, ongoing consumption and proteolytic degradation (e.g., by neutrophilic elastase) levels of all three coagulation inhibitors are low. Also, significant downregulation of thrombomodulin and endothelial protein C receptor (EPCR) in inflammatory conditions will cause impaired conversion of protein C to activated protein C. In addition, at the time of the greatest activation of coagulation in sepsis, endogenous fibrinolysis is largely turned off. After the acute release of plasminogen activators (i.e., tissue-type plasminogen activator (t-PA) and urokinase-type plasminogen activator (u-PA)) from storage sites in vascular endothelial cells during inflammatory conditions, the increase in plasminogen activation and subsequent plasmin generation is annihilated by a sustained increase in plasminogen activator inhibitor type 1 (PAI-1) [38]. Of interest, studies have shown that a functional mutation in the PAI-1 gene, the 4G/5G polymorphism, not only affected the plasma levels of PAI-1 but was also linked to the clinical outcome of Gram-negative sepsis. Patients with the 4G/4G genotype had significantly higher PAI-1 concentrations and an increased mortality [39]. Other studies showed that the PAI-1 polymorphism increased the risk of developing septic shock from meningococcal infection [40].

4.4 Inflammation and the Coagulopathy of Sepsis

Like virtually all systemic inflammatory effects of infection, the derangement of the hemostatic system in sepsis is orchestrated by several cytokines. Most pro-inflammatory cytokines have been demonstrated to initiate coagulation activation in vitro. In sepsis high levels of cytokines can be found in the circulation of affected patients and investigational infection or experimental endotoxemia results in the transient increase in plasma levels of these cytokines [27]. The cytokine tumor necrosis factor (TNF) is the first mediator that becomes detectable, followed by an increase in serum levels of several interleukins (IL), of which IL-6 and IL-1 are prominent. Simultaneously, anti-inflammatory cytokines (such as IL-10) may have an inhibitory role in the activation of coagulation.

As TNF is the principal cytokine to become detectable in the circulation upon bacteremia and this cytokine has potent procoagulant effects, it was initially believed that hemostatic activation in sepsis was mediated by TNF. However, in several trials using different strategies to block TNF activity, it was shown that endotoxin induction of TNF could be completely abrogated, whereas activation of coagulation was not affected, albeit that the effects on coagulation inhibitors and fibrinolysis seemed to be regulated by TNF [27]. Also, in animals infused with a lethal dose of *E. coli*, an anti-TNF antibody had little or no effect on fibrinogen consumption or clinical outcome [41]. In line with this, clinical trials with an anti-TNF monoclonal antibody in septic patients did not show any advantage [42]. Interestingly, it was demonstrated in subsequent studies that strategies that blocked IL-6 caused a complete inhibition of endotoxin-induced activation of coagulation [43]. Also, studies in cancer patients with recombinant IL-6 showed that following the infusion of this cytokine, marked thrombin generation occurred [44]. Hence, these results suggest that IL-6 rather than TNF is important as a mediator for cytokine-induced coagulation activation. Whereas IL-1 is a potent agonist of tissue factor expression in vitro, its role has not been fully elucidated in vivo. Administration of an IL-1 receptor antagonist partly blocked the procoagulant response in experimental sepsis models and inhibited thrombin generation in patients [45]. However, most of the alterations in coagulation occur well before IL-1 becomes detectable in the circulation, leaving a potential role of IL-1 in the coagulopathy of sepsis an unsettled issue.

Coagulation factors and anticoagulant proteins do not only play a role in hemostatic activation but also interact with specific cell receptors leading to activation of signaling pathways (Fig. 4.1). Specifically, protease interactions that modulate inflammatory processes may be important in sepsis. The most significant pathway by which coagulation factors regulate inflammation is by binding to protease-activated receptors (PARs). PARs are transmembrane G-protein-coupled receptors, and four different types (PAR 1–4) have been recognized [46]. A typical property of PARs is that they serve as their own ligand. Proteolytic cleavage by an activated coagulation factor leads to exposure of a neo-amino terminus that is capable of activating the same receptor (and presumably adjacent receptors), leading to transmembrane signaling. PAR-1, PAR-3, and PAR4 are receptors that are activated by thrombin, while PAR-2 is triggered by the tissue factor/factor VIIa complex, factor Xa, and trypsin. PAR-1 is also a receptor for the tissue factor/factor VIIa complex and factor Xa.

It has become apparent that there is a significant cross talk between coagulation inhibitors and inflammatory mediators as well. Antithrombin can serve as a regulator of inflammation, e.g., by direct binding to inflammatory cells, thereby reducing cytokine and chemokine receptor expression [47]. Also, there is ample evidence that the protein C system importantly regulates inflammatory activity [48]. Activated protein C has been demonstrated to attenuate endotoxin-induced production of TNF-α, IL-1β, IL-6, and IL-8 by monocytes/macrophages [49]. In addition, activated protein C blocks cytokine release and leukocyte activation in experimental bacteremia in vivo [50]. Inhibition of the protein C pathway by a monoclonal antibody aggravates the inflammatory response, as shown by enhanced levels of pro-inflammatory cytokines and increased leukocyte activation and tissue damage [51]. Mice with a heterozygous protein C deficiency due to targeted disruption of the protein C gene have not only a stronger hemostatic response to experimental endotoxemia but also show marked differences in inflammatory responses (e.g., higher levels of circulating pro-inflammatory cytokines) [52].

4.5 Diagnosis of the Coagulopathy in Sepsis

There are several other causes for coagulation changes in septic patients. A low platelet count is almost invariably present in patients with severe sepsis, but thrombocytopenia may also be due to other (potentially concurrently present) conditions, such as immune thrombocytopenia, heparin-induced thrombocytopenia, thrombotic microangiopathies, or medication-induced bone marrow depression [53]. It is crucial to adequately diagnose these differential causes of thrombocytopenia, as they may necessitate specific management strategies [20]. Laboratory assays can be useful in differentiating the coagulopathy in sepsis from various other hemostatic conditions, such as vitamin K deficit or liver insufficiency. As these disorders may be present at the same time with sepsis-associated coagulopathy, this differentiation is not always easy [54, 55].

According to the contemporary thinking about sepsis-associated coagulopathy, the assessment of soluble fibrin in plasma appears to be important [56]. Generally, the sensitivity of assays for soluble fibrin for sepsis-associated coagulopathy is better than the specificity. Some clinical investigations have shown that at certain concentrations of soluble fibrin sepsis-associated coagulopathy is highly probable [22]. Most of the clinical trials show a sensitivity of 90–100% but simultaneously a rather low specificity [57]. Fibrin degradation products (FDPs) may be assayed by specific ELISAs or by latex agglutination assays, enabling quick and bedside determination in urgent cases. None of the available tests for fibrin degradation products distinguishes degradation products of cross-linked fibrin or fibrinogen degradation, which may cause falsely abnormal results [58]. The specificity of high levels of fibrin split products is therefore modest, and a series of other clinical situations, such as trauma, recent surgery, inflammation, or venous thromboembolism, may cause elevated FDPs. More modern tests are specifically targeted at the determination of neo-antigens on degraded cross-linked fibrin. Typically these assays react with an epitope related to plasmin-degraded cross-linked γ-chain, resulting in fragment D-dimer. These tests better distinguish degradation of cross-linked fibrin from fibrinogen or fibrinogen degradation products [59].

Ongoing coagulation activation results in depletion of coagulation factors in septic patients. Also, reduced synthesis, e.g., caused by impaired liver function or vitamin K deficiency, and loss of coagulation factors, due to massive bleeding, may be important. Measurement of fibrinogen levels has been widely promoted as a helpful tool for the diagnosis of coagulation abnormalities in sepsis, but in fact this is not very helpful in most cases [10, 60]. Fibrinogen acts as an acute-phase reactant, and despite considerable turnover, plasma concentrations can be well within the normal range. In a consecutive series of patients, the sensitivity of a low fibrinogen level for the diagnosis of DIC was less than 30%, and hypofibrinogenemia was established in extreme cases of Gram-negative septicemia only. Sequential assessment of fibrinogen might be more helpful and yield diagnostic insight.

Thrombelastography is increasingly employed in critically ill patients with a hypercoagulable state, including those with DIC [61, 62]. Procoagulant as well as anticoagulant states in DIC as indicated with thrombelastography was demonstrated to have a good correlation with clinically important organ dysfunction and survival although its advantage over usual coagulation assays has not yet been confirmed [63–65]. In a systematic review of 2 randomized controlled trials and 16 observational studies in patients with sepsis, it was demonstrated that thrombelastography was helpful in correctly identifying the endogenous fibrinolytic state [66]. The authors also found a correlation between hypocoagulability in sepsis and increased mortality. The accurate use of thrombelastography for the diagnosis of DIC has not been rigorously evaluated, although supporters believe that the assay may be helpful for appraising the state of coagulation in patients with critical illness [67, 68].

Based on retrospective analyses of databases from critically ill patients, composite scores for the diagnosis of sepsis-associated coagulopathy have been devised by the International Society on Thrombosis and Hemostasis (ISTH) [69]. The system is based on readily available laboratory tests, i.e., platelet count, prothrombin time, D-dimer, and fibrinogen levels. A diagnosis of DIC is compatible with a score of 5 or more points. The prothrombin time expressed in seconds in the scoring system may be replaced by the INR, making consistency between centers and standardization easier [70]. Validation analyses have shown a high diagnostic accuracy of the scoring system [71, 72]. The intensity of the coagulopathy as judged by this composite score is strongly associated with survival rates in critically ill patients [73]. Combining predictive intensive care measurement systems such as Acute Physiology and Chronic Health Evaluation (APACHE-II) with the DIC score seems to be a potent method to predict the prognosis in septic patients. Similar composite scores have been designed and studied in Japan [74]. The most relevant discrepancies between the ISTH and Japanese scores are a higher sensitivity and a higher proportion of patients with hemato-oncological diseases that are diagnosed with DIC by the Japanese systems [75, 76].

4.6 Supportive Treatment of Coagulation Abnormalities in Sepsis

The foundation of the treatment of septic coagulopathy is adequate management of the sepsis, e.g., by appropriate antibiotics and source control. However, in many situations, adjunctive supportive treatment, aimed at the replacement of organ function, is necessary. Likewise, coagulation may need supportive measures as the coagulopathy may proceed even after adequate sepsis treatment has been initiated. Some studies show that adjunctive interventions aimed at the derangement of coagulation may positively influence morbidity and mortality. The increase in the understanding of the various pathways that are important in coagulopathy of sepsis has indeed been helpful in the development of such adjunctive management strategies.

Low levels of platelets and coagulation factors may increase the risk of bleeding. However, plasma or platelet substitution therapy should not be instituted on the basis of laboratory results alone; it is indicated only in patients with active bleeding and in those requiring an invasive procedure or otherwise at risk for bleeding complications [77]. The presumed efficacy of treatment with plasma, fibrinogen, cryoprecipitate, or platelets is not based on randomized controlled trials but appears to be rational therapy in bleeding patients or in patients at risk for bleeding with a significant depletion of these hemostatic factors [37]. It may be required to use large volumes of plasma to restore normal concentrations of coagulation factors. Coagulation factor concentrates, such as prothrombin complex concentrate, may overcome this impediment, but these agents may lack important factors (e.g., factor V). Moreover, in older literature, caution is advocated with the use of prothrombin complex concentrates in systemic coagulation activation, as it may aggravate the coagulopathy due to small traces of activated factors in the concentrate. It is, however, less likely that this is still the case for the concentrates that are currently in use. Specific deficiencies in coagulation factors, such as fibrinogen, may be corrected by administration of purified coagulation factor concentrates [37].

Experimental studies have shown that heparin can at least partly inhibit the activation of coagulation in sepsis [78]. Uncontrolled case series in patients with sepsis and DIC have claimed to be successful. However, an advantageous effect of heparin on clinically important outcome events in patients with DIC has never been clearly demonstrated in controlled clinical trials [79], although there is cumulating evidence that heparin might be beneficial [80, 81]. In addition, there are several studies showing that critically ill patients with sepsis need adequate prophylaxis for venous thromboembolism, usually with (low molecular weight) heparin [82, 83]. Therapeutic doses of heparin are indicated in patients with clinically overt thromboembolism or extensive fibrin deposition, like purpura fulminans or acral ischemia. Patients with sepsis may benefit from prophylaxis to prevent venous thromboembolism, which may not be achieved with standard low-dose subcutaneous heparin [84].

Restoration of the levels of physiological anticoagulants in sepsis may be a rational approach [85]. Based on successful preclinical studies, the use of antithrombin concentrates has been examined mainly in randomized controlled trials in patients with severe sepsis. All trials have shown some beneficial effect in terms of improvement of laboratory parameters, shortening of the duration of the coagulopathy, or even improvement in organ function. In several small clinical trials, the use of very high doses of antithrombin concentrate showed even a modest reduction in mortality, however, without being statistically significant. A large-scale, multicenter, randomized controlled trial also showed no significant reduction in mortality of patients with sepsis [86]. Interestingly, post hoc subgroup analyses of this study indicated some benefit in patients who did not receive concomitant heparin and in those with the most severe coagulopathy [87]. Recent propensity-adjusted retrospective data from Japan demonstrated a significant benefit of antithrombin-treated patients with severe infection and sepsis [88, 89]. However these observations still need prospective validation.

Adjunctive therapy with activated protein C (APC) has also been widely studied. A phase III trial of APC concentrate in patients with sepsis was prematurely stopped because of efficacy in reducing mortality in these patients [23]. All-cause mortality at 28 days after inclusion was 24.7% in the APC group versus 30.8% in the control group (a 19.4% relative risk reduction). And there was also an improvement of coagulation abnormalities and reduced organ failure in APC-treated patients. Of note, patients with the most severe coagulopathy benefited most from this treatment [73]. However, a series of negative trials in specific populations of patients with severe sepsis led to scepticism regarding the use of APC in sepsis, and meta-analyses of published literature concluded that the basis for treatment with APC, even in patients with a high disease severity, was not very strong or even insufficient [90]. On top of that, there was uncertainty regarding the bleeding risk of APC in patients with severe sepsis. The last large placebo-controlled trial in patients with severe sepsis and septic shock was prematurely stopped due to the lack of any significant benefit of APC [91]. Subsequently, the manufacturer of APC has decided to withdraw the product from the market, which has resulted in a revision of current guidelines for treatment of DIC [92].

The most promising intervention at this moment is recombinant soluble thrombomodulin. Several preclinical studies in experimental sepsis models have shown that soluble thrombomodulin is capable of improving the derangement of coagulation and may restore organ dysfunction [93]. In phases I–II clinical studies, the pharmacokinetic profile of recombinant soluble thrombomodulin was determined [94]. In a subsequent phase III randomized double-blind clinical trial in patients with DIC, administration of the soluble thrombomodulin had a significantly better effect on bleeding manifestations and coagulation parameters than heparin, but the mortality rate at 28 days was similar in the two study groups [95]. When limiting these results to patients with severe infection and sepsis, DIC resolution rates were 67.5% in thrombomodulin-treated patients and 55.6% in the control group, and 28-day mortality rates were 21.4% and 31.6%, respectively. Subsequently, soluble thrombomodulin was evaluated in a phase II/III clinical study in 750 patients with sepsis and disseminated intravascular coagulation [96]. Twenty-eight-day mortality was 17.8% in the thrombomodulin group and 21.6% in the placebo group. Markers of coagulation activation were lower in the thrombomodulin group than in the placebo group. There were no differences between groups in bleeding or thrombotic events. The promising results with recombinant soluble thrombomodulin are supported by retrospective data in large series of Japanese patients and are currently being evaluated in a large international multicenter trial [97, 98].

4.7 New Pathways and Targets in the Management of DIC

In view of the overwhelming evidence for the central role of impaired natural anticoagulant pathways in the pathogenesis of DIC, much attention has been focused on the restoration of physiological anticoagulation as (adjunctive) treatment of DIC [6]. However, despite the fact that these interventions (such as recombinant human-activated protein C or antithrombin concentrate) have shown efficacy in reversing the coagulopathy, they have not resulted in an improvement on clinically relevant outcomes, such as survival or improvement of organ dysfunction [99]. One of the factors responsible for this may be that all these anticoagulants are clearly limited by the potential risk of major hemorrhage in critically ill patients. Therefore, it has been hypothesized that molecules that have less anticoagulant properties but have retained their anti-inflammatory effects may be promising new agents for the management of DIC. For example, non-anticoagulant heparin inhibits the expression and function of adhesion molecules, such as P-selectin and L-selectin. Moreover, this compound directly affects pro-inflammatory mediators, such as nuclear factor (NF)-κβ and cytokines, and attenuates endothelial cell dysfunction through the nitric oxide system. Non-anticoagulant heparin has a strong affinity for extracellular histones that result from cellular destruction during severe inflammation and that are robustly associated with endothelial dysfunction, organ failure, and death during sepsis [100]. Binding of this non-anticoagulant heparin to histones strongly inhibited cytotoxic activity in vitro and translated to impaired inflammation and improved survival in animal models of systemic infection and inflammation. Similarly, recent experiments indicate a beneficial effect of activated protein C variants that have lost their anticoagulant properties [101].

Another interesting new target may the glycocalyx covering the endothelial surface of the vascular bed [102]. The endothelium of the capillary bed is the most important interface in which the interaction between inflammation and coagulation takes place. All physiologic anticoagulant systems and various adhesion molecules that may modulate both inflammation and coagulation are connected to the endothelium. In sepsis, endothelial glycosaminoglycans present in the glycocalyx are downregulated by pro-inflammatory cytokines, thereby impairing the functions of antithrombin (AT), tissue factor pathway inhibitor (TFPI), leukocyte adhesion, and leukocyte transmigration. Because the glycocalyx also plays a role in other endothelial functions, including maintenance of the vascular barrier function, nitric oxide-mediated vasodilation, and antioxidant activity, all these processes can be impaired in DIC. Moreover, specific disruption of the glycocalyx results in thrombin generation and platelet adhesion within a few minutes. Novel interventions aimed at restoration of the glycocalyx may potentially maintain adequate physiological anticoagulation to balance activated coagulation in DIC [103].

References

1. Angus DC, van der Poll T. Severe sepsis and septic shock. N Engl J Med. 2013;369(9):840–51.
2. Martin GS, Mannino DM, Eaton S, Moss M. The epidemiology of sepsis in the United States from 1979 through 2000. N Engl J Med. 2003;348(16):1546–54.
3. Angus DC, Linde-Zwirble WT, Lidicker J, Clermont G, Carcillo J, Pinsky MR. Epidemiology of severe sepsis in the United States: analysis of incidence, outcome, and associated costs of care. Crit Care Med. 2001;29(7):1303–10.
4. van der Poll T, van de Veerdonk FL, Scicluna BP, Netea MG. The immunopathology of sepsis and potential therapeutic targets. Nat Rev Immunol. 2017;17(7):407–20.
5. Levi M, van der Poll T. Coagulation and sepsis. Thromb Res. 2017;149:38–44.
6. Gando S, Levi M, Toh CH. Disseminated intravascular coagulation. Nat Rev. 2016;2:16037.
7. Levi M. The coagulant response in sepsis. Clin Chest Med. 2008;29(4):627–42.
8. Levi M, ten Cate H. Disseminated intravascular coagulation. N Engl J Med. 1999;341(8): 586–92.
9. Miller DL, Welty-Wolf K, Carraway MS, Ezban M, Ghio A, Suliman H, et al. Extrinsic coagulation blockade attenuates lung injury and proinflammatory cytokine release after intratracheal lipopolysaccharide. Am J Respir Cell Mol Biol. 2002;26(6):650–8.
10. Levi M, ten Cate H, van der Poll T. Disseminated intravascular coagulation: state of the art. Thromb Haemost. 1999;82:695–705.
11. Ratnoff OD, Nebehay WG. Multiple coagulative defects in a patient with the Waterhouse-Friderichsen syndrome. Ann Intern Med. 1962;56:627.
12. Wheeler AP, Bernard GR. Treating patients with severe sepsis. N Engl J Med. 1999;340(3):207–14.
13. Levi M, de Jonge E, van der Poll T. Sepsis and disseminated intravascular coagulation. J Thromb Thrombolysis. 2003;16(1–2):43–7.
14. Vanderschueren S, De Weerdt A, Malbrain M, Vankersschaever D, Frans E, Wilmer A, et al. Thrombocytopenia and prognosis in intensive care. Crit Care Med. 2000;28(6):1871–6.
15. Strauss R, Wehler M, Mehler K, Kreutzer D, Koebnick C, Hahn EG. Thrombocytopenia in patients in the medical intensive care unit: bleeding prevalence, transfusion requirements, and outcome. Crit Care Med. 2002;30(8):1765–71.
16. Akca S, Haji Michael P, de Medonca A, Suter PM, Levi M, Vincent JL. The time course of platelet counts in critically ill patients. Crit Care Med. 2002;30:753–6.
17. Mavrommatis AC, Theodoridis T, Orfanidou A, Roussos C, Christopoulou-Kokkinou V, Zakynthinos S. Coagulation system and platelets are fully activated in uncomplicated sepsis. Crit Care Med. 2000;28(2):451–7.
18. Folman CC, Linthorst GE, van Mourik J, van Willigen G, de Jonge E, Levi M, et al. Platelets release thrombopoietin (Tpo) upon activation: another regulatory loop in thrombocytopoiesis? Thromb Haemost. 2000;83(6):923–30.
19. Francois B, Trimoreau F, Vignon P, Fixe P, Praloran V, Gastinne H. Thrombocytopenia in the sepsis syndrome: role of hemophagocytosis and macrophage colony-stimulating factor. Am J Med. 1997;103(2):114–20.

20. Warkentin TE, Aird WC, Rand JH. Platelet-endothelial interactions: sepsis, HIT, and antiphospholipid syndrome. Hematology Am Soc Hematol Educ Program. 2003;1:497–519.
21. MacLeod JB, Lynn M, McKenney MG, Cohn SM, Murtha M. Early coagulopathy predicts mortality in trauma. J Trauma. 2003;55(1):39–44.
22. Shorr AF, Thomas SJ, Alkins SA, Fitzpatrick TM, Ling GS. D-dimer correlates with proinflammatory cytokine levels and outcomes in critically ill patients. Chest. 2002;121(4):1262–8.
23. Bernard GR, Vincent JL, Laterre PF, LaRosa SP, Dhainaut JF, Lopez-Rodriguez A, et al. Efficacy and safety of recombinant human activated protein C for severe sepsis. N Engl J Med. 2001;344(10):699–709.
24. Gando S, Nanzaki S, Sasaki S, Kemmotsu O. Significant correlations between tissue factor and thrombin markers in trauma and septic patients with disseminated intravascular coagulation. Thromb Haemost. 1998;79(6):1111–5.
25. Levi M, van der Poll T, Buller HR. The bidirectional relationship between coagulation and inflammation. Circulation. 2004;109:2698–704.
26. Aird WC. Vascular bed-specific hemostasis: role of endothelium in sepsis pathogenesis. Crit Care Med. 2001;29(7 Suppl):S28–34.
27. Levi M, van der Poll T. Inflammation and coagulation. Crit Care Med. 2010;38(2 Suppl):S26–34.
28. Taylor FB Jr, Chang A, Ruf W, Morrissey JH, Hinshaw L, Catlett R, et al. Lethal E. coli septic shock is prevented by blocking tissue factor with monoclonal antibody. Circ Shock. 1991;33(3):127–34.
29. Levi M, ten Cate H, Bauer KA, van der Poll T, Edgington TS, Buller HR, et al. Inhibition of endotoxin-induced activation of coagulation and fibrinolysis by pentoxifylline or by a monoclonal anti-tissue factor antibody in chimpanzees. J Clin Investig. 1994;93(1):114–20.
30. Osterud B, Flaegstad T. Increased tissue thromboplastin activity in monocytes of patients with meningococcal infection: related to an unfavourable prognosis. Thromb Haemost. 1983;49(1):5–7.
31. Franco RF, de Jonge E, Dekkers PE, Timmerman JJ, Spek CA, van Deventer SJ, et al. The in vivo kinetics of tissue factor messenger RNA expression during human endotoxemia: relationship with activation of coagulation. Blood. 2000;96(2):554–9.
32. Giesen PL, Rauch U, Bohrmann B, Kling D, Roque M, Fallon JT, et al. Blood-borne tissue factor: another view of thrombosis. Proc Natl Acad Sci U S A. 1999;96(5):2311–5.
33. Osterud B, Rao LV, Olsen JO. Induction of tissue factor expression in whole blood – lack of evidence for the presence of tissue factor expression on granulocytes. Thromb Haemost. 2000;83:861–7.
34. Rauch U, Bonderman D, Bohrmann B, Badimon JJ, Himber J, Riederer MA, et al. Transfer of tissue factor from leukocytes to platelets is mediated by CD15 and tissue factor. Blood. 2000;96(1):170–5.
35. Zimmerman GA, McIntyre TM, Prescott SM, Stafforini DM. The platelet-activating factor signaling system and its regulators in syndromes of inflammation and thrombosis. Crit Care Med. 2002;30(5 Suppl):S294–301.
36. Shebuski RJ, Kilgore KS. Role of inflammatory mediators in thrombogenesis. J Pharmacol Exp Ther. 2002;300(3):729–35.
37. Levi M, van der Poll T. Coagulation in patients with severe sepsis. Semin Thromb Hemost. 2015;41(1):9–15.
38. Biemond BJ, Levi M, ten CH, van dP, Buller HR, Hack CE, et al. Plasminogen activator and plasminogen activator inhibitor I release during experimental endotoxaemia in chimpanzees: effect of interventions in the cytokine and coagulation cascades. Clin Sci. 1995;88(5):587–94.
39. Hermans PW, Hibberd ML, Booy R, Daramola O, Hazelzet JA, de GR, et al. 4G/5G promoter polymorphism in the plasminogen-activator-inhibitor-1 gene and outcome of meningococcal disease. Meningococcal Research Group. Lancet. 1999;354(9178):556–60.
40. Westendorp RG, Hottenga JJ, Slagboom PE. Variation in plasminogen-activator-inhibitor-1 gene and risk of meningococcal septic shock. Lancet. 1999;354(9178):561–3.

41. Hinshaw LB, Tekamp-Olson P, Chang AC, Lee PA, Taylor FB Jr, Murray CK, et al. Survival of primates in LD100 septic shock following therapy with antibody to tumor necrosis factor (TNF alpha). Circ Shock. 1990;30(3):279–92.
42. Abraham E, Wunderink R, Silverman H, Perl TM, Nasraway S, Levy H, et al. Efficacy and safety of monoclonal antibody to human tumor necrosis factor alpha in patients with sepsis syndrome. A randomized, controlled, double-blind, multicenter clinical trial. TNF-alpha MAb Sepsis Study Group. JAMA. 1995;273(12):934–41.
43. van der Poll T, Levi M, Hack CE, ten Cate H, van Deventer S, Eerenberg AJ, et al. Elimination of interleukin 6 attenuates coagulation activation in experimental endotoxemia in chimpanzees. J Exp Med. 1994;179(4):1253–9.
44. Stouthard JM, Levi M, Hack CE, Veenhof CH, Romijn HA, Sauerwein HP, et al. Interleukin-6 stimulates coagulation, not fibrinolysis, in humans. Thromb Haemost. 1996;76(5):738–42.
45. Boermeester MA, van Leeuwen P, Coyle SM, Wolbink GJ, Hack CE, Lowry SF, et al. Interleukin-1 blockade attenuates mediator release and dysregulation of the hemostatic mechanism during human sepsis. Arch Surg. 1995;130(7):739–48.
46. Coughlin SR. Thrombin signalling and protease-activated receptors. Nature. 2000;407(6801):258–64.
47. Kaneider NC, Forster E, Mosheimer B, Sturn DH, Wiedermann CJ. Syndecan-4-dependent signaling in the inhibition of endotoxin-induced endothelial adherence of neutrophils by antithrombin. Thromb Haemost. 2003;90(6):1150–7.
48. Esmon CT. New mechanisms for vascular control of inflammation mediated by natural anticoagulant proteins. J Exp Med. 2002;196(5):561–4.
49. Yuksel M, Okajima K, Uchiba M, Horiuchi S, Okabe H. Activated protein C inhibits lipopolysaccharide-induced tumor necrosis factor-alpha production by inhibiting activation of both nuclear factor-kappa B and activator protein-1 in human monocytes. Thromb Haemost. 2002;88(2):267–73.
50. Murakami K, Okajima K, Uchiba M, Johno M, Nakagaki T, Okabe H, et al. Activated protein C attenuates endotoxin-induced pulmonary vascular injury by inhibiting activated leukocytes in rats. Blood. 1996;87(2):642–7.
51. Taylor FB Jr, Stearns-Kurosawa DJ, Kurosawa S, Ferrell G, Chang AC, Laszik Z, et al. The endothelial cell protein C receptor aids in host defense against Escherichia coli sepsis. Blood. 2000;95(5):1680–6.
52. Levi M, Dorffler-Melly J, Reitsma PH, Buller HR, Florquin S, van der Poll T, et al. Aggravation of endotoxin-induced disseminated intravascular coagulation and cytokine activation in heterozygous protein C deficient mice. Blood. 2003;101:4823–7.
53. Baughman RP, Lower EE, Flessa HC, Tollerud DJ. Thrombocytopenia in the intensive care unit. Chest. 1993;104(4):1243–7.
54. Levi M, de Jonge E, Meijers J. The diagnosis of disseminated intravascular coagulation. Blood Rev. 2002;16(4):217–23.
55. Levi M, Toh CH, Thachil J, Watson HG. Guidelines for the diagnosis and management of disseminated intravascular coagulation. Br J Haematol. 2009;145(1):24–33.
56. Dempfle CE, Pfitzner SA, Dollman M, Huck K, Stehle G, Heene DL. Comparison of immunological and functional assays for measurement of soluble fibrin. Thromb Haemost. 1995;74(2):673–9.
57. Horan JT, Francis CW. Fibrin degradation products, fibrin monomer and soluble fibrin in disseminated intravascular coagulation. Semin Thromb Hemost. 2001;27(6):657–66.
58. Prisco D, Paniccia R, Bonechi F, Francalanci I, Abbate R, Gensini GF. Evaluation of new methods for the selective measurement of fibrin and fibrinogen degradation products. Thromb Res. 1989;56(4):547–51.
59. Shorr AF, Trotta RF, Alkins SA, Hanzel GS, Diehl LF. D-dimer assay predicts mortality in critically ill patients without disseminated intravascular coagulation or venous thromboembolic disease. Intensive Care Med. 1999;25(2):207–10.
60. Levi M, Meijers JC. DIC: which laboratory tests are most useful. Blood Rev. 2011;25(1):33–7.

61. Dempfle CE, Borggrefe M. Point of care coagulation tests in critically ill patients. Semin Thromb Hemost. 2008;34(5):445–50.
62. Levi M, Hunt BJ. A critical appraisal of point-of-care coagulation testing in critically ill patients. J Thromb Haemost. 2015;13(11):1960–7.
63. Johansson PI, Stensballe J, Vindelov N, Perner A, Espersen K. Hypocoagulability, as evaluated by thrombelastography, at admission to the ICU is associated with increased 30-day mortality. Blood Coagul Fibrinolysis. 2010;21(2):168–74.
64. Park MS, Martini WZ, Dubick MA, Salinas J, Butenas S, Kheirabadi BS, et al. Thromboelastography as a better indicator of hypercoagulable state after injury than prothrombin time or activated partial thromboplastin time. J Trauma. 2009;67(2):266–75.
65. Collins PW, Macchiavello LI, Lewis SJ, Macartney NJ, Saayman AG, Luddington R, et al. Global tests of haemostasis in critically ill patients with severe sepsis syndrome compared to controls. Br J Haematol. 2006;135(2):220–7.
66. Muller MC, Meijers JC, Vroom MB, Juffermans NP. Utility of thromboelastography and/or thromboelastometry in adults with sepsis: a systematic review. Crit Care. 2014;18(1):R30.
67. Brenner T, Schmidt K, Delang M, Mehrabi A, Bruckner T, Lichtenstern C, et al. Viscoelastic and aggregometric point-of-care testing in patients with septic shock – cross-links between inflammation and haemostasis. Acta Anaesthesiol Scand. 2012;56(10):1277–90.
68. Daudel F, Kessler U, Folly H, Lienert JS, Takala J, Jakob SM. Thromboelastometry for the assessment of coagulation abnormalities in early and established adult sepsis: a prospective cohort study. Crit Care. 2009;13(2):R42.
69. Taylor FB Jr, Toh CH, Hoots WK, Wada H, Levi M. Towards definition, clinical and laboratory criteria, and a scoring system for disseminated intravascular coagulation. Thromb Haemost. 2001;86(5):1327–30.
70. Kim HK, Hong KH, Toh CH. Application of the international normalized ratio in the scoring system for disseminated intravascular coagulation. J Thromb Haemost. 2010;8(5):1116–8.
71. Bakhtiari K, Meijers JC, de Jonge E, Levi M. Prospective validation of the international society of thrombosis and haemostasis scoring system for disseminated intravascular coagulation. Crit Care Med. 2004;32:2416–21.
72. Toh CH, Hoots WK. The scoring system of the scientific and standardisation committee on disseminated intravascular coagulation of the International Society on thrombosis and haemostasis: a five year overview. J Thromb Haemost. 2007;5:604–6.
73. Dhainaut JF, Yan SB, Joyce DE, Pettila V, Basson BR, Brandt JT, et al. Treatment effects of drotrecogin alfa (activated) in patients with severe sepsis with or without overt disseminated intravascular coagulation. J Thromb Haemost. 2004;2:1924–33.
74. Wada H, Gabazza EC, Asakura H, Koike K, Okamoto K, Maruyama I, et al. Comparison of diagnostic criteria for disseminated intravascular coagulation (DIC): diagnostic criteria of the International Society of Thrombosis and Hemostasis and of the Japanese Ministry of Health and Welfare for overt DIC. Am J Hematol. 2003;74(1):17–22.
75. Wada H, Thachil J, Di NM, Mathew P, Kurosawa S, Gando S, et al. Guidance for diagnosis and treatment of DIC from harmonization of the recommendations from three guidelines. J Thromb Haemost. 2013;11:761–7.
76. Levi M. Settling the score for disseminated intravascular coagulation. Crit Care Med. 2005;33(10):2417–8.
77. Levi M. Platelets in critical illness. Semin Thromb Hemost. 2016;42(3):252–7.
78. du Toit HJ, Coetzee AR, Chalton DO. Heparin treatment in thrombin-induced disseminated intravascular coagulation in the baboon. Crit Care Med. 1991;19(9):1195–200.
79. Feinstein DI. Diagnosis and management of disseminated intravascular coagulation: the role of heparin therapy. Blood. 1982;60(2):284–7.
80. Zarychanski R, Abou-Setta AM, Kanji S, Turgeon AF, Kumar A, Houston DS, et al. The efficacy and safety of heparin in patients with sepsis: a systematic review and metaanalysis. Crit Care Med. 2015;43(3):511–8.
81. Levi M. The dual face of heparin in severe infection. Blood. 2014;123(7):947–8.
82. Boonyawat K, Crowther M. Venous thromboembolism prophylaxis in critically ill patients. Semin Thromb Hemost. 2015;41(1):68–74.

83. Levi M, Levy M, Williams MD, Douglas I, Artigas A, Antonelli M, et al. Prophylactic heparin in patients with severe sepsis treated with drotrecogin alfa (activated). Am J Respir Crit Care Med. 2007;176(5):483–90.
84. Dorffler-Melly J, de Jonge E, Pont AC, Meijers J, Vroom MB, Buller HR, et al. Bioavailability of subcutaneous low-molecular-weight heparin to patients on vasopressors. Lancet. 2002;359(9309):849–50.
85. Levy JH, Sniecinski RM, Welsby IJ, Levi M. Antithrombin: anti-inflammatory properties and clinical applications. Thromb Haemost. 2016;115(4):712–28.
86. Warren BL, Eid A, Singer P, Pillay SS, Carl P, Novak I, et al. Caring for the critically ill patient. High-dose antithrombin III in severe sepsis: a randomized controlled trial. JAMA. 2001;286(15):1869–78.
87. Kienast J, Juers M, Wiedermann CJ, Hoffmann JN, Ostermann H, Strauss R, et al. Treatment effects of high-dose antithrombin without concomitant heparin in patients with severe sepsis with or without disseminated intravascular coagulation. J Thromb Haemost. 2006;4(1):90–7.
88. Tagami T, Matsui H, Horiguchi H, Fushimi K, Yasunaga H. Antithrombin and mortality in severe pneumonia patients with sepsis-associated disseminated intravascular coagulation: an observational nationwide study. J Thromb Haemost. 2014;12(9):1470–9.
89. Iba T, Saitoh D, Wada H, Asakura H. Efficacy and bleeding risk of antithrombin supplementation in septic disseminated intravascular coagulation: a secondary survey. Crit Care. 2014;18(5):497.
90. Levi M. Activated protein C in sepsis: a critical review. Curr Opin Hematol. 2008;15(5):481–6.
91. Ranieri VM, Thompson BT, Barie PS, Dhainaut JF, Douglas IS, Finfer S, et al. Drotrecogin Alfa (activated) in adults with septic shock. N Engl J Med. 2012;366(22):2055–64.
92. Thachil J, Toh CH, Levi M, Watson HG. The withdrawal of activated protein C from the use in patients with severe sepsis and DIC [amendment to the BCSH guideline on disseminated intravascular coagulation]. Br J Haematol. 2012;157(4):493–4.
93. Levi M, van der Poll T. Thrombomodulin in sepsis. Minerva Anestesiol. 2013;79(3):294–8.
94. Tsuruta K, Yamada Y, Serada M, Tanigawara Y. Model-based analysis of covariate effects on population pharmacokinetics of thrombomodulin alfa in patients with disseminated intravascular coagulation and normal subjects. J Clin Pharmacol. 2011;51(9):1276–85.
95. Saito H, Maruyama I, Shimazaki S, Yamamoto Y, Aikawa N, Ohno R, et al. Efficacy and safety of recombinant human soluble thrombomodulin (ART-123) in disseminated intravascular coagulation: results of a phase III, randomized, double-blind clinical trial. J Thromb Haemost. 2007;5(1):31–41.
96. Vincent JL, Ramesh MK, Ernest D, LaRosa SP, Pachl J, Aikawa N, et al. A randomized, double-blind, placebo-controlled, Phase 2b study to evaluate the safety and efficacy of recombinant human soluble thrombomodulin, ART-123, in patients with sepsis and suspected disseminated intravascular coagulation. Crit Care Med. 2013;41(9):2069–79.
97. Yamakawa K, Aihara M, Ogura H, Yuhara H, Hamasaki T, Shimazu T. Recombinant human soluble thrombomodulin in severe sepsis: a systematic review and meta-analysis. J Thromb Haemost. 2015;13(4):508–19.
98. Levi M. Recombinant soluble thrombomodulin: coagulation takes another chance to reduce sepsis mortality. J Thromb Haemost. 2015;13(4):505–7.
99. Levi M, Schultz M, van der Poll T. Sepsis and thrombosis. Semin Thromb Hemost. 2013;39(5):559–66.
100. Wildhagen KC, Garcia de FP, Reutelingsperger CP, Schrijver R, Areste C, Ortega-Gomez A, et al. Non-anticoagulant heparin prevents histone-mediated cytotoxicity in vitro and improves survival in sepsis. Blood. 2014;123(7):1098–101.
101. Kerschen EJ, Fernandez JA, Cooley BC, Yang XV, Sood R, Mosnier LO, et al. Endotoxemia and sepsis mortality reduction by non-anticoagulant activated protein C. J Exp Med. 2007;204(10):2439–48.
102. Schouten M, Wiersinga WJ, Levi M, van Der PT. Inflammation, endothelium, and coagulation in sepsis. J Leukoc Biol. 2008;83(3):536–45.
103. Nieuwdorp M, Meuwese MC, Mooij HL, van Lieshout MH, Hayden A, Levi M, et al. Tumor necrosis factor-alpha inhibition protects against endotoxin-induced endothelial glycocalyx perturbation. Atherosclerosis. 2009;202(1):296–303.

The Endocrine System in Sepsis

5

Nicholas Heming, Sivanthiny Sivanandamoorthy,
Paris Meng, and Djillali Annane

5.1 The Endocrine System

5.1.1 Introduction

The endocrine system plays a major role in coordinating body functions, through the production and dissemination of chemical messengers [1]. The endocrine system maintains biological homeostasis by regulating water and electrolytes balance, metabolism, growth and development, as well as reproduction. The endocrine system is composed of glands which release hormones in response to nervous or hormonal signals. Hormones are specialized chemical compounds which are delivered through the bloodstream and bind to specialized cellular receptors, thereby modifying the cellular function of target cells. In vertebrates, endocrine glands include the pituitary, pineal, adrenal, thyroid, and parathyroid glands as well as the islets of Langerhans in the pancreas, intestinal mucosa, ovary, and testis. Apart from these specialized glands, hormones may also be produced by organs having a specific physiological role that may also exhibit secondary endocrine functions such as the heart or the kidneys (Fig. 5.1). Hormones are divided into three different types: peptides or proteins (e.g., growth hormone, insulin, glucagon), derivatives of the amino acid tyrosine (e.g., thyroid and adrenal medullary hormones), and steroids, derived from cholesterol (e.g., adrenal cortex and sexual hormones). Protein hormones are usually synthesized on the endoplasmic reticulum as inactive preprohormones which are subsequently cleaved into prohormones and then hormones and

N. Heming · S. Sivanandamoorthy · P. Meng · D. Annane (✉)
General Intensive Care Unit, Raymond Poincaré Hospital, Garches, France

School of Medicine Simone Veil, University of Versailles, Versailles, France

University Paris Saclay, Versailles, France
e-mail: nicholas.heming@aphp.fr; sivanthiny.sivanandamoorthy@aphp.fr; paris.meng@aphp.fr; djillali.annane@aphp.fr

W. J. Wiersinga, C. W. Seymour (eds.), *Handbook of Sepsis*,
https://doi.org/10.1007/978-3-319-73506-1_5

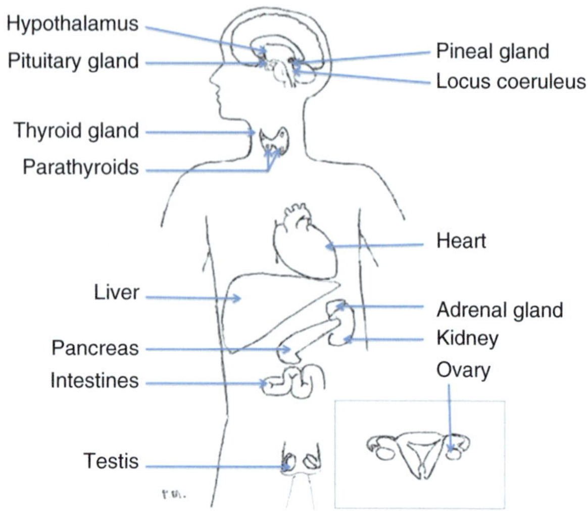

Fig. 5.1 Main organs involved in the synthesis and release of hormones

stored in vesicles until needed. Exocytosis of the vesicles is induced by an increase in cellular calcium concentration or an increase in cyclic adenosine monophosphate (cAMP) concentration leading to activation of a protein kinase. Amine hormones are formed in the cytoplasm of glandular cells. Thyroid hormones are stored within the thyroid gland, bound to the thyroglobulin. Epinephrine and norepinephrine are synthesized and stored in preformed vesicles in the adrenal medulla. Steroid hormones are mainly synthetized from cholesterol. There is very little steroid hormone storage; however the cholesterol ester precursors are stored in cytoplasmic vesicles, ready to be rapidly mobilized. Since steroid hormones are lipophilic, steroid hormone synthesis is followed by rapid diffusion into the bloodstream. The main hormones are listed by organ in Table 5.1.

5.1.2 Hormone Secretion Control Mechanisms

Duration of action of hormones varies widely. For instance, the release of catecholamines occurs seconds after a neuronal impulse, and full effect occurs within minutes. Steroids acting through the genomic pathway start having a physiological action several hours after their release into the circulation. By opposition, other hormones such as thyroid or growth hormones are fully effective after several months. Hormone production is a closely controlled phenomenon. Hormone production is controlled through negative feedback mechanisms where, after release of a hormone, products resulting of the cellular action of this hormone inhibit further production of the hormone. Hormone regulatory mechanisms may occur during synthesis (whether during transcription or translation) or at the time of release.

Rarely, hormones may induce positive feedback. For example, before ovulation, stimulation of the anterior pituitary by estrogens induces a brisk increase of luteinizing hormone, which in turn stimulates estrogen production.

Hormone secretions also undergo periodic variations, induced by the diurnal cycle, the stage of development, or the onset of senescence. A well-known example

Table 5.1 List of main hormones, including site of production, targets, and their function

Organ	Hormones	Target tissues	Main functions
Anterior pituitary	Adrenocorticotropic hormone (ACTH)	Adrenal cortex	Regulates satiety Produces glucocorticoids and mineralocorticoids
	Follicle-stimulating hormone (FSH)	Female: Graafian follicles Male: Sertoli cells of the testes	Reproduction: – Female: initiates follicular growth – Male: enhances androgen-binding protein and acts in the spermatogenesis
	Luteinizing hormone (LH)	Female: granulosa cells and theca cells Male: Leydig of the testes	Reproduction: – Females: triggers ovulation and maintains luteal function during the first 2 weeks of menstruation – Males: ↗ testosterone production
	Growth hormone (GH)	Liver, chondrocyte	Anabolism: protein synthesis, reduction of liver uptake of glucose Growth during childhood ↗ Calcium retention and bone mineralization Stimulates the immune system
	Melanocyte-stimulating hormone (MSH)	Melanocyte	↗ Melanin synthesis
	Prolactin	Mammary glands	Development of female breast ↗ Lactation
	Thyroid-stimulating hormone (TSH)	Thyroid	Produces triiodothyronine (T3) and thyroxin (T4)

(continued)

Table 5.1 (continued)

Organ	Hormones	Target tissues	Main functions
Posterior pituitary	Oxytocin	Brain, mammary glands, endometrium, myometrium, kidneys, heart	Brain actions: – Sexual arousal – Social behavior – Behavior – ↗ Trust and ↘ fear Peripheral actions: – Letdown reflex in lactating – Uterine contraction – ↘ Diuresis and stimulates sodium excretion – Embryonic development of the heart
	Vasopressin/antidiuretic hormone (ADH)	Kidneys, anterior pituitary gland, vessels, pancreas, adrenal gland	V1a receptor: – Vasoconstriction, gluconeogenesis, platelet aggregation, and release of factor VII and von Willebrand factor – ↗ Aldosterone synthesis – ↗ Cortisol synthesis V1b receptor: – ↗ Corticotropin release, prolactin release, GH release, – ↗ Atrial natriuretic peptides synthesis – ↗ Insulin synthesis V2 receptor: regulates plasmatic osmolality and volemia by reabsorption of free water in the collecting duct cells (kidneys)
Thyroid	Triiodothyronine (T3) Thyroxine (T4)	Whole body	↗ Metabolism ↗ Growth Metabolic effects: – ↗ Carbohydrate metabolism, fat metabolism – ↘ Cholesterol, phospholipid, and triglyceride plasma levels
	Calcitonin	Bone, intestine, kidney, central nervous system	↘ Blood calcium levels Regulates vitamin D and bone mineral metabolism
Parathyroid	Parathyroid hormone (PTH)	Bone, kidneys, gastrointestinal tract	↗ Blood calcium concentration by enhancing calcium release from the bone, calcium reabsorption from renal tubules, and calcium absorption in the intestine

Atrial myocytes of the heart	Atrial natriuretic peptide (ANP)	Kidneys, vessels, adrenal, adipose tissue	↘ Cardiac output, blood volume, central venous pressure, arterial blood pressure ↗ Elimination of sodium
Cardiac ventricles	Brain natriuretic peptide (BNP)	Kidneys, vessels, adrenal, adipose tissue	↗ Renal sodium secretion and excretion ↗ Lipolysis
Pancreas: beta cells	Insulin	Liver, muscle, adipocyte	Promotes glucose entry in many cells ↘ Gluconeogenesis, proteinolysis, lipolysis ↗ Fatty acid and glycogen synthesis
Pancreas: alpha cells	Glucagon	Liver	↗ Blood glucose level by increasing glycogenolysis and gluconeogenesis
Hypothalamus cells and cells of pancreas, intestine, stomach	Somatostatin	Pancreas	Suppresses gastro-intestinal hormone secretion ↘ Insulin and glucagon secretion ↘ GH and TSH release
Liver	Angiotensinogen	Plasma	Releases aldosterone Vasoconstriction
	Insulin-like growth factor	Muscle, cartilage, bone, liver, kidneys, nerves, skin, lung	Regulates cell proliferation and apoptosis
Adrenal medulla	Cortisol	Liver, vessels, immune system, hippocampus	Anti-inflammatory and immunosuppressive actions Metabolism: – ↗ Hepatic gluconeogenesis and glycogenolysis – ↗ Peripheral insulin resistance – ↗ Free fatty acid and amino acid Cardiovascular: – Maintains vascular tone – Maintains endothelial and vascular permeability
	Aldosterone	Collecting ducts of the kidneys	Reabsorption of sodium and excretion of potassium

(continued)

Table 5.1 (continued)

Organ	Hormones	Target tissues	Main functions
Kidneys	Renin	Plasma	Activates the renin-angiotensin-aldosterone system by cleaving angiotensinogen to angiotensin I
	Calcitriol	Intestinal epithelium	↗ Calcium absorption from the gastrointestinal tract
	Erythropoietin	Bone marrow	↗ Erythrocyte production
Ovary, placenta	Estrogen	Uterus, coagulation system, liver, gastrointestinal tract	Development of female secondary sexual characteristics Regulates the menstrual cycle ↗ Lipid metabolism, protein synthesis, fluid balance
	Progesterone	Endometrium, vaginal epithelium, brain, smooth muscle, immune system, thyroid, bone	Reproduction Involved in myelinization, synaptic function
Placenta	Human chorionic gonadotropin (HCG)	Bone, gastrointestinal tract, kidneys	Maintains the corpus luteum and progesterone production during pregnancy
Testes	Testosterone	Bone, muscles, sex organs	Development of male secondary sexual characteristics Anabolism: ↗ muscle mass, ↗ bone density and maturation

Adrenal medulla	Epinephrine, norepinephrine	Blood vessels, heart, pancreas, liver, kidney, uterus, bronchi, seminal tract, detrusor, gastrointestinal tract, adipose tissue, skeletal muscle, salivary gland	Alpha1-adrenergic receptor: – Vasoconstriction – Contraction of smooth muscle, bronchoconstriction – Mydriasis – Contraction of urethral sphincter Alpha 2-adrenergic receptor: – Vasoconstriction of the coronary arteries and other arteries – Venoconstriction – ↘ Lipolysis – Suppression of the release of norepinephrine – Platelet aggregation Beta1-adrenergic receptor: – ↗ Chronotropic, inotropic, bathmotropic, and dromotropic effect – Lipolysis – Release renin Beta2-adrenergic receptor: – ↗ Chronotropic and inotropic effect – Vasodilatation – Relaxation of the smooth muscle like bronchodilation – Insulin and glucagon secretion – Glycogenolysis – ↗ Muscle mass and contraction skeletal Beta3-adrenergic receptor: – Thermogenesis in skeletal muscle – Enhances lipolysis

is the circadian rhythm of glucocorticoid secretion. Indeed, the secretory rates of CRF, ACTH, and cortisol are high in the early morning but low in the evening.

5.1.3 Organization of the Endocrine System

5.1.3.1 The Adrenergic System

Catecholamines include epinephrine, norepinephrine, and dopamine. Epinephrine is secreted by the chromaffin cells of the adrenal medulla and by some neurons of the central nervous system (CNS), while norepinephrine is produced in the locus coeruleus located in the pons. The amino acid tyrosine is the substrate for the biosynthesis of all catecholamines. The tyrosine hydroxylase catalyzes the transformation of tyrosine to 3,4-dihydroxy-L-phenylalanine (L-DOPA), in a rate-limiting reaction. L-DOPA is decarboxylated by the DOPA decarboxylase to form dopamine. Dopamine is subsequently oxidized by dopamine β-hydroxylase into norepinephrine. The terminal step in catecholamine biosynthesis is catalyzed by the phenylethanolamine N-methyltransferase which converts norepinephrine to epinephrine [2]. Stress is the major physiologic triggers of epinephrine release [3]. ACTH and the sympathetic nervous system stimulate the synthesis of epinephrine precursors by enhancing the activity of tyrosine hydrolase and dopamine beta-hydrolase, involved in catecholamine synthesis as well as the release of epinephrine. Catecholamines do not exert negative feedback in order to downregulate its own synthesis.

5.1.3.2 The Pituitary Hypothalamic Axis

The hypothalamus is organized into three regions: an anterior region, a medial region, and the posterior region. The pituitary gland is divided into two lobes: an anterior lobe (adenohypophysis), derived from an invagination of the oral ectoderm, and a posterior lobe (neurohypophysis), which is an extension of the hypothalamus, originating from the neuroectoderm. Hypothalamic-derived peptides release stimulating peptides, including corticotropin-releasing hormone (CRH), gonadotropin-releasing hormone (GnRH), growth hormone-releasing hormone (GHRH), thyrotropin-releasing hormone (TRH), as well as inhibiting factors such as GH-inhibitory hormone (somatostatin) and prolactin-inhibiting hormone. Hypothalamic cells are directly connected to the neurohypophysis and secrete releasing hormones in synchronous pulses, into the vessels of the pituitary stalk, which stimulate or inhibit the secretion of adenohypophysis hormones. The anterior pituitary produces adrenocorticotropic hormone (ACTH), gonadotropic hormones (follicle-stimulating hormone (FSH), luteinizing hormone (LH)), growth hormone (GH), melanocyte-stimulating hormone (MSH), prolactin (PRL), and thyroid-stimulating hormone (TSH). The posterior pituitary stores and secretes neurohormones such as oxytocin, a peptide hormone produced by the paraventricular nuclei of the hypothalamus and vasopressin (Fig. 5.2).

5.1.3.3 The Adrenal Glands

The adrenal glands lie at the superior pole of the kidneys. Each adrenal gland is composed of a central part, the adrenal medulla, and a peripheral part, the adrenal

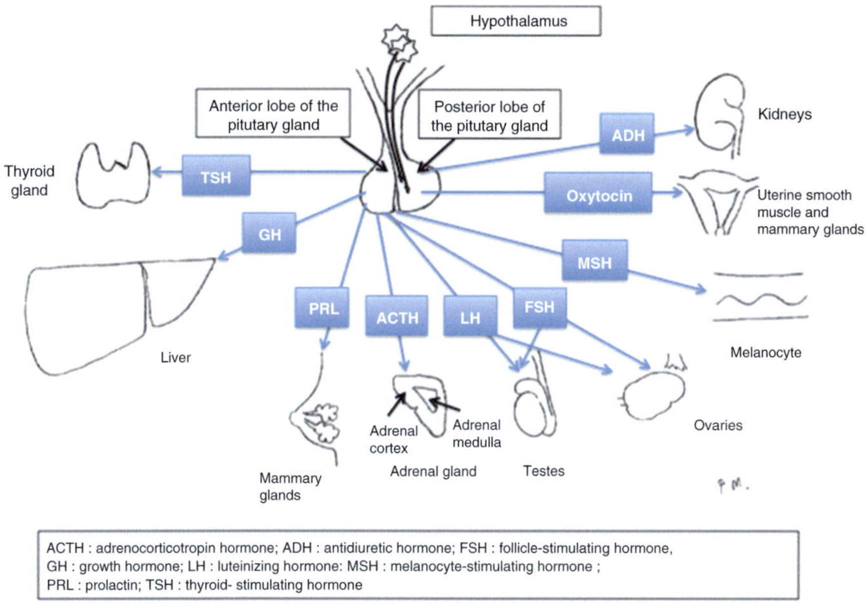

Fig. 5.2 Hypothalamic-pituitary controls of endocrine organs and tissues

cortex. The adrenal medulla is closely connected to the sympathetic system and secretes epinephrine and norepinephrine in response to sympathetic stimulation. Epinephrine and norepinephrine control cardiac output and blood pressure and stimulate glycogenesis.

The adrenal cortex produces a different group of hormones called corticosteroids as well as small quantities of androgenic hormones. ACTH produced by the pituitary gland stimulates adrenal steroid synthesis. Corticosteroids are derived from cholesterol. Corticosteroids are divided into glucocorticoids (cortisol, corticosterone) and mineralocorticoids (aldosterone). Circulating adrenocortical hormones are bound to plasma proteins (cortisol-binding globulin and albumin) and are metabolized in the liver. Aldosterone is produced in response to increased extracellular potassium concentration, while increased sodium concentration in the extracellular fluid decreases the production of aldosterone. The renin-angiotensin induces an increased production of aldosterone, while ACTH is necessary for the synthesis of aldosterone but has little command on the rate of synthesis. Both cortisol and aldosterone bind to a specific intracellular receptor protein, forming a complex which is transferred to the nucleus where it interacts with cellular DNA, promoting the expression of specific mRNA. Aldosterone promotes reabsorption of sodium and secretion of potassium at the renal tubular epithelial cells, leading to increased extracellular volume. Cortisol stimulates gluconeogenesis and mobilizes proteins and fatty acids for use in stressful situations. Cortisol also has anti-inflammatory effects as well as causes resolution of inflammation. ACTH stimulates cortisol production, by activating the adenylyl cyclase, leading to increased cellular concentrations of cyclic AMP.

5.1.3.4 Vasopressin

Vasopressin, also known as the antidiuretic hormone, is a small peptide containing nine amino acids, synthesized as a precursor containing neurophysin II by the hypothalamus and stored in the posterior pituitary gland. Osmotic or hypovolemic stimuli induce vasopressin to be released into the circulation. The V_2 vasopressin receptor is mainly expressed in the ascending loop and collecting duct cells of the kidney. Upon binding of vasopressin, the receptor, through coupled G-proteins, activates the adenylyl cyclase, leading to the expression of the aquaporin water channels, leading to reabsorption of free water [4]. V_1 receptors are implicated in regulating the production of cortisol, aldosterone, GH, insulin, and prolactin.

5.1.3.5 Insulin

Insulin is a peptide hormone which is produced by the beta cells of the pancreatic islets. Synthesized as pre-proinsulin, proinsulin is converted into insulin and C-peptide and stored in secretory granules awaiting release by fusion of secretory granules with the plasma membrane, following an increase in intracellular calcium concentration or cyclic AMP signaling. Blood glucose concentration is regulated by insulin secretion. High blood glucose concentration stimulates the beta cells to secrete insulin, whereas a low blood glucose level induces the secretion of glucagon by the pancreatic alpha cells [5].

5.1.3.6 The Thyroid Gland

Thyroid hormones are synthesized from the tyrosine amino acid, thyroglobulin (TG), and iodine in the thyroid gland. Thyroid hormone production is composed into 80% of thyroxin (T4) and 20% of triiodothyronine (T3). In peripheral tissue, such as the liver, the less active prohormone T4 is converted to the active T3 and the metabolically inactive reverse T3 (rT3) by deiodinases, in equal quantities. Thyroid hormones are secreted in the bloodstream, where they bind to transport proteins. The half-life is 7 days for T4 and 24 h for T3. Thyroid hormone production is regulated by TSH synthesized in the anterior pituitary gland, which is regulated by TRH from the hypothalamus. A negative feedback loop by thyroid hormones, on the hypothalamus and pituitary gland, maintains homeostasis.

5.1.3.7 The Somatotropic Axis

The two main elements of the somatotropic axis are the GH, a peptide hormone, secreted by the anterior pituitary, and insulin-like growth factor type I (IGF-I), a peptide hormone, secreted mainly by the liver. Secretion of GH is pulsatile and is maximal during slow-wave sleep (stages III and IV). Circulating GH is partially linked to a binding protein, GH-binding protein (GHBP), in fact the extra membrane fraction of the GH receptor [6]. GH exerts its effects on tissue growth via IGF-I. A high proportion (about 99%) of circulating IGF-I is bound to proteins, including the IGF-binding protein (IGFBP) family, of which six proteins are known (IGFBP-1 to IGFBP-6).

Regulation of GH synthesis involves the growth hormone-releasing hormone (GHRH) which stimulates GH production, while somatostatin inhibits GH production [7]. Ghrelin, a gastric hormone, stimulates the production of GH directly and indirectly (by stimulating GHRH and inhibiting somatostatin) [8]. Hypoglycemia stimulates the production of GH by stimulation of the production of GHRH (alpha-adrenergic pathway) and inhibition of somatostatin. Glucose intake inhibits GH production by increasing somatostatin (beta-adrenergic) tone. Amino acids (L-arginine and L-ornithine) are potent secretagogues of GH via somatostatin inhibition. Adult sexual steroids stimulate the production of GH during puberty by increasing the amplitude of GH peaks. The regulation of the production of IGF-I and IGFBP-3 is controlled by GH, the nutritional status, and insulinemia [9, 10]. Malnutrition is associated with lower levels of IGF-I and IGFBP-3 and a decrease in the GH receptors. During obesity, GH production is lowered but IGF-I and IGFBP-3 levels are normal.

5.1.3.8 Sex Hormones

The female monthly sexual cycle is driven by cyclic changes in secreted hormones. The pulsatile secretion of GnRH regulates the production by the anterior pituitary of FSH and LH, both heterodimeric glycoproteins. During the follicular phase of the ovarian cycle, the predominant hormone is FSH. FSH targets follicles, stimulating their maturation and production of increasingly higher levels of estrogen. Paradoxically, FSH levels are only slightly reduced in response to high levels of estrogens, highlighting a lack of negative feedback of estrogens on FSH. At the end of the follicular phase, toward the 14th day of the cycle, a surge in estrogen level triggers FSH and LH peaks through positive feedback mechanisms, leading to ovulation. During the following luteal phase, LH stimulates the transformation of the follicle into a corpus luteum. As a result, progesterone and estrogen levels increase, inducing a reduction of hypothalamic progesterone and estrogen receptor expression until estrogen exposure becomes undetectable. This change in hypothalamic sensitivity to circulating estrogens shifts the GnRH secretion to a lower rate and inhibits LH and FSH secretion. At the end of the luteal phase, the corpus luteum degenerates leading to reduced levels of circulating progesterone and estrogen, which in turn triggers menstruation, and stimulates the secretion of LH and FSH, thereby signaling the beginning of a new cycle. Through both positive and negative feedback mechanisms, the secretion of gonadotropins is cyclic [11].

Testosterone, the male sex hormone, is produced by the interstitial cells of Leydig in the testes, in response to LH stimulation throughout adulthood. Testosterone in turn exhibits inhibitory effects on the secretion of LH and GnRH.

5.2 The Endocrine Response to Stress

Stress is defined as a state of disharmony, where vital physiological systems do not function in an optimal manner. Stress is elicited by many different triggers, physical, such as following infection, burns, trauma, or surgery, or psychological. Stress signals are neurosensory, blood-borne, or mediated through limbic pathways. The response to stress varies according to the nature, duration, and intensity of the stressor which drives physiological changes (involving the cardiovascular, respiratory, endocrine, or immune systems) in order to reestablish homeostasis. The response to life-threatening stress is usually divided into three phases: an acute phase, an established organ dysfunction phase, and a phase of recovery.

The acute phase stress response is characterized by the release of the stress hormones, cortisol, catecholamines, vasopressin, glucagon, and GH. The synthesis and liberation of these hormones is aimed at maintaining an adequate blood volume, cardiac output, and tissue oxygenation as well as mobilizing reserves for the immediate production of energy. Initially, oxygen consumption and energy expenditure are increased. At the same time, nonessential functions such as growth or the reproductive functions are suspended. Critical illness is also associated with insulin resistance, where normal concentrations of insulin are unable to correctly regulate blood glucose levels. This state is partly explained by the effect of cytokines on insulin resistance as well as by increased gluconeogenesis.

Sometime after the acute phase, during the established organ dysfunction phase, the hormonal profile alters substantially. Some endocrine changes seem to be adaptive, such as the low T3 syndrome, which may play a role in reducing energy requirements. Low T3 syndrome associates a decrease in the concentration of the T3 due to a decrease of peripheral conversion of T4 to T3 as well as an increased concentration of rT3, an inactive form of T3. Additionally, several pro-inflammatory cytokines (IL-1, IL-6, and TNF-α) suppress the thyroid axis. Other endocrine changes are maladaptive such as the critical illness-related corticosteroid insufficiency (CIRCI), where patients exhibit reduced adrenal responsiveness to ACTH and relatively low cortisol levels. These endocrine changes are somewhat induced by hormonal modifications observed during the acute phase. Indeed, cortisol produced during the acute phase suppresses the secretion of GH, gonadotropins, and TSH.

The recovery phase is an anabolic phase occurring up to 2 months after resolution of the acute inflammatory phase. The main hormones implicated in wound healing are the growth factors IGF-1 and GH. IGF-1 promotes muscle protein synthesis, as well as the proliferation of fibroblasts and keratinocytes, leading to increased tissue formation of collagen.

5.3 Endocrine Alterations During Sepsis

5.3.1 The Adrenergic System

A major activation of the adrenergic system is observed during sepsis, which in turn may be worsened by the administration of exogenous catecholamines. Myocardial depression, defined by a low left ventricular ejection fraction, may occur in up to 50% of cases of septic shock [12]. Myocardial depression may occur through multiple pathways, including autonomic dysregulation, metabolic changes, mitochondrial dysfunction, as well as the consequence of increased catecholamine concentrations and possibly microvascular dysfunction [13]. Adrenergic stimulation of an already failing heart increases the cardiac work and consumption of oxygen. The membrane expression of β-adrenergic receptors is reduced during sepsis. Heart rate variability, which offers an insight into the vagal to sympathetic balance, is impaired during sepsis and may be associated with an unfavorable outcome [14, 15]. Catecholamines may promote bacterial growth and virulence, while at the same time negatively affecting the efficacy and survival of immune cells [16, 17]. Adrenergic stimulation favors insulin resistance and the associated hyperglycemia. β-Adrenergic blockade has been shown to be beneficial in experimental models of sepsis as well as in one single-center human study [18–20].

5.3.2 The Hypothalamic-Pituitary-Adrenal Axis

Sepsis impedes the function of the hypothalamic-pituitary-adrenal axis through multiple mechanisms. The first such mechanism is through altered CRH/ACTH synthesis. Direct ischemic or hemorrhagic damage to the hypothalamus or the pituitary gland may occur during sepsis, thereby altering CRH/ACTH synthesis [21]. Pro-inflammatory cytokines, such as IL-1, are readily produced during sepsis and interact with the hypothalamus/pituitary inducing a biphasic hormonal response characterized by an initial transient increase followed by a progressive decline in anterior pituitary ACTH concentration [22–24]. Sepsis-related decrease in ACTH synthesis occurs in both rodents and humans and is insufficiently compensated by the production of ACTH's natural secretagogues [25]. This condition is also coined as critical illness-related corticosteroid insufficiency and may in the severest forms of sepsis affect up to 60% of patients [26, 27]. Indeed, ACTH levels are significantly lower in septic than in healthy subjects. Additionally, altered ACTH synthesis in response to metyrapone is observed in roughly 50% of septic patients [26].

Sepsis may also be associated with altered steroidogenesis. One of the most well-known causes of altered steroidogenesis occurs after necrosis or hemorrhage of both adrenal glands, also known as the Waterhouse-Friderichsen syndrome [28, 29]. Altered steroidogenesis may occur without any structural damage being done to the adrenal glands. Since cortisol storage in the adrenals is limited, adequate hormonal response to stress relies on de novo cortisol synthesis. Approximately 50% of septic shock patients exhibit decreased cortisol synthesis as well as an inadequate response to the administration of metyrapone [26]. Steroidogenesis may be compromised during any stage of steroid biosynthesis. Histological examination of the adrenal cortex of both animals and humans with sepsis found marked depletion in lipid droplets, suggesting deficiency in esterified cholesterol storage, the first compound to enter the steroidogenesis pathway, possibly mediated by a deficiency in adrenal scavenger receptor B1 (SRB1) [30–32]. A pharmacological inhibitor of steroidogenesis is etomidate, a commonly used drug in intensive care units, emergency rooms, and operating theaters, which inhibits the last enzymatic step in cortisol synthesis and is associated with an increased risk of adrenal insufficiency (OR 19.98; 95% CI 3.95–101.11) up to 6 h post-dosing as well as a small increase in organ dysfunction [33]. Finally, peripheral resistance to glucocorticoids occurs during sepsis. A number of factors may prevent the peripheral bioactivity of cortisol. Sepsis is associated with a marked reduction in plasma levels of corticosteroid-binding globulin (CBG) and albumin [26, 34]. Reduced concentration of cortisol carriers leads to increased plasma concentration of free cortisol. One of the physiological means by which patients seek to withstand severe illness might be by reducing cortisol clearance from plasma, thereby diminishing cortisol inactivation [35]. However, since CBG-bound cortisol is specifically released at sites of inflammation, via neutrophil elastase-dependent mechanisms, the net effect of sepsis-associated reduced CBG and albumin levels is a reduced cortisol delivery to local sites of inflammation [36, 37]. Th2 cell-derived cytokines, such as IL-2 or IL-4, may upregulate the 11β-hydroxysteroid dehydrogenase type 2 (11β-HSD-2), thereby promoting the metabolism of cortisol to the less active component cortisone [38]. Finally, the glucocorticoid receptor (GR)-α may be inhibited at a cellular level, through a decreased capacity of binding, altered capacity to translocate or a loss of the capacity to form dimers [39–41].

5.3.2.1 Corticosteroids in Septic Shock

The use of corticosteroids remains controversial. There is a general agreement that corticosteroids improve shock, organ dysfunction, and length of hospital stay. Their effects on survival and on the risk of secondary infections remain controversial.

Corticosteroids participate in restoring effective blood volume, through activation of mineralocorticoid receptors in the kidney leading to sodium retention. They also contribute to restoring systemic vascular resistance. Indeed, increasing sodium and water content in a vessel's interstitium results in increased stiffness of the vessel wall. Corticosteroids enhance vascular contractile and blood pressure responses to α-1 agonists, through nongenomic effects such as the modulation of α-1 agonists' receptor second messenger and ATP-sensitive K channels [42–44]. Patients with septic shock and a blunted response to a bolus of ACTH exhibit lower systemic vascular resistance and a greater blood pressure response to norepinephrine after a hydrocortisone bolus than patients with an intact HPA axis [43]. Corticosteroids may also improve the microcirculation in septic shock [45]. A systematic review included the findings of 12 trials reporting the effects of corticosteroids on shock reversal by 1 week to be 1.31 (95% CI 1.14–1.51; *P* value = 0.0001) [46]. Corticosteroids inhibit iNOS expression in the renal cortex, restoring an adequate oxygen supply to the kidney [47]. Corticosteroids may attenuate sepsis-associated brain dysfunction by preventing a breakdown of the blood-brain barrier [48]. The same systematic review included the findings of eight trials reporting the effects of corticosteroids on the reduction of the SOFA of −1.53 (−2.04 to −1.03; *P* value <0.00001) [46]. Corticosteroids skew T cells toward a Th2 profile, favoring the production of anti-inflammatory cytokines. Data from 19 trials found the RR for superinfection to be 1.02 (0.87–1.20; *P* value = 0.81) [46]. Most animal models of sepsis found the administration of corticosteroids to be associated with survival benefits [49]. The RR of dying at 28 days of sepsis or septic shock after having received corticosteroids was 0.87 (0.76–1.00, *P* value = 0.05). Current international guidelines recommend restricting the use of hydrocortisone to vasopressor-dependent septic shock [27, 50].

5.3.3 Vasopressin

In patients with septic shock, circulating levels of vasopressin peak within the first 24 h and then decline over time [51]. Vasopressin supplementation failed to improve mortality in a large multicenter randomized trial [52]. A recent trial found no improvement in the number of kidney failure-free days when comparing norepinephrine to vasopressin in septic shock, although the requirement for renal replacement therapy was lower in the vasopressin group [53]. Mortality rates were similar between both groups.

5.3.4 Insulin

Insulin resistance is a hallmark of critical illness. Hyperglycemia is associated with mortality. Several trials sought to determine whether controlling blood glucose levels was associated with a better outcome. A German multicenter study, comparing intensive insulin therapy to conventional treatment, was conducted in severe sepsis. The rate of death at 28 days and the intensity of organ failure were similar between the intensive insulin therapy group (target blood glucose levels 80–110 mg/dL) and the conventional treatment group (target blood glucose levels 180–200 mg/dL). This trial was stopped prematurely because patients in the intensive therapy group suffered from more episodes of hypoglycemia [54]. A French multicenter study in septic shock found similar results [55]. Mortality rates did not differ between the intensive insulin and the conventional treatment arm although there were significantly more episodes of hypoglycemia in the intensive treatment arm. Current guidelines recommend the administration of insulin in order to control hyperglycemia during severe sepsis or septic shock aiming at obtaining a target blood glucose <180 mg/dL [50].

5.3.5 Thyroid Hormones

Critically ill patients suffer from the so called sick euthyroid illness, characterized by low T3 levels associated with low TSH and T4 levels [56]. These modifications may be considered adaptive, aimed at sparing energy during a stressful period. Seeking to artificially correct the hormone levels in patients diagnosed with sick euthyroid illness may be associated with increased harm, as demonstrated in series of small trials in the critically ill [57–59].

The daily administration of 300 μg of T4, over a 2-day period, in patients suffering from acute renal failure contributed to lowering TSH levels. There was no effect on the severity of acute renal failure, and mortality rates were 43% in T4-treated patients versus 13% in the control group [58]. The administration of T3 to patients undergoing coronary artery bypass surgery resulted in an increased cardiac output and lowered systemic vascular resistance without any effect on patient-centered outcome [59].

5.3.6 Growth Hormone

Critical illness, including sepsis, is marked by protein catabolism and muscle wasting. This is even more common in patents requiring prolonged stays in the ICU. GH improves nitrogen balance and tissue healing. Two independent multicenter international trials have investigated the benefits and risks of recombinant human GH in patients requiring prolonged intensive care [60]. The two studies included a total of 532 patients who had spent more than 5 days in the ICU. Treatment was administered daily throughout the ICU stay for a maximum of 21 days and led to increased levels of IGF-1, but increased in-hospital mortality (39% in the treatment group vs. 20% in the placebo group for the Finnish study and 44% in the treatment group vs. 18% in the placebo group for the European study).

5.3.7 Androgens

Patients suffering from prolonged critical illness exhibit low serum concentrations of testosterone, of LH, and of GnRH [61]. The administration of synthetic androgens induces a gain in muscle mass and strength and improves respiratory function in COPD patients and HIV-associated wasting syndromes [62, 63]. Treating severe burn victims by testosterone reduced protein catabolism [64]. Data on other subgroups of patients and on patient-centered outcomes are still scarce.

Overall the only endocrine condition during sepsis which is assessable to treatment is critical illness-related corticosteroid insufficiency which can be treated in the event of septic shock with hydrocortisone (iv bolus of 50 mg q6) combined to fludrocortisone (oral dose of 50 μg per day) given for 7 days.

References

1. Guyton AC, Hall JE. Textbook of medical physiology. Philadelphia: Saunders; 2005.
2. Kirshner N, Goodall M. The formation of adrenaline from noradrenaline. Biochim Biophys Acta. 1957;24:658–9.
3. Lehninger principles of biochemistry (9781429234146) | Macmillan Learning [Internet]. [Cited 2017 Oct 1]. http://www.macmillanlearning.com/catalog/Product/lehningerprinciplesofbiochemistry-sixthedition-nelson
4. Nielsen S, Chou CL, Marples D, Christensen EI, Kishore BK, Knepper MA. Vasopressin increases water permeability of kidney collecting duct by inducing translocation of aquaporin-CD water channels to plasma membrane. Proc Natl Acad Sci U S A. 1995;92:1013–7.
5. Fu Z, Gilbert ER, Liu D. Regulation of insulin synthesis and secretion and pancreatic Beta-cell dysfunction in diabetes. Curr Diabetes Rev. 2013;9:25–53.

6. Baumann G. Growth hormone-binding proteins: state of the art. J Endocrinol. 1994;141:1–6.
7. Tannenbaum GS, Painson JC, Lapointe M, Gurd W, McCarthy GF. Interplay of somatostatin and growth hormone-releasing hormone in genesis of episodic growth hormone secretion. Metabolism. 1990;39:35–9.
8. Kojima M, Hosoda H, Date Y, Nakazato M, Matsuo H, Kangawa K. Ghrelin is a growth-hormone-releasing acylated peptide from stomach. Nature. 1999;402:656–60.
9. Giustina A, Veldhuis JD. Pathophysiology of the neuroregulation of growth hormone secretion in experimental animals and the human. Endocr Rev. 1998;19:717–97.
10. Thissen JP, Ketelslegers JM, Underwood LE. Nutritional regulation of the insulin-like growth factors. Endocr Rev. 1994;15:80–101.
11. Channing CP, Schaerf FW, Anderson LD, Tsafriri A. Ovarian follicular and luteal physiology. Int Rev Physiol. 1980;22:117–201.
12. Parker MM, Shelhamer JH, Bacharach SL, Green MV, Natanson C, Frederick TM, et al. Profound but reversible myocardial depression in patients with septic shock. Ann Intern Med. 1984;100:483–90.
13. Rudiger A, Singer M. Mechanisms of sepsis-induced cardiac dysfunction. Crit Care Med. 2007;35:1599–608.
14. Godin PJ, Fleisher LA, Eidsath A, Vandivier RW, Preas HL, Banks SM, et al. Experimental human endotoxemia increases cardiac regularity: results from a prospective, randomized, crossover trial. Crit Care Med. 1996;24:1117–24.
15. Korach M, Sharshar T, Jarrin I, Fouillot JP, Raphaël JC, Gajdos P, et al. Cardiac variability in critically ill adults: influence of sepsis. Crit Care Med. 2001;29:1380–5.
16. Lyte M, Freestone PPE, Neal CP, Olson BA, Haigh RD, Bayston R, et al. Stimulation of Staphylococcus epidermidis growth and biofilm formation by catecholamine inotropes. Lancet. 2003;361:130–5.
17. van der Poll T, Coyle SM, Barbosa K, Braxton CC, Lowry SF. Epinephrine inhibits tumor necrosis factor-alpha and potentiates interleukin 10 production during human endotoxemia. J Clin Invest. 1996;97:713–9.
18. Suzuki T, Morisaki H, Serita R, Yamamoto M, Kotake Y, Ishizaka A, et al. Infusion of the beta-adrenergic blocker esmolol attenuates myocardial dysfunction in septic rats. Crit Care Med. 2005;33:2294–301.
19. Aboab J, Sebille V, Jourdain M, Mangalaboyi J, Gharbi M, Mansart A, et al. Effects of esmolol on systemic and pulmonary hemodynamics and on oxygenation in pigs with hypodynamic endotoxin shock. Intensive Care Med. 2011;37:1344–51.
20. Morelli A, Ertmer C, Westphal M, Rehberg S, Kampmeier T, Ligges S, et al. Effect of heart rate control with esmolol on hemodynamic and clinical outcomes in patients with septic shock: a randomized clinical trial. JAMA. 2013;310:1683–91.
21. Annane D, Pastores S, Arlt W, Balk RA, Beishuizen A, Briegel J, et al. Critical illness-related corticosteroid insufficiency (CIRCI): a narrative review from a multispecialty task force of the Society of Critical Care Medicine (SCCM) and the European Society of Intensive Care Medicine (ESICM). Intensive Care Med. 2017;43(12):1781–92. https://doi.org/10.1007/s00134-017-4914-x.
22. Parsadaniantz SM, Batsché E, Gegout-Pottie P, Terlain B, Gillet P, Netter P, et al. Effects of continuous infusion of interleukin 1 beta on corticotropin-releasing hormone (CRH), CRH receptors, proopiomelanocortin gene expression and secretion of corticotropin, beta-endorphin and corticosterone. Neuroendocrinology. 1997;65:53–63.
23. Parsadaniantz SM, Levin N, Lenoir V, Roberts JL, Kerdelhué B. Human interleukin 1β: Corticotropin releasing factor and ACTH releasing and gene expression in the male rat: in vivo and in vitro studies: human interleukin 1β. J Neurosci Res. 1994;37:675–82.
24. Cortes-Puch I, Hicks CW, Sun J, Solomon SB, Eichacker PQ, Sweeney DA, et al. Hypothalamic-pituitary-adrenal axis in lethal canine Staphylococcus aureus pneumonia. AJP Endocrinol Metab. 2014;307:E994–1008.
25. Polito A, Sonneville R, Guidoux C, Barrett L, Viltart O, Mattot V, et al. Changes in CRH and ACTH synthesis during experimental and human septic shock. PLoS One. 2011;6:e25905.

26. Annane D, Maxime V, Ibrahim F, Alvarez JC, Abe E, Boudou P. Diagnosis of adrenal insufficiency in severe sepsis and septic shock. Am J Respir Crit Care Med. 2006;174:1319–26.
27. Annane D, Pastores S, Rochwerg B, Arlt W, Balk RA, Beishuizen A, et al. Guidelines for the diagnosis and management of Critical Illness-Related Corticosteroid Insufficiency (CIRCI) in critically ill patients (Part I): Society of Critical Care Medicine (SCCM) and European Society of Intensive Care Medicine (ESICM) 2017. Crit Care Med. 2017;45(12):2078–88. https://doi.org/10.1097/CCM.0000000000002737.
28. Waterhouse R. A case of suprarenal apoplexy. Lancet. 1911;177:577–8.
29. Friderichsen C. Nebennierenapoplexie bei kleinen Kindern. Jahrb Kinderh. 1918;87:109–25.
30. Wang N, Weng W, Breslow JL, Tall AR. Scavenger receptor BI (SR-BI) is up-regulated in adrenal gland in apolipoprotein A-I and hepatic lipase knock-out mice as a response to depletion of cholesterol stores. In vivo evidence that SR-BI is a functional high density lipoprotein receptor under feedback control. J Biol Chem. 1996;271:21001–4.
31. Polito A, Lorin de la Grandmaison G, Mansart A, Louiset E, Lefebvre H, Sharshar T, et al. Human and experimental septic shock are characterized by depletion of lipid droplets in the adrenals. Intensive Care Med. 2010;36:1852–8.
32. Gilibert S, Galle-Treger L, Moreau M, Saint-Charles F, Costa S, Ballaire R, et al. Adrenocortical scavenger receptor class B type I deficiency exacerbates endotoxic shock and precipitates sepsis-induced mortality in mice. J Immunol. 2014;193:817–26.
33. Bruder EA, Ball IM, Ridi S, Pickett W, Hohl C. Single induction dose of etomidate versus other induction agents for endotracheal intubation in critically ill patients. In: The Cochrane Collaboration, editor. Cochrane Database Syst. Rev. [Internet]. Chichester: John Wiley & Sons, Ltd; 2015. [Cited 2017 Aug 1]. http://doi.wiley.com/10.1002/14651858.CD010225.pub2.
34. Beishuizen A, Thijs LG, Vermes I. Patterns of corticosteroid-binding globulin and the free cortisol index during septic shock and multitrauma. Intensive Care Med. 2001;27:1584–91.
35. Boonen E, Vervenne H, Meersseman P, Andrew R, Mortier L, Declercq PE, et al. Reduced cortisol metabolism during critical illness. N Engl J Med. 2013;368:1477–88.
36. Pemberton PA, Stein PE, Pepys MB, Potter JM, Carrell RW. Hormone binding globulins undergo serpin conformational change in inflammation. Nature. 1988;336:257–8.
37. Hammond GL, Smith CL, Paterson NAM, Sibbald WJ. A role for corticosteroid-binding globulin in delivery of cortisol to activated neutrophils*. J Clin Endocrinol Metab. 1990;71:34–9.
38. Rook G, Baker R, Walker B, Honour J, Jessop D, Hernandez-Pando R, et al. Local regulation of glucocorticoid activity in sites of inflammation: insights from the study of tuberculosis. Ann N Y Acad Sci. 2006;917:913–22.
39. Stith RD, McCallum RE. Down regulation of hepatic glucocorticoid receptors after endotoxin treatment. Infect Immun. 1983;40:613–21.
40. Kamiyama K, Matsuda N, Yamamoto S, Takano K -i, Takano Y, Yamazaki H, et al. Modulation of glucocorticoid receptor expression, inflammation, and cell apoptosis in septic guinea pig lungs using methylprednisolone. AJP Lung Cell Mol Physiol. 2008;295:L998–1006.
41. Kleiman A, Hubner S, Rodriguez Parkitna JM, Neumann A, Hofer S, Weigand MA, et al. Glucocorticoid receptor dimerization is required for survival in septic shock via suppression of interleukin-1 in macrophages. FASEB J. 2012;26:722–9.
42. Annane B, Sebille L, Mathieu R, et al. Impaired pressor sensitivity to noradrenaline in septic shock patients with and without impaired adrenal function reserve: Pressor response to noradrenaline and adrenal function. Br J Clin Pharmacol. 2002;46:589–97.
43. Liu J, Haigh RM, Jones CT. Enhancement of noradrenaline-induced inositol polyphosphate formation by glucocorticoids in rat vascular smooth muscle cells. J Endocrinol. 1992;133:405–11.
44. d'Emmanuele di Villa Bianca R, Lippolis L, Autore G, Popolo A, Marzocco S, Sorrentino L, et al. Dexamethasone improves vascular hyporeactivity induced by LPS *in vivo* by modulating ATP-sensitive potassium channels activity. Br J Pharmacol. 2003;140:91–6.
45. Büchele GL, Silva E, Ospina-Tascón GA, Vincent J-L, De Backer D. Effects of hydrocortisone on microcirculatory alterations in patients with septic shock. Crit Care Med. 2009;37:1341–7.

46. Annane D, Bellissant E, Bollaert PE, Briegel J, Keh D, Kupfer Y. Corticosteroids for treating sepsis. Cochrane Database Syst Rev. 2015;12:CD002243.
47. Johannes T, Mik EG, Klingel K, Dieterich H-J, Unertl KE, Ince C. Low-dose dexamethasone-supplemented fluid resuscitation reverses endotoxin-induced acute renal failure and prevents cortical microvascular hypoxia. Shock. 2009;31:521–8.
48. Förster C, Burek M, Romero IA, Weksler B, Couraud P-O, Drenckhahn D. Differential effects of hydrocortisone and TNFα on tight junction proteins in an *in vitro* model of the human blood-brain barrier: hydrocortisone and BBB properties in brain endothelial cell line. J Physiol. 2008;586:1937–49.
49. Annane D. Corticosteroids for severe sepsis: an evidence-based guide for physicians. Ann Intensive Care. 2011;1:7.
50. Rhodes A, Evans LE, Alhazzani W, Levy MM, Antonelli M, Ferrer R, et al. Surviving sepsis campaign: international guidelines for management of sepsis and septic shock: 2016. Intensive Care Med. 2017;43:304–77.
51. Sharshar T, Blanchard A, Paillard M, Raphael JC, Gajdos P, Annane D. Circulating vasopressin levels in septic shock. Crit Care Med. 2003;31:1752–8.
52. Russell JA, Walley KR, Singer J, Gordon AC, Hébert PC, Cooper DJ, et al. Vasopressin versus norepinephrine infusion in patients with septic shock. N Engl J Med. 2008;358:877–87.
53. Gordon AC, Mason AJ, Thirunavukkarasu N, Perkins GD, Cecconi M, Cepkova M, et al. Effect of early vasopressin vs norepinephrine on kidney failure in patients with septic shock: the VANISH randomized clinical trial. JAMA. 2016;316:509–18.
54. Brunkhorst FM, Engel C, Bloos F, Meier-Hellmann A, Ragaller M, Weiler N, et al. Intensive insulin therapy and pentastarch resuscitation in severe sepsis. N Engl J Med. 2008;358:125–39.
55. COIITSS Study Investigators, Annane D, Cariou A, et al. Corticosteroid treatment and intensive insulin therapy for septic shock in adults: a randomized controlled trial. JAMA. 2010;303:341–8.
56. Plikat K, Langgartner J, Buettner R, Bollheimer LC, Woenckhaus U, Schölmerich J, et al. Frequency and outcome of patients with nonthyroidal illness syndrome in a medical intensive care unit. Metabolism. 2007;56:239–44.
57. Brent GA, Hershman JM. Thyroxine therapy in patients with severe nonthyroidal illnesses and low serum thyroxine concentration. J Clin Endocrinol Metab. 1986;63:1–8.
58. Acker CG, Singh AR, Flick RP, Bernardini J, Greenberg A, Johnson JP. A trial of thyroxine in acute renal failure. Kidney Int. 2000;57:293–8.
59. Klemperer JD, Klein I, Gomez M, Helm RE, Ojamaa K, Thomas SJ, et al. Thyroid hormone treatment after coronary-artery bypass surgery. N Engl J Med. 1995;333:1522–7.
60. Takala J, Ruokonen E, Webster NR, Nielsen MS, Zandstra DF, Vundelinckx G, et al. Increased mortality associated with growth hormone treatment in critically ill adults. N Engl J Med. 1999;341:785–92.
61. Sharshar T, Bastuji-Garin S, De Jonghe B, Stevens RD, Polito A, Maxime V, et al. Hormonal status and ICU-acquired paresis in critically ill patients. Intensive Care Med. 2010;36:1318–26.
62. Schols AM, Soeters PB, Mostert R, Pluymers RJ, Wouters EF. Physiologic effects of nutritional support and anabolic steroids in patients with chronic obstructive pulmonary disease. A placebo-controlled randomized trial. Am J Respir Crit Care Med. 1995;152:1268–74.
63. Strawford A, Barbieri T, Van Loan M, Parks E, Catlin D, Barton N, et al. Resistance exercise and supraphysiologic androgen therapy in eugonadal men with HIV-related weight loss: a randomized controlled trial. JAMA. 1999;281:1282–90.
64. Ferrando AA, Sheffield-Moore M, Wolf SE, Herndon DN, Wolfe RR. Testosterone administration in severe burns ameliorates muscle catabolism. Crit Care Med. 2001;29:1936–42.

6 Sepsis Biomarkers

Jean-Louis Vincent and Christophe Lelubre

Key Points

- Accurate and early diagnosis of sepsis enables rapid initiation of appropriate therapy and thus improves outcomes.
- Biomarkers may be used to aid diagnosis, provide indication of disease severity and prognosis, and guide antibiotic therapy.
- Currently available biomarkers are not specific for sepsis and are raised in other inflammatory processes, making them more useful to rule out than to rule in a diagnosis of infection.
- Biomarker levels should never be used in isolation, but can provide complementary information as part of a full clinical patient workup.

6.1 Introduction

Sepsis is a condition of life-threatening organ dysfunction caused by a dysregulated host response to infection [1]. Potentially affecting as many as 20 million individuals globally each year [2], the consequences of sepsis include prolonged intensive care unit (ICU) and hospital lengths of stay, long-term morbidity, and increased short-term and long-term risk of death [3]. Despite many years of active and intense research, no specific interventions have been identified for the treatment of sepsis,

---

The authors have no conflicts of interest to declare related to this manuscript.

J.-L. Vincent, M.D., Ph.D. (✉)
Department of Intensive Care, Erasme Hospital, Université Libre de Bruxelles, Brussels, Belgium
e-mail: jlvincent@intensive.org

C. Lelubre, M.D.
Laboratoire de Médecine Expérimentale (ULB 222 Unit), Université Libre de Bruxelles, CHU de Charleroi, A. Vésale Hospital, Montigny-Le-Tilleul, Belgium

W. J. Wiersinga, C. W. Seymour (eds.), *Handbook of Sepsis*,
https://doi.org/10.1007/978-3-319-73506-1_6

and management relies on adequate resuscitation and organ support combined with eradication of the infecting microorganism with antibiotics and source control [4].

The most important aspect of management for patients with sepsis is to institute appropriate measures as soon as possible in the course of the disease. But identifying sepsis can be complicated, especially early in its course when signs and symptoms are nonspecific and present in many individuals without as well as those with sepsis. Moreover, microbiological information may not be available because cultures are still pending or remain negative in part because some patients with suspected sepsis are already receiving antimicrobial therapy and in part because microorganisms are not always present in the blood. Identifying sepsis may also be difficult in specific populations, such as neonates, and in specific circumstances, such as polytrauma or pancreatitis.

Because sepsis is a clinical picture corresponding to the effects of organ dysfunction due to an infection [1], no specific test can identify it. However, the host response associated with infection can be easily quantified. Indeed, as we have begun to unravel the pathophysiology and mechanisms of sepsis, some of the multiple molecules involved in the complex systemic response to organisms have been identified and proposed as potential (bio)markers or indicators of sepsis. Some of these biomarkers are known to play key roles in the immune response, while others are more innocent bystanders. Either way, their concentrations change as a reflection of the host response, providing an indication of the presence or severity of sepsis.

Biomarkers can have three important roles:

1. To identify (or rule out) sepsis. Biomarkers are often promoted as being of use to identify the presence of sepsis, but they are actually better at ruling out sepsis than at confirming it. Indeed, none of the markers currently available is 100% specific for sepsis, and given the complexity of the sepsis response and the fact that similar inflammatory responses are mounted in response to other conditions, such as major trauma and surgery, it is unlikely that any biomarker specific for sepsis will ever be identified. Nonetheless, biomarkers, if sensitive enough, may be useful for ruling out a diagnosis of sepsis, according to the "SnNOut" principle (a test with a high *sensitivity*, if *negative*, rules *out* the diagnosis) [5].
2. To evaluate the severity (and prognosis) of sepsis. For example, greater increases in the concentration of a biomarker can indicate more severe disease, which may be useful in patient triage, especially when making decisions about the need for ICU admission.
3. To evaluate a patient's response to therapy. This use necessitates repeated measures of biomarker levels to evaluate trends over time. Decreasing biomarker levels can indicate that a patient is responding to treatment, whereas increasing levels suggest a need to review and perhaps change treatment.

More than 170 biomarkers have been studied for potential use in septic patients [6]. In this chapter, we will discuss the two most widely used and studied biomarkers of sepsis, C-reactive protein (CRP) and procalcitonin (PCT), and briefly present some promising candidate biomarkers for the future, and then consider in more depth the potential role(s) of sepsis biomarkers in the intensive care unit (ICU) and emergency department.

6.2 Biomarkers

6.2.1 C-Reactive Protein

CRP is an acute-phase protein first described in 1930 by Tillett and Francis [7]. CRP is a member of the pentraxin family [8] and is synthesized principally by hepatocytes in response to stimulation by cytokines, notably interleukin (IL)-6.

CRP concentrations are increased in many inflammatory conditions and are used across medical specialties as a general indicator of inflammation and to follow disease status and response to treatment in various conditions, including rheumatoid arthritis [9]. CRP concentrations are therefore readily available at low cost. CRP has a half-life of approximately 19 h, and levels begin to rise after 12–24 h, peaking within 2–3 days [10]. CRP concentrations should not be used as a marker of infection in patients with fulminant hepatic failure [11].

6.2.2 Procalcitonin

PCT, another acute-phase protein, is a 116-amino acid prohormone of calcitonin and is primarily expressed in the C-cells of the thyroid gland. However, during sepsis, PCT is produced by multiple tissues in response to inflammatory cytokines and bacterial endotoxins [12], resulting in increased concentrations. PCT was first proposed as a biomarker in 1993 [13]. Although PCT concentrations are increased in other inflammatory conditions, such as pancreatitis or after polytrauma or major surgery [14–16], PCT levels during systemic bacterial infections are typically higher than in these noninfectious inflammatory states. PCT levels begin to rise within 3–4 h and peak within 6–24 h, which is earlier than CRP [10]. However, whereas CRP levels are unaffected by renal failure or renal replacement therapy (RRT), PCT levels are raised in patients with renal failure and those receiving RRT, so that higher cutoffs are needed if PCT is being used as a biomarker of sepsis in such patients [17].

6.2.3 CD64

CD64 is an immunoglobulin Fcγ receptor (Fcγ-RIII) expressed on monocytes and eosinophils, which mediates phagocytosis of bacteria and other microorganisms. Neutrophils normally have low levels of CD64 antigen on their membrane, but expression (assessed by a FACS [fluorescence-activated cell sorting] analysis) is increased within 4–6 h after activation by inflammatory cytokines, not only in infectious processes but also in many other conditions, including cardiopulmonary bypass [18]. In 468 ICU patients, a cutoff admission CD64 expression of 230 median fluorescence intensity (MFI) identified sepsis with a sensitivity of 89% and specificity of 87% [19]. Interestingly, the presence of a normal CD64 expression combined with a normal CRP value ruled out sepsis with a probability of 99%. In a meta-analysis of eight studies assessing CD64 expression for sepsis diagnosis, the pooled sensitivity was 0.76 (95% CI 0.73–0.78) and the pooled specificity was 0.85 (95% CI 0.82–0.87) [20]. de Jong et al. recently reported that although CD64 expression was a good indicator of disease severity, it was not a good predictor of 28-day mortality [21].

6.2.4 Adrenomedullin

Adrenomedullin is a circulating 52-amino acid peptide that is highly conserved across evolution. It is expressed mainly in endothelial and vascular smooth muscle cells and has multiple functions including vasodilatory activity. It has an in vivo half-life of just over 20 min. Concentrations of adrenomedullin increase in patients with sepsis and are independently and strongly associated with mortality [22–24].

6.2.5 sTREM-1

Triggering receptor expressed on myeloid cells-1 (TREM-1), a member of the immunoglobulin superfamily, is involved in the innate immune response. Present on the surface of polymorphonuclear cells and mature monocytes, TREM expression is upregulated during bacterial and fungal infection [25] and soluble TREM (sTREM-1) released into the bloodstream. Levels are also increased in other body fluids, such as cerebrospinal fluid (CSF) and urine. sTREM has demonstrated good diagnostic and prognostic ability in some patients with sepsis, although a meta-analysis of nine studies reported only moderate sensitivity and specificity to predict mortality (0.75 [95% CI 0.61–0.86] and 0.66 [95% CI 0.54–0.75], respectively) [26].

6.2.6 Presepsin

Presepsin (soluble CD14) is a glycoprotein receptor involved in the activation of Toll-like receptor 4 in response to the binding of lipopolysaccharide. Plasma levels of presepsin rise early during sepsis, and it has a half-life of 4–5 h. Presepsin has been shown to have diagnostic and prognostic value in patients with sepsis [27–29]. In a meta-analysis of eight studies assessing presepsin for the diagnosis of sepsis, the pooled sensitivity and specificity were 0.86 (95% CI 0.79–0.91) and 0.78 (95% CI 0.68–0.85), respectively [30]. Similar results were reported in a subsequent meta-analysis of 18 studies [31].

6.3 Application of Sepsis Biomarkers in Clinical Practice

In this section, we will concentrate on the two biomarkers that have been largely investigated in clinical studies, CRP and PCT, but the same possible applications will also apply to the other potential biomarkers mentioned earlier.

6.3.1 First Application: Recognition or Exclusion of Infection

Sepsis markers can be used to diagnose infection. As mentioned earlier, this is important because any infection needs prompt therapy with appropriate antibiotics and source control when indicated. Especially in patients with sepsis, any delay in diagnosis retards initiation of appropriate treatment, which is associated with worse outcomes [32].

Importantly, although we generally refer to these biomarkers as sepsis markers, the more correct term is infection markers or even host response markers. Infection typically includes some host response, not only fever and the associated tachycardia but also altered white blood cell count and changes in the concentrations of these "sepsis" markers. However, these markers are very sensitive, so that elevated concentrations reflect not only infection but also other types of host responses to trauma, surgery (which is after all a special form of "programmed" trauma), pancreatitis, etc. Indeed, the sepsis response is essentially triggered by pathogen-associated molecular patterns (PAMPs), molecules, such as endotoxin, lipoteichoic acid, and nucleic acid motifs, which are derived from microorganisms. These PAMPs bind to pattern recognition receptors (PRRs) on macrophages, polymorphonuclear, and endothelial cells, causing an increase in the transcription of genes involved in inflammatory responses and leading to the release of the inflammatory mediators of sepsis. Importantly, damage-associated molecular patterns (DAMPs) released by cellular injury, for example, postsurgery, trauma, or burns, can induce the same inflammatory reaction through the same receptors [33]. This explains why biomarker levels can increase in both sepsis and other inflammatory conditions and why a fever should not always be treated with antibiotics. In addition, many critically ill patients have some degree of gut hypoperfusion, which may be responsible for translocation of bacteria and their products, again leading to an inflammatory response [34]. This event can occur in situations where infection is not predominant (e.g., in trauma) but may again contribute to the "infection-like" host reaction.

This lack of specificity for an infectious source of the inflammatory response has an important consequence: biomarkers are more useful to rule out than to rule in infection. Indeed, unless very high, concentrations of sepsis markers are not actually very good at identifying an infection or distinguishing infection from other causes of inflammation. Because of this low specificity, the so-called "SpPIn" rule (a test with a high *specificity*, if *positive*, rules *in* the diagnosis) may not be applicable for the diagnosis of sepsis [5]. However, as discussed earlier, low biomarker concentrations can be used to exclude the presence of infection (Fig. 6.1). This ability for a diagnostic test to rule out a diagnosis may be assessed by several indices

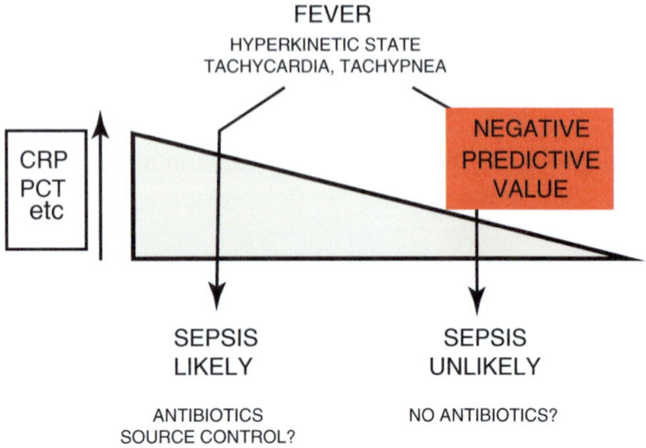

Fig. 6.1 Biomarkers are more useful to rule out than to rule in infection

including a low negative likelihood ratio (best if close to zero), which is a combination of sensitivity and specificity in a single parameter [5].

CRP has been widely studied for its potential as a diagnostic biomarker of sepsis. Ugarte et al. reported a sensitivity of 71.8% and specificity of 66.6% for diagnosis of infection in 190 adult ICU patients, with a CRP cutoff value of 7.9 mg/dL [35]. In 112 ICU patients, Povoa et al. [36] reported a sensitivity of 93.4% and a specificity of 86.1% for infection using a CRP cutoff of >8.7 mg/dL. In surgical ICU patients, Santonocito et al. reported that CRP levels increased more in the first few days after major surgery in infected than in non-infected patients [37].

Because many, especially elderly, patients will already have a raised CRP concentration prior to ICU admission, an increase in CRP concentrations over time may be more reliable to identify infection. Povoa et al. measured CRP concentrations daily in a small cohort of ICU patients and reported that a maximum daily CRP variation >4.1 mg/dL predicted development of nosocomial infection with a sensitivity of 92.1% and specificity of 71.4% [38].

Several studies have suggested that PCT may be a better diagnostic indicator than CRP [39, 40]. However, in patients with acute exacerbations of chronic obstructive pulmonary disease (COPD), Daniels et al. reported that CRP was a better marker of infection than PCT [41]. Similarly, Gaini et al. reported that CRP was better than PCT as a diagnostic marker for infection in patients with suspected community-acquired pneumonia [42]. In a recent study of 1572 episodes of suspected sepsis, Ljungström et al. reported that CRP had greater sensitivity than PCT but much lower specificity [43].

In addition to aiding with diagnosis of infection versus other cause of inflammation, attempts have been made to use biomarker levels to distinguish between different types of infection. In a recent systematic review of 59 studies that used biomarkers to distinguish between bacterial and nonbacterial infections, none of the markers studied, including CRP and PCT, consistently showed high diagnostic performance [44]. Nevertheless, most studies included in the review reported higher CRP and PCT concentrations in patients with bacterial infections than in those with infections of other, mostly viral, causes [44]. Other biomarkers have been much less widely studied, and it is difficult to draw any conclusions regarding their ability to differentiate between bacterial and nonbacterial infections.

6.3.2 Second Application: Evaluation of the Severity of Disease and Prognosis

For many biomarkers, the degree of change in concentration is proportional to the severity of the disease and, therefore, to the risk of death. Biomarkers could therefore potentially provide useful information for patient triage, particularly in terms of need for ICU admission. Lobo et al. [45] reported that ICU patients with serum CRP levels >10 mg/dL at ICU admission were more likely to develop organ dysfunction than patients with CRP levels <1 mg/dL and had higher mortality rates (36 vs. 21%, $p < 0.05$). Raised CRP levels may also be associated with worse longer-term outcomes. For example, in nonsurgical ICU patients, Grander et al. reported that the maximum ICU concentration during the ICU stay and the discharge CRP concentration were both independently associated with post-ICU mortality in ICU survivors [46]. However, in a mixed medical-surgical ICU, Al-Subaie et al. reported that discharge CRP concentrations were not different in patients who were later readmitted to the ICU or died in the hospital after ICU discharge compared to other patients [47].

In ICU patients with sepsis, Giamarellos-Bourboulis et al. reported higher mortality rates in those with PCT concentrations >0.85 ng/mL than in those with PCT ≤ 0.85 ng/mL (OR for death, 2.404; 95% CI, 1.385–4.171, $p = 0.002$) [48]. In patients with healthcare-associated pneumonia, PCT concentrations were significantly higher in 30-day non-survivors than in survivors [49]. In a meta-analysis of 23 studies, Liu et al. reported that an elevated PCT concentration was associated with an increased risk of death, with a pooled relative risk of 2.60 (95% CI 2.05–3.30, $I^2 = 63.5\%$) [50].

Importantly, changes in biomarker concentrations over time are again more valuable than single measurements. In the study by Lobo et al. [45], a decrease in CRP concentration after 48 h in patients with CRP concentrations >10 mg/dL on ICU admission was associated with a mortality rate of 15%, whereas an increase in CRP was associated with a mortality rate of 61% ($p < 0.05$). Karlsson et al. [51] reported in patients with sepsis that although PCT concentrations were similar in hospital survivors and non-survivors, mortality rates were higher in patients whose PCT concentration decreased by less than 50% over 72 h than in those whose levels decreased by more than 50% (30 vs. 12%, $p = 0.007$). In a retrospective analysis of 409 ICU survivors, patients in whom CRP concentrations decreased by less than 25% between 48 and 24 h prior to discharge had increased mortality (23 vs. 11%, $p = 0.002$) and post-ICU length of stay (26 [7–43] vs. 11 [5–27] days, $p = 0.036$) than those in whom it decreased by more than 25% [52]. In a prospective multicenter study of 289 patients, Georgopoulou et al. [53] reported that patients in whom the PCT on day 3 was decreased by more than 30% or was less than 0.25 ng/mL had a mortality of 12% compared to 30% in patients in whom PCT on day 3 was greater than 0.25 ng/mL or had decreased less than 30% ($p < 0.0001$). In another recent multicenter prospective study across 13 American ICUs, failure to decrease PCT by at least 80% from baseline to day 4 was an independent predictor of 28-day mortality in Cox regression analysis (hazard ratio 1.97 [95% CI, 1.18–3.30; $p < 0.009$]) after adjusting for relevant confounders [54].

Few studies have directly compared the prognostic properties of different biomarkers. In an early study comparing CRP to PCT, we reported that PCT had a stronger prognostic value than CRP [35]. Hoeboer and Groeneveld similarly reported that PCT was more predictive of septic shock, organ failure, and mortality in febrile critically ill patients [55].

6.3.3 Third Application: Therapeutic Guidance

If sepsis markers reflect the development and severity of the host response, then logically they should be expected to provide information regarding patient response to therapy. A persistently raised biomarker concentration could suggest that source control is suboptimal or that the chosen antimicrobial regime is not adequately covering the causative pathogen(s). Similarly decreasing biomarker concentrations may suggest resolution of infection (Fig. 6.2), enabling antibiotics to be stopped. Adjusting antibiotic therapy according to biomarker concentrations could thus potentially help reduce adverse effects and costs and reduce the development of antimicrobial resistance. However, the potential risks associated with this approach include poorer control of infection with increased risk of relapse.

In 50 adult ICU patients with sepsis, Schmit and Vincent [56] reported that CRP concentrations decreased more rapidly in patients with a favorable response to empiric antibiotics than in patients who required a change in antibiotic therapy. Similarly, in patients with ventilator-associated pneumonia, serum CRP levels at 96 h were significantly lower in patients with appropriate than in those with inappropriate empirical treatment [57], and in patients with community-acquired pneumonia, those in whom CRP levels decreased by less than 60% by day 3 after admission had an increased risk of having received inappropriate empiric antibiotic

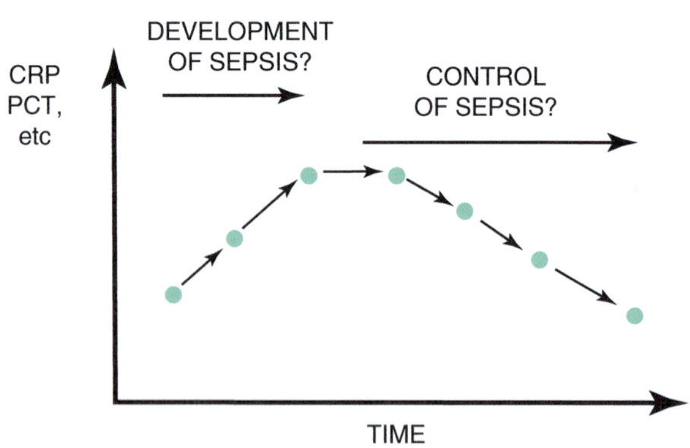

Fig. 6.2 Biomarker concentrations increase as sepsis develops, but decrease as sepsis resolves with effective treatment

treatment [58]. However, use of CRP levels to guide therapy has rarely been tested in adult patients with sepsis. In a randomized controlled study by Oliveira et al. evaluating the effects of CRP- and PCT-guided algorithms to guide antibiotic discontinuation in patients with sepsis, CRP and PCT were similar in their ability to reduce antibiotic duration [59].

Several studies using PCT-guided antibiotic therapy have been conducted in different groups of critically ill patients including those with community-acquired pneumonia [60], lower respiratory tract infections [61, 62], suspected infection [63, 64], and with sepsis [65–69]. Most studies have reported reduced antibiotic duration in patients managed using PCT algorithms to reduce antibiotic usage, with no negative impact on outcomes. However, a recent retrospective analysis suggested that PCT use was associated with increased antibiotic days and incidence of *Clostridium difficile* infection, with no change in mortality [70]. Moreover, studies using algorithms to *escalate* antibiotic therapy have suggested harmful effects of this approach [71]. The most recent meta-analysis of studies that tested PCT-guided antibiotic decisions for adults with sepsis or septic shock included ten randomized controlled trials and concluded that "Up-to-date evidence of very low to moderate quality, with insufficient sample power per outcome, does not clearly support the use of procalcitonin-guided antimicrobial therapy to minimize mortality, mechanical ventilation, clinical severity, reinfection or duration of antimicrobial therapy of patients with septic conditions" [72]. The latest Surviving Sepsis Campaign guidelines state: "We suggest that procalcitonin levels can be used to support the discontinuation of empiric antibiotics in patients who initially appeared to have sepsis, but subsequently have limited clinical evidence of infection (weak recommendation, low quality of evidence)" [4].

6.4 Practical Limitations and Challenges of Biomarkers

Any biomarker value needs to be interpreted in the context of a full clinical history and examination and the presence of other signs and symptoms of infection. This aspect is true for all three potential biomarker roles. For example, no one would diagnose sepsis simply based on an elevated CRP or PCT concentration—these values offer support to the diagnosis when other signs are present, such as fever, unexplained organ dysfunction, etc. Similarly, no one would guess the severity of disease or likely outcome based on a biomarker concentration or even a trend in concentrations without taking into account the multiple other factors that can indicate severity and impact on outcomes. And finally, no one would suggest stopping antibiotic therapy in a patient with sepsis based purely on a (still somewhat random) biomarker concentration, without considering the clinical status and evolution of the patient and bacteriological factors, including the causative microorganism [73]. Indeed, although PCT-guided therapy may be associated with reduced antibiotic exposure, there is no consensus on cutoff points at which antibiotics could be safely stopped or on which algorithm of the many that have been tested is most effective. Such decisions must be made at an individual patient level.

Another challenge with the use of biomarkers is the complexity of the sepsis response, which varies among individuals and within individuals over time, making it unlikely that any one biomarker will ever be sufficient to diagnose sepsis, evaluate prognosis, or guide treatment. Combinations of biomarkers may prove more useful, but which biomarkers should be included in such panels is far from clear and will likely vary according to the intended use of the biomarkers: diagnosis, prognosis, or therapeutic guidance. In emergency department, patients suspected of having community-acquired infections, a combination of six biomarkers (soluble urokinase-type plasminogen activator, sTREM-1, macrophage migration inhibitory factor, CRP, PCT, and neutrophil count), had a significantly greater area under the curve (AUC) for bacterial infection than did any of the individual markers [74]. Similarly, Gibot et al. reported that a combined score of PCT, sTREM-1, and the CD64 index diagnosed sepsis better than any of the individual biomarkers [75]. In the study by Dimoula et al. [19], the combination of CRP with CD64 expression had greater diagnostic power than either biomarker alone.

Finally, the economics of biomarker use must not be neglected. de Jong et al. [64] reported that antibiotic costs were reduced by about 34 euros per patient when using a PCT-guided algorithm for antibiotic use. In addition to reduced antibiotic costs, other cost savings associated with biomarker use may include shorter ICU and hospital stays, reduced adverse effects of antibiotics, and reduced development of antibiotic resistance. In a retrospective, propensity score-matched multivariable analysis, Balk et al. [76] reported that patients in whom a PCT test was performed on the first day of ICU admission had significantly lower hospital and ICU lengths of stay, as well as decreased total, ICU, and pharmacy costs of care. However, these potential cost savings need to be balanced against the costs of the biomarker tests, which, apart from CRP, are still considerable. In a small study, Deliberato et al. reported a net cost saving of $388 per patient after taking into account costs of PCT testing. And in a meta-analysis of 18 studies of PCT-guided antibiotic therapy in adults and children, cost-effectiveness acceptability curves showed that PCT-guided treatment had a probability of ≥84% of being cost-effective for the settings and populations considered [77].

Conclusion

Biomarkers reflect the magnitude of the host response to an aggression. Importantly, the host response is not entirely specific for infection, because the same molecular mechanisms are involved in different types of injury, including the damage associated with trauma, postsurgery, burns, etc. Hence, there will never be a biomarker that is 100% sensitive and 100% specific for infection or even one that approaches the considerable sensitivity and specificity of troponin for acute myocardial infarction. There will, therefore, never be a perfect marker to answer the question "is this patient infected?". CRP is not a perfect biomarker for sepsis, but the advantages of PCT are only moderate. Panels of biomarkers may be better than individual biomarkers to aid diagnosis, but which combinations of biomarkers are likely to be of greatest use remains a matter of ongoing research. Whichever biomarker(s) is used, levels must be interpreted in the context of the full clinical picture and never in isolation.

References

1. Singer M, Deutschman CS, Seymour CW, et al. The third international consensus definitions for sepsis and septic shock (Sepsis-3). JAMA. 2016;315:801–10.
2. Fleischmann C, Scherag A, Adhikari NK, et al. Assessment of global incidence and mortality of hospital-treated sepsis. Current estimates and limitations. Am J Respir Crit Care Med. 2016;193:259–72.
3. Shankar-Hari M, Rubenfeld GD. Understanding long-term outcomes following sepsis: implications and challenges. Curr Infect Dis Rep. 2016;18:37.
4. Rhodes A, Evans LE, Alhazzani W, et al. Surviving sepsis campaign: International Guidelines for Management of Sepsis and Septic Shock: 2016. Crit Care Med. 2017;45:486–552.
5. Pewsner D, Battaglia M, Minder C, et al. Ruling a diagnosis in or out with "SpPIn" and "SnNOut": a note of caution. BMJ. 2004;329:209–13.
6. Pierrakos C, Vincent JL. Sepsis biomarkers: a review. Crit Care. 2010;14:R15.
7. Tillett WS, Francis T. Serological reactions in pneumonia with a non-protein somatic fraction of pneumococcus. J Exp Med. 1930;52:561–71.
8. Thompson D, Pepys MB, Wood SP. The physiological structure of human C-reactive protein and its complex with phosphocholine. Structure. 1999;7:169–77.
9. National Institute for Health and Care Excellence. Rheumatoid arthritis: national clinical guideline for management and treatment in adults. London: Royal College of Physicians; 2009.
10. Markanday A. Acute phase reactants in infections: evidence-based review and a guide for clinicians. Open Forum Infect Dis. 2015;2:ofv098.
11. Silvestre JP, Coelho LM, Povoa PM. Impact of fulminant hepatic failure in C-reactive protein? J Crit Care. 2010;25:657–12.
12. Muller B, White JC, Nylen ES, et al. Ubiquitous expression of the calcitonin-i gene in multiple tissues in response to sepsis. J Clin Endocrinol Metab. 2001;86:396–404.
13. Assicot M, Gendrel D, Carsin H, et al. High serum procalcitonin concentrations in patients with sepsis and infection. Lancet. 1993;341:515–8.
14. Mofidi R, Suttie SA, Patil PV, et al. The value of procalcitonin at predicting the severity of acute pancreatitis and development of infected pancreatic necrosis: systematic review. Surgery. 2009;146:72–81.
15. Meisner M, Adina H, Schmidt J. Correlation of procalcitonin and C-reactive protein to inflammation, complications, and outcome during the intensive care unit course of multiple-trauma patients. Crit Care. 2006;10:R1.
16. Meisner M, Rauschmayer C, Schmidt J, et al. Early increase of procalcitonin after cardiovascular surgery in patients with postoperative complications. Intensive Care Med. 2002;28:1094–102.
17. Grace E, Turner RM. Use of procalcitonin in patients with various degrees of chronic kidney disease including renal replacement therapy. Clin Infect Dis. 2014;59:1761–7.
18. Djebara S, Biston P, Fosse E, et al. Time course of CD64, a leukocyte activation marker, during cardiopulmonary bypass surgery. Shock. 2017;47:158–64.
19. Dimoula A, Pradier O, Kassengera Z, et al. Serial determinations of neutrophil CD64 expression for the diagnosis and monitoring of sepsis in critically ill patients. Clin Infect Dis. 2014;58:820–9.
20. Wang X, Li ZY, Zeng L, et al. Neutrophil CD64 expression as a diagnostic marker for sepsis in adult patients: a meta-analysis. Crit Care. 2015;19:245.
21. de Jong E, de Lange DW, Beishuizen A, et al. Neutrophil CD64 expression as a longitudinal biomarker for severe disease and acute infection in critically ill patients. Int J Lab Hematol. 2016;38:576–84.
22. Marino R, Struck J, Maisel AS, et al. Plasma adrenomedullin is associated with short-term mortality and vasopressor requirement in patients admitted with sepsis. Crit Care. 2014; 18:R34.

23. Caironi P, Latini R, Struck J, et al. Circulating biologically active adrenomedullin (bio-ADM) predicts hemodynamic support requirement and mortality during sepsis. Chest. 2017;152:312–20.
24. Simon TP, Martin L, Doemming S, et al. Plasma adrenomedullin in critically ill patients with sepsis after major surgery: a pilot study. J Crit Care. 2017;38:68–72.
25. Bouchon A, Facchetti F, Weigand MA, et al. TREM-1 amplifies inflammation and is a crucial mediator of septic shock. Nature. 2001;410:1103–7.
26. Su L, Liu D, Chai W, et al. Role of sTREM-1 in predicting mortality of infection: a systematic review and meta-analysis. BMJ Open. 2016;6:e010314.
27. Behnes M, Bertsch T, Lepiorz D, et al. Diagnostic and prognostic utility of soluble CD 14 subtype (presepsin) for severe sepsis and septic shock during the first week of intensive care treatment. Crit Care. 2014;18:507.
28. Yu H, Qi Z, Hang C, et al. Evaluating the value of dynamic procalcitonin and presepsin measurements for patients with severe sepsis. Am J Emerg Med. 2017;35:835–41.
29. Matera G, Quirino A, Peronace C, et al. Soluble CD14 subtype-a new biomarker in predicting the outcome of critically ill septic patients. Am J Med Sci. 2017;353:543–51.
30. Zhang X, Liu D, Liu YN, et al. The accuracy of presepsin (sCD14-ST) for the diagnosis of sepsis in adults: a meta-analysis. Crit Care. 2015;19:323.
31. Wu CC, Lan HM, Han ST, et al. Comparison of diagnostic accuracy in sepsis between presepsin, procalcitonin, and C-reactive protein: a systematic review and meta-analysis. Ann Intensive Care. 2017;7:91.
32. Kumar A, Haery C, Paladugu B, et al. The duration of hypotension before the initiation of antibiotic treatment is a critical determinant of survival in a murine model of Escherichia coli septic shock: association with serum lactate and inflammatory cytokine levels. J Infect Dis. 2006;193:251–8.
33. Zhang Q, Raoof M, Chen Y, et al. Circulating mitochondrial DAMPs cause inflammatory responses to injury. Nature. 2010;464:104–7.
34. de Jong PR, Gonzalez-Navajas JM, Jansen NJ. The digestive tract as the origin of systemic inflammation. Crit Care. 2016;20:279.
35. Ugarte H, Silva E, Mercan D, et al. Procalcitonin used as a marker of infection in the intensive care unit. Crit Care Med. 1999;27:498–504.
36. Povoa P, Coelho L, Almeida E, et al. C-reactive protein as a marker of infection in critically ill patients. Clin Microbiol Infect. 2005;11:101–8.
37. Santonocito C, De Loecker I, Donadello K, et al. C-reactive protein kinetics after major surgery. Anesth Analg. 2014;119:624–9.
38. Povoa P, Coelho L, Almeida E, et al. Early identification of intensive care unit-acquired infections with daily monitoring of C-reactive protein: a prospective observational study. Crit Care. 2006;10:R63.
39. Uzzan B, Cohen R, Nicolas P, et al. Procalcitonin as a diagnostic test for sepsis in critically ill adults and after surgery or trauma: a systematic review and meta-analysis. Crit Care Med. 2006;34:1996–2003.
40. Castelli GP, Pognani C, Cita M, et al. Procalcitonin as a prognostic and diagnostic tool for septic complications after major trauma. Crit Care Med. 2009;37:1845–9.
41. Daniels JM, Schoorl M, Snijders D, et al. Procalcitonin vs C-reactive protein as predictive markers of response to antibiotic therapy in acute exacerbations of COPD. Chest. 2010;138:1108–15.
42. Gaini S, Koldkjaer OG, Pedersen C, et al. Procalcitonin, lipopolysaccharide-binding protein, interleukin-6 and C-reactive protein in community-acquired infections and sepsis: a prospective study. Crit Care. 2006;10:R53.
43. Ljungstrom L, Pernestig AK, Jacobsson G, et al. Diagnostic accuracy of procalcitonin, neutrophil-lymphocyte count ratio, C-reactive protein, and lactate in patients with suspected bacterial sepsis. PLoS One. 2017;12:e0181704.
44. Kapasi AJ, Dittrich S, Gonzalez IJ, et al. Host biomarkers for distinguishing bacterial from non-bacterial causes of acute febrile illness: a comprehensive review. PLoS One. 2016;11:e0160278.

45. Lobo SM, Lobo FR, Bota DP, et al. C-reactive protein levels correlate with mortality and organ failure in critically ill patients. Chest. 2003;123:2043–9.
46. Grander W, Dunser M, Stollenwerk B, et al. C-reactive protein levels and post-ICU mortality in nonsurgical intensive care patients. Chest. 2010;138:856–62.
47. Al-Subaie N, Reynolds T, Myers A, et al. C-reactive protein as a predictor of outcome after discharge from the intensive care: a prospective observational study. Br J Anaesth. 2010;105:318–25.
48. Giamarellos-Bourboulis EJ, Tsangaris I, Kanni T, et al. Procalcitonin as an early indicator of outcome in sepsis: a prospective observational study. J Hosp Infect. 2011;77:58–63.
49. Hong DY, Park SO, Kim JW, et al. Serum procalcitonin: an independent predictor of clinical outcome in health care-associated pneumonia. Respiration. 2016;92:241–51.
50. Liu D, Su L, Han G, et al. Prognostic value of procalcitonin in adult patients with sepsis: a systematic review and meta-analysis. PLoS One. 2015;10:e0129450.
51. Karlsson S, Heikkinen M, Pettila V, et al. Predictive value of procalcitonin decrease in patients with severe sepsis: a prospective observational study. Crit Care. 2010;14:R205.
52. Ranzani OT, Prada LF, Zampieri FG, et al. Failure to reduce C-reactive protein levels more than 25% in the last 24 hours before intensive care unit discharge predicts higher in-hospital mortality: a cohort study. J Crit Care. 2012;27:525–15.
53. Georgopoulou AP, Savva A, Giamarellos-Bourboulis EJ, et al. Early changes of procalcitonin may advise about prognosis and appropriateness of antimicrobial therapy in sepsis. J Crit Care. 2011;26:331–7.
54. Schuetz P, Birkhahn R, Sherwin R, et al. Serial procalcitonin predicts mortality in severe sepsis patients: results from the multicenter procalcitonin MOnitoring SEpsis (MOSES) study. Crit Care Med. 2017;45:781–9.
55. Hoeboer SH, Groeneveld AB. Changes in circulating procalcitonin versus C-reactive protein in predicting evolution of infectious disease in febrile, critically ill patients. PLoS One. 2013;8:e65564.
56. Schmit X, Vincent JL. The time course of blood C-reactive protein concentrations in relation to the response to initial antimicrobial therapy in patients with sepsis. Infection. 2008;36:213–9.
57. Lisboa T, Seligman R, Diaz E, et al. C-reactive protein correlates with bacterial load and appropriate antibiotic therapy in suspected ventilator-associated pneumonia. Crit Care Med. 2008;36:166–71.
58. Bruns AH, Oosterheert JJ, Hak E, et al. Usefulness of consecutive C-reactive protein measurements in follow-up of severe community-acquired pneumonia. Eur Respir J. 2008;32:726–32.
59. Oliveira CF, Botoni FA, Oliveira CR, et al. Procalcitonin versus C-reactive protein for guiding antibiotic therapy in sepsis: a randomized trial. Crit Care Med. 2013;41:2336–43.
60. Christ-Crain M, Stolz D, Bingisser R, et al. Procalcitonin guidance of antibiotic therapy in community-acquired pneumonia: a randomized trial. Am J Respir Crit Care Med. 2006;174:84–93.
61. Christ-Crain M, Jaccard-Stolz D, Bingisser R, et al. Effect of procalcitonin-guided treatment on antibiotic use and outcome in lower respiratory tract infections: cluster-randomised, single-blinded intervention trial. Lancet. 2004;363:600–7.
62. Schuetz P, Christ-Crain M, Thomann R, et al. Effect of procalcitonin-based guidelines vs standard guidelines on antibiotic use in lower respiratory tract infections: the ProHOSP randomized controlled trial. JAMA. 2009;302:1059–66.
63. Bouadma L, Luyt CE, Tubach F, et al. Use of procalcitonin to reduce patients' exposure to antibiotics in intensive care units (PRORATA trial): a multicentre randomised controlled trial. Lancet. 2010;375:463–74.
64. de Jong E, van Oers JA, Beishuizen A, et al. Efficacy and safety of procalcitonin guidance in reducing the duration of antibiotic treatment in critically ill patients: a randomised, controlled, open-label trial. Lancet Infect Dis. 2016;16:819–27.
65. Nobre V, Harbarth S, Graf JD, et al. Use of procalcitonin to shorten antibiotic treatment duration in septic patients: a randomized trial. Am J Respir Crit Care Med. 2008;177:498–505.

66. Schroeder S, Hochreiter M, Koehler T, et al. Procalcitonin (PCT)-guided algorithm reduces length of antibiotic treatment in surgical intensive care patients with severe sepsis: results of a prospective randomized study. Langenbeck's Arch Surg. 2009;394:221–6.
67. Shehabi Y, Sterba M, Garrett PM, et al. Procalcitonin algorithm in critically ill adults with undifferentiated infection or suspected sepsis: a randomized controlled trial. Am J Respir Crit Care Med. 2014;190:1102–10.
68. Bloos F, Trips E, Nierhaus A, et al. Effect of sodium selenite administration and procalcitonin-guided therapy on mortality in patients with severe sepsis or septic shock: a randomized clinical trial. JAMA Intern Med. 2016;176:1266–76.
69. Deliberato RO, Marra AR, Sanches PR, et al. Clinical and economic impact of procalcitonin to shorten antimicrobial therapy in septic patients with proven bacterial infection in an intensive care setting. Diagn Microbiol Infect Dis. 2013;76:266–71.
70. Chu DC, Mehta AB, Walkey AJ. Practice patterns and outcomes associated with procalcitonin use in critically ill patients with sepsis. Clin Infect Dis. 2017;64:1509–15.
71. Jensen JU, Hein L, Lundgren B, et al. Procalcitonin-guided interventions against infections to increase early appropriate antibiotics and improve survival in the intensive care unit: a randomized trial. Crit Care Med. 2011;39:2048–58.
72. Andriolo BN, Andriolo RB, Salomao R, et al. Effectiveness and safety of procalcitonin evaluation for reducing mortality in adults with sepsis, severe sepsis or septic shock. Cochrane Database Syst Rev. 2017;1:CD010959.
73. Vincent JL, Teixeira L. Sepsis biomarkers: value and limitations. Am J Respir Crit Care Med. 2014;190:1081–2.
74. Kofoed K, Andersen O, Kronborg G, et al. Use of plasma C-reactive protein, procalcitonin, neutrophils, macrophage migration inhibitory factor, soluble urokinase-type plasminogen activator receptor, and soluble triggering receptor expressed on myeloid cells-1 in combination to diagnose infections: a prospective study. Crit Care. 2007;11:R38.
75. Gibot S, Bene MC, Noel R, et al. Combination biomarkers to diagnose sepsis in the critically ill patient. Am J Respir Crit Care Med. 2012;186:65–71.
76. Balk RA, Kadri SS, Cao Z, et al. Effect of procalcitonin testing on health-care utilization and costs in critically ill patients in the United States. Chest. 2017;151:23–33.
77. Westwood M, Ramaekers B, Whiting P, et al. Procalcitonin testing to guide antibiotic therapy for the treatment of sepsis in intensive care settings and for suspected bacterial infection in emergency department settings: a systematic review and cost-effectiveness analysis. Health Technol Assess. 2015;19:v–xxv. 1–236

Part III

Sepsis Management

International Clinical Practice Guidelines

7

Radu Postelnicu, Andrew Rhodes, and Laura Evans

Key Points

- Clinical practice guidelines are propositions developed methodologically to help physicians in their decisions concerning the appropriateness of care in a given clinical setting.
- They lead to improvement in health outcomes by advancing the quality of clinical decisions, as they empower physicians to choose treatments of proven benefit and to abandon those that may cause no benefit or harm.
- The Surviving Sepsis Campaign guidelines were developed to provide guidance for clinicians caring for adult patients with sepsis or septic shock.
- The most recent SCC guidelines recommend the implementation of bundles in improving the quality of care of patients.

7.1 Introduction

Recent years have witnessed an exponential growth of scientific data and published material, with the number of indexed Medline publications rising from 2500 to more than 5000 per month [1]. This huge quantity of information makes it difficult

R. Postelnicu, M.D. · L. Evans, M.D. (✉)
Division of Pulmonary, Critical Care, and Sleep Medicine, New York University School of Medicine, Bellevue Hospital, New York, NY, USA
e-mail: radu.postelnicu@nyumc.org; laura.evans@nyumc.org

A. Rhodes, M.B.B.S.
Department of Intensive Care Medicine, St. George's University Hospital, London, UK
e-mail: andrewrhodes@nhs.net

W. J. Wiersinga, C. W. Seymour (eds.), *Handbook of Sepsis*,
https://doi.org/10.1007/978-3-319-73506-1_7

for physicians to integrate related information into daily practice. It has been estimated that between 30 and 50% of patients do not receive health care in accordance with best practice [2, 3]. Translating research into clinical practice to improve health-care decision-making is a major concern and is the spotlight of quality improvement programs around the world. Clinical practice guidelines (CPG) are one of the tools that have been developed to solve this problem.

CPGs are an important mechanism that can influence clinical practice. Many local, national, and international societies develop tools to identify relevant clinical areas, reviewing applicable evidence, formulating specific clinical questions and recommendations that they believe clinicians and their patients should follow. As a result, guideline panels have grown in size, which also poses a specific challenge in decision-making. In this chapter, we review the methodologic considerations for the development of international clinical practice guidelines while focusing on the Surviving Sepsis Campaign guidelines and the key points in their recommendations.

7.2 Background

Sepsis is a frequently fatal condition that affects more than one million patients a year in the United States alone [4]. Based on a better understanding of the pathobiology of infection, the Society of Critical Care Medicine (SCCM) and the European Society of Intensive Care Medicine (ESICM) updated definitions of sepsis and septic shock in 2015. Sepsis is defined as a life-threatening organ dysfunction caused by a dysregulated host response to infection. Septic shock can be defined as a subset of sepsis in which underlying circulatory, cellular, and metabolic abnormalities are profound enough to cause a substantial increase in mortality [5].

The Barcelona Declaration in 2002 established the formation of the Surviving Sepsis Campaign (SSC)—a collaboration by the SCCM and the ESCIM to reduce mortality from sepsis and septic shock. The aim was to harness the support of governments, health agencies, the public, and other health-care professionals to decrease the relative mortality of sepsis by 25% over the following 5 years [6]. The Barcelona Declaration outlined a six-point action plan designed to improve the management of sepsis: building awareness of the problem, improving diagnosis and recognition, defining and increasing the use of appropriate treatment and care, educating health-care professionals, improving counseling and post-intensive care unit care, and developing guidelines of care [6]. The initial SSC guidelines were first published in 2004 and revised in 2008, 2012, and 2016 [7–13]. The mortality of patients with sepsis has improved over time [14]. In an observational study that included 29,470 patients in sepsis worldwide, every quarter of participation in the SSC initiative was associated with a significant decrease in the odds of hospital mortality (odds ratio, 0.96; 95%CI, 0.95–0.97; $P < 0.001$) [15]. The developed guidelines followed a rigorous process which will be discussed in this chapter (Fig. 7.1). Since guidelines are rarely integrated into practice in a timely fashion, the SSC recommends the use of bundles, which simplify the intricate processes of care in patients with sepsis and septic shock.

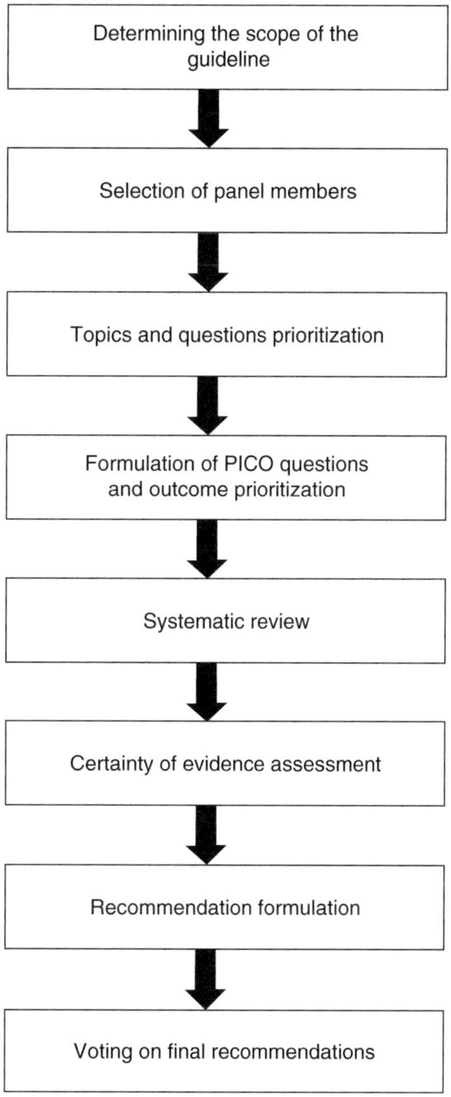

Fig. 7.1 The Surviving Sepsis Campaign guideline development process

7.3 Guideline Development

Health-care professionals rely heavily on the translation of evidence into CPG [16]. The United States Institute of Medicine (IOM) defines CPG as "statements that include recommendations intended to optimize patient care that are informed by a systematic review of evidence and an assessment of the benefits and harms of alternative care options" [17]. The number of guidelines developed by medical societies has increased exponentially in the last few decades. Clinicians, patients, and other stakeholders struggle with numerous and sometimes contradictory guidelines of variable quality [18].

Until the 1990s, most guidelines were established based on expert opinion only [19]. While the advantages of this approach were simplicity and rapidity, it was later determined that these recommendations were in contradiction with systematic reviews. Reliable and valid recommendations require a rigorous methodological approach combining systematic review of the results of clinical research with discussed and explicit expert judgment [20]. CPG rely on evidence-based medicine (EBM) or factual medicine, which aims at conscientious, explicit, and judicious use of currently available evidence for making and carrying out decisions about patient care [21]. International collaboration offers additional opportunities to enhance guideline development [22].

7.3.1 Guideline Development Group

The guideline development group reviews the evidence, translates it into practice recommendations, writes the guideline, and assures that the recommendations are not biased by being based on factors other than the best available scientific evidence. These groups should include diverse stakeholders, such as content experts, health-care professionals, and methodologists, with skills in evidence appraisal and synthesis. It is important that the groups involve experts from a single discipline, as groups without multidisciplinary membership have been associated with recommendations that are not evidence based [23–27]. A dysfunctional group may also yield unreliable recommendations [28].

Guideline chairs and members are charged with weighing published evidence, transforming knowledge into recommendations, illuminating areas of continuing controversy, discarding outdated or disproven guidance, and eventually developing the guidelines document. All of this requires deep engagement, diversity of opinion, and substantial investment of time. In the updated version of the SSC guidelines, the selection of committee members was based on expertise in specific aspects of sepsis. The guideline was generated by 55 international experts representing 25 international organizations involved in the care of patients with sepsis and providing 93 recommendations on early management of sepsis and septic shock. The resulting large and diverse panels present opportunities for decision-making, such as ensuring that all participants have a voice and can influence the results of the debate, dealing with disagreements, achieving consensus, ensuring transparency, and resolving situations in which consensus is not possible. Co-chairs were appointed by the SCCM and ESICM governing bodies, and each sponsoring organization appointed a representative who had sepsis expertise. The SCC Guidelines Committee Oversight Group and the co-chairs were responsible for appointing additional committee members and to balance continuity and provide new perspectives with the previous committee's membership and to address content needs.

7.3.2 Management of Potential Conflict of Interest

Conflicts of interest are a set of circumstances that create a risk that professional judgment or actions regarding a primary interest will be unduly influenced by secondary interest [29]. Members of a guideline development group should disclose any personal or household financial and nonfinancial COI relationships related to the guideline topic. Several systematic reviews have highlighted the influence of conflicts of interest on the opinion of experts and the conclusions of systematic reviews and guidelines [30]. In 44 CPG in Europe and North America involving 199 experts, 81% had some relationship with the pharmaceutical industry, 58% had received some financial support, and 38% had a consultation role or were employed by industry [31]. This highlights the importance of an explicit and transparent procedure in the declaration made by the members of the working group concerning the potential conflicts of interest with the main topic of CPG. An effective and neutral chair is critical and should lead the group to ensure balanced contributions from all members. The chair should facilitate discussion and consensus and have general knowledge of the topic.

The updated SSC guidelines did not have any industry input, and the panelists did not receive any honoraria. Each member was required to complete a personal disclosure of potential COI upon joining the guidelines panel and then annually. If there was a risk of potential COI, these members had limited voting opportunities on the topics pertinent to the COI, or they were assigned to a different group.

7.3.3 Question Development

Practice guideline development starts with identification of a clinical problem or question. The updated SSC guidelines focus on early management of patients with sepsis or septic shock. The SCC guideline development group was divided into five different sections: hemodynamics, infection, adjunctive therapies, metabolic, and ventilation. The group designations developed into the internal work structure of the guidelines committee. For each question, the co-chairs and group heads defined the relevant population, alternative management strategies (intervention and comparator), and the outcomes (e.g., population, intervention, comparator, and outcome [PICO] format). Through discussion via e-mail, teleconferences, and face-to-face meetings, topics were prioritized and organized.

Each clinical question provided the framework for formulating study inclusion and exclusion criteria and guided the search for relevant evidence (systematic reviews and original studies). Panels typically restricted included studies to randomized controlled trials (RCTs) for intervention questions but included observational studies when there was a paucity of RCT data addressing an intervention and for questions of risk assessment. The decision regarding question inclusion was reached by discussion and consensus among the guideline panel leaders with input from panel members and the methodology team within each group. Questions from the previous version of the SSC guidelines were reviewed, and those that were considered important and clinically relevant were retained. Questions that were considered less important or of low priority to clinicians were omitted, and new questions that were considered high priority were added (Fig. 7.2).

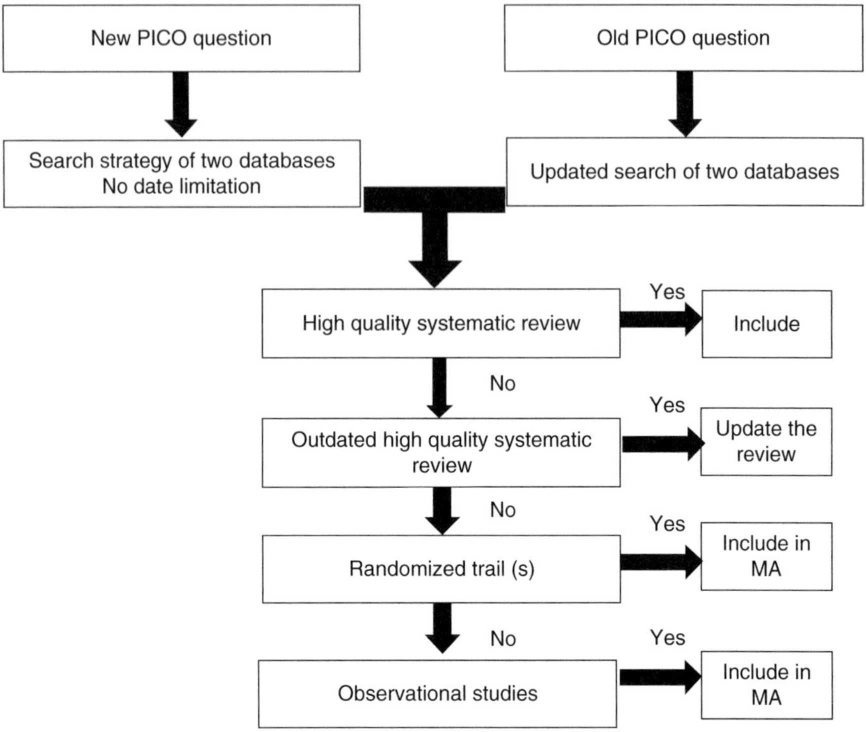

Fig. 7.2 The Surviving Sepsis Campaign guideline question development pathway

7.3.4 Decision-Making Process

Group consensus is critical in any guideline development process. It is required to select and interpret evidence, to translate evidence into recommendations, and, in settings when there is no clear evidence, to determine how to handle these situations. Most organizations use formal consensus processes, such as Delphi, nominal group technique, or formal balloting. Formal methods have been shown to result in a less biased and more evidence-based process than informal methods [24, 26, 32]. A guideline should clearly define a quorum and document the consensus process [33–35]. The SSC guidelines required 80% agreement on the developed topics from 75% of the panel members. In settings where consensus was not met, reformulation and revoting of the topics was required.

7.3.5 Grading of Recommendations

Trustworthy guidelines are based on high-quality systematic reviews of evidence [36–39]. Guideline development groups synthesize and grade evidence using a standardized approach. There are several different grading systems available; however, the Grading of Recommendations Assessment, Development, and Evaluation (GRADE) system is increasingly being adopted by guideline developers worldwide [40, 41]. This method uses structured approaches to collect, analyze, and summarize the relevant evidence and to use that evidence to produce and grade recommendations.

The GRADE methodology is based on assessment of evidence according to six categories: (1) risk of bias, (2) inconsistency, (3) indirectness, (4) imprecision, (5) publication bias, and (6) other criteria, followed by assessment of the balance between benefit and harm, patients' values and preferences, cost and resources, and feasibility and acceptability of the intervention [41–46]. GRADE classifies quality of evidence as high, moderate, low, or very low. It also allows the quality of evidence derived from observational data to be upgraded from low to moderate or high categories and the quality of evidence coming from randomized trials to be downgraded depending on the details of design and execution of the studies. This approach to determining the quality of evidence requires subjective judgment and thus invites differences of opinion.

A strong recommendation reflects the collective opinion of the guideline development group that the desirable effects of the intervention (e.g., beneficial health outcomes, less burden on staff and patients, and cost savings) will clearly outweigh the undesirable effects (e.g., harms, more burden, and greater costs) [47]. Alternatively, a weak recommendation suggests that the desirable effects will outweigh the undesirable ones, but the panel is not certain about trade-offs. This situation occurs when key evidence is of low quality or the benefits and downsides are closely matched [47].

In order to explore the range and distribution of the opinions held by SSC guideline development group within the GRADE framework, a GRADE grid was designed and implemented. This grid allows members of the panel to record their views about the balance between the benefits and disadvantages of specific interventions, after review of the available evidence. This assessment is then mapped to the strength of recommendation for each intervention, which should be assigned on the basis of evaluation of the evidence, benefits and harms, consistency, clinical effect, and generalizability and applicability, as well as patient preferences. Clear identification of the quality of evidence and strength of clinical recommendations increases the trustworthiness and improves the implementation of clinical guidelines [48–50].

Guideline development groups assess whether the desirable effects of adherence outweigh the undesirable effects, and the strength of a recommendation reflects the degree of confidence in that balance assessment. A strong recommendation in favor of an intervention conveys the certainty the desirable effects of adherence to a recommendation will clearly outweigh the undesirable effects [51]. A weak recommendation in favor of an intervention indicates the conclusion that the desirable effects of adherence to a recommendation probably will outweigh the undesirable effects. This occurs due to low-quality evidence—and thus uncertainty remains regarding the benefits and risks—or the benefits and downsides are closely balanced. In the SSC guidelines, a strong recommendation is worded as "we recommend" and a weak

Table 7.1 Factors determining strong versus weak recommendations

What should be considered	Recommended process
High or moderate quality of evidence	The higher the quality of evidence, the more likely a strong recommendation
Certainty about the balance of benefits vs. harms and burdens	– A larger difference between the desirable and undesirable consequences and the certainty around that difference, the more likely a strong recommendation – The smaller the net benefit and the lower the certainty for that benefit, the more likely a weak recommendation
Certainty in, or similar, values	The more certainty or similarity in values and preferences, the more likely a strong recommendation
Resource implications	The lower the cost of an intervention compared to the alternative and other costs related to the decision (i.e., fewer resources consumed), the more likely a strong recommendation

recommendation as "we suggest." There are several different factors which need to be considered in determining strong versus weak recommendations, such as the quality of evidence, certainty about the balance of benefits versus harms and burdens, certainty in the values, and the resource implications (Table 7.1).

Describing a recommendation as strong implies that many patients would accept that intervention and a majority of clinicians should use it in most situations. Circumstances may exist in which a strong recommendation cannot or should not be followed for an individual because of that patient's preferences or clinical characteristics that make the recommendation less applicable. A strong recommendation does not imply standard of care. Additionally, best practice statements (BPS) represent ungraded strong recommendations and are used under strict criteria. An instance where a BPS would be appropriate includes situations when the benefit or harm is unequivocal, but the evidence is hard to summarize or assess using GRADE methodology [52].

7.4 Surviving Sepsis Campaign Guideline Recommendations

7.4.1 Utilization of Surviving Sepsis Campaign Bundles

International guideline recommendations are rarely integrated into practice in a timely fashion. In order to overcome this impedance, the SSC guidelines recommend the use of bundles to simplify the complex processes of care in patients with sepsis and septic shock. This development of a practical working plan aims to more easily convert recommendations into practice [53]. Bundles as set of elements of care, when distilled from evidence-based guidelines and implemented into a group, have an effect on outcomes beyond implementing the individual elements alone [54]. The SSC bundles are an important vehicle in aiding and tracking implementation of the SSC guidelines. The SSC bundles have undergone revisions over time based on the best available evidence. The most recent update is shown in Table 7.2.

Table 7.2 The Surviving Sepsis Campaign bundles

To be completed within 3 h	To be completed within 6 h
Measure lactate level	Apply vasopressors (for hypotension that does not respond to initial fluid resuscitation) to maintain a mean arterial pressure ≥ 65 mmHg
Obtain blood culture prior to antibiotics	In the event of persistent hypotension after initial fluid administration (MAP <65 mmHg) or if initial lactate was ≥4 mmol/L, reassess volume status and tissue perfusion and document findings according to attached table
Administer broad-spectrum antibiotics	Re-measure lactate if initial lactate is elevated
Administer 30 mL/kg crystalloid for hypotension or lactate level ≥ 4 mmol/L	

Increased compliance with sepsis bundles in the United States is associated with a decrease in mortality from sepsis and septic shock to less than 10% [55]. Investigators have shown comparable results in other developed countries such as the United Kingdom and Spain [56, 57]. The SSC recently published outcomes of bundle implementation over a 7.5-year period and showed that participation in the SSC alone improved mortality [58]. Additionally, hospitals with higher guideline compliance also had reduced hospital and ICU length of stay [58]. These results revealed the sustainability of better outcomes with increased compliance. Similar results are seen in developing countries such as India, Brazil, and China [59–61]. Compliance with SCC bundles has also been shown to reduce hospital care costs, with a reduction in up to $5000 per patient in the United States [62]. Consistent adherence to the SSC bundles can be further extrapolated to cost savings in the billions of dollars in all patients with sepsis and septic shock. However, adherence to guidelines remains low, specifically among internal medicine and emergency room physicians at the forefront of managing patients with sepsis and septic shock [63]. Well-described barriers to implementation of evidence-based guidelines include lack of familiarity, lack of agreement, and an inability to overcome the inertia of existing behavior [64]. Utilization of a performance improvement program is strongly associated with improved bundle compliance [65]. Furthermore, initiatives such as educational programs, clinical decision support tools, and dedicated medical staff have been introduced worldwide, which have augmented compliance with bundle implementation [65]. A multifaceted approach using early recognition strategies, multidisciplinary educational sessions, and continuous performance assessment may have an exponential value [66, 67].

7.4.2 Educational Programs

Educational programs may vary according to institutional practices, but they should include training of physicians and nursing staff in the definitions of sepsis and septic shock, their early recognition, and benefits of timely management. The aim of such educational processes should be to affect a culture change to support the immediate treatment of sepsis and septic shock in the same manner as a trauma, stroke, or myocardial infarction. Such training can be delivered in various innovative ways—from an e-learning package to simulation-based courses [68, 69]. Its efficacy should be assessed by measuring bundle compliance rates. Regular reinforcements should be scheduled to assure the program's sustainability and to avoid a gradual decline in health-care provider awareness. Outcome measures and process-of-care variables (e.g., bundle compliance) should be assessed regularly to determine the effectiveness of each educational program. Implementation of educational programs based on the SCC guidelines broadens awareness, enhances interdisciplinary collaboration, improves bundle compliance, and also leads to improved mortality [57, 70].

7.4.3 Clinical Decision Support Tools

Early detection of sepsis is often difficult, as its presentation may be subtle and insidious. Even after the implementation of educational programs, the diagnosis can be delayed. Additional factors such as excessive workload, patient acuity, and high patient care responsibilities are well-defined barriers to early detection and SCC guideline adherence [71]. Physiologic deterioration often precedes clinical deterioration, and the recognition of this concept has led to the development of early warning systems to enhance early identification of patients who are at high risk for decompensation [72]. Use of an early warning and response system which monitors real-time laboratory values and vital signs has been shown to improve early sepsis care and may reduce sepsis mortality [73]. An early warning system that brings an interdisciplinary team to the bedside should integrate the patient's vital signs and laboratory values into the electronic medical record and establish a threshold for triggering the alert. The National Early Warning Score (NEWS) incorporates respiration rate, oxygen saturation, temperature, systolic blood pressure, pulse rate, and level of consciousness and is used in the emergency department to rapidly identify patients with sepsis and septic shock [72]. The Prehospital Early Sepsis Detection (PRESEP) score assesses vital signs and blood sugar levels and can be utilized in the prehospital setting [74]. In the emergency department or hospital wards, commonly used early warning scores may be more accurate than bedside tools such as qSOFA or SIRS in predicting in-hospital mortality and ICU transfer in patients with suspected infection [75]. Implementation of an early warning system improves early sepsis care and has an important role in optimizing timely compliance with the SSC bundles [71, 74]. However, there are no comparative studies of early warning systems that demonstrate a clear and significant difference between them.

7.4.4 Dedicated Medical Staff

Early identification and standardized management of sepsis is the cornerstone of the SSC guidelines, and hospital-based systems should be established to facilitate prompt identification of these patients [76]. Institutional support is crucial in cultivating an environment of early recognition and management of patients with sepsis [76]. Infrastructural platforms must be enabled by administrators and implemented by health-care providers [77]. Development of quality improvement and performance initiative projects should be utilized to provide continuous feedback to health-care workers. This can ultimately lead to a reduction in sepsis-related mortality, ICU length of stay, and an increase in cost savings [78, 79]. Once a patient with sepsis has been identified, a dedicated *sepsis response team* may be deployed to enhance compliance with the SSC bundles. This sepsis response team is essentially a specialized *rapid response team*, organized and equipped to provide early goal-directed therapy [80]. The *sepsis response team* can be equipped with fluids, antibiotics, and the means to obtain venous access in order to expedite timely management of these patients. These teams can deliver protocolized care in early sepsis and lead to the appropriate utilization of the sepsis resuscitation bundle. Such a team should be multidisciplinary and include a critical care physician, hospitalist physician, and nursing staff. If institutional resources permit, the addition of a pharmacist responder has also been shown to improve bundle compliance [81].

Conclusion

Clinical practice guidelines are propositions developed methodologically to help the physician and the patient in their decisions concerning the appropriateness of care in a given clinical setting. They can apply to prevention, diagnostic procedures, treatments, or follow-up policies of a given disease or group of diseases. CPG evaluate the present state of knowledge of a particular clinical setting, based on the critical appraisal of scientific data, and judgment of a group of experts, and delineate management strategies for the patients concerned. They lead to improvement in health outcomes by advancing the quality of clinical decisions, as they empower physicians to choose treatments of proven benefit and to abandon those that may cause no benefit or harm.

The SSC guidelines were developed to provide guidance for clinicians caring for adult patients with sepsis or septic shock. They are intended to be best practice and are not created to represent standard of care. The most recent SCC guidelines recommend the implementation of bundles in improving the quality of care of patients. Achieving compliance with the guidelines is dependent on the institutional support and can include educational programs, early warning system utilization, and sepsis response teams.

References

1. Fervers B, Carretier J, Bataillard A. Clinical practice guidelines. J Visc Surg. 2010; 147(6):e341–9.
2. McGlynn EA, Asch SM, Adams J, Keesey J, Hicks J, DeCristofaro A, et al. The quality of health care delivered to adults in the United States. N Engl J Med. 2003;348(26):2635–45.
3. Grol R. Successes and failures in the implementation of evidence-based guidelines for clinical practice. Med Care. 2001;39(8 Suppl 2):II46–54.

4. De Backer D, Dorman T. Surviving sepsis guidelines: a continuous move toward better care of patients with sepsis. JAMA. 2017;317(8):807–8.
5. Singer M, Deutschman CS, Seymour C, et al. The third international consensus definitions for sepsis and septic shock (sepsis-3). JAMA. 2016;315(8):801–10.
6. Slade E, Tamber PS, Vincent JL. The surviving sepsis campaign: raising awareness to reduce mortality. Crit Care. 2003;7(1):1–2.
7. Dellinger RP, Carlet JM, Masur H, Gerlach H, Calandra T, Cohen J, et al. Surviving sepsis campaign guidelines for management of severe sepsis and septic shock. Crit Care Med. 2004;32(3):858–73.
8. Dellinger RP, Levy MM, Rhodes A, Annane D, Gerlach H, Opal SM, et al. Surviving sepsis campaign: international guidelines for management of severe sepsis and septic shock, 2012. Intensive Care Med. 2013;39(2):165–228.
9. Dellinger RP, Levy MM, Rhodes A, Annane D, Gerlach H, Opal SM, et al. Surviving Sepsis Campaign: international guidelines for management of severe sepsis and septic shock: 2012. Crit Care Med. 2013;41(2):580–637.
10. Dellinger RP, Levy MM, Carlet JM, Bion J, Parker MM, Jaeschke R, et al. Surviving sepsis campaign: international guidelines for management of severe sepsis and septic shock: 2008. Crit Care Med. 2008;36(1):296–327.
11. Dellinger RP, Levy MM, Carlet JM, Bion J, Parker MM, Jaeschke R, et al. Surviving sepsis campaign: international guidelines for management of severe sepsis and septic shock: 2008. Intensive Care Med. 2008;34(1):17–60.
12. Rhodes A, Evans LE, Alhazzani W, Levy MM, Antonelli M, Ferrer R, et al. Surviving sepsis campaign: international guidelines for management of sepsis and septic shock: 2016. Intensive Care Med. 2017;43(3):304–77.
13. Rhodes A, Evans LE, Alhazzani W, Levy MM, Antonelli M, Ferrer R, et al. Surviving sepsis campaign: international guidelines for management of sepsis and septic shock: 2016. Crit Care Med. 2017;45(3):486–552.
14. Kaukonen KM, Bailey M, Suzuki S, Pilcher D, Bellomo R. Mortality related to severe sepsis and septic shock among critically ill patients in Australia and New Zealand, 2000–2012. JAMA. 2014;311(13):1308–16.
15. Levy MM, Rhodes A, Phillips GS, Townsend SR, Schorr CA, Beale R, et al. Surviving sepsis campaign: association between performance metrics and outcomes in a 7.5-year study. Crit Care Med. 2015;43(1):3–12.
16. Institute of Medicine (US) Committee to Advise the Public Health Service on Clinical Practice Guidelines. Introduction and Background. In: Field MJ, Lohr KN, editors. Clinical Practice Guidelines: Directions for a New Program. Washington, DC: The National Academies Press; 1990. p. 19–32.
17. AGREE Collaboration. Development and validation of an international appraisal instrument for assessing the quality of clinical practice guidelines: the AGREE project. Qual Saf Health Care. 2003;12(1):18–23.
18. Owens DK. Spine update. Patient preferences and the development of practice guidelines. Spine (Phila Pa 1976). 1998;23(9):1073–9.
19. Grimshaw J, Russell I. Achieving health gain through clinical guidelines. I: developing scientifically valid guidelines. Qual Health Care. 1993;2(4):243–8.
20. Woolf SH, Grol R, Hutchinson A, Eccles M, Grimshaw J. Clinical guidelines: potential benefits, limitations, and harms of clinical guidelines. BMJ. 1999;318(7182):527–30.
21. Isaac CA, Franceschi A. EBM: evidence to practice and practice to evidence. J Eval Clin Pract. 2008;14(5):656–9.
22. Nease RF Jr, Owens DK. A method for estimating the cost-effectiveness of incorporating patient preferences into practice guidelines. Med Decis Mak. 1994;14(4):382–92.
23. Fretheim A, Schunemann HJ, Oxman AD. Improving the use of research evidence in guideline development: 3. Group composition and consultation process. Health Res Policy Syst. 2006;4:15.

24. Hutchings A, Raine R. A systematic review of factors affecting the judgments produced by formal consensus development methods in health care. J Health Serv Res Policy. 2006;11(3):172–9.
25. Kahan JP, Park RE, Leape LL, Bernstein SJ, Hilborne LH, Parker L, et al. Variations by specialty in physician ratings of the appropriateness and necessity of indications for procedures. Med Care. 1996;34(6):512–23.
26. Murphy E, Dingwall R, Greatbatch D, Parker S, Watson P. Qualitative research methods in health technology assessment: a review of the literature. Health Technol Assess. 1998;2(16):iii–x. 1–274.
27. Shekelle PG, Woolf SH, Eccles M, Grimshaw J. Clinical guidelines: developing guidelines. BMJ. 1999;318(7183):593–6.
28. Pagliari C, Grimshaw J, Eccles M. The potential influence of small group processes on guideline development. J Eval Clin Pract. 2001;7(2):165–73.
29. Institute of Medicine (US) Committee on Conflict of Interest in Medical Research, Education, and Practice. Conflicts of Interest and Development of Clinical Practice Guidelines. In Lo B, Field MJ, editors. Conflict of Interest in Medical Research, Education, and Practice. Washington, DC: The National Academies Press; 2009. p. 189–215.
30. Jorgensen AW, Hilden J, Gotzsche PC. Cochrane reviews compared with industry supported meta-analyses and other meta-analyses of the same drugs: systematic review. BMJ. 2006;333(7572):782.
31. Choudhry NK, Stelfox HT, Detsky AS. Relationships between authors of clinical practice guidelines and the pharmaceutical industry. JAMA. 2002;287(5):612–7.
32. Shekelle PG, Schriger DL. Evaluating the use of the appropriateness method in the Agency for Health Care Policy and Research Clinical Practice Guideline Development process. Health Serv Res. 1996;31(4):453–68.
33. Fink A, Kosecoff J, Chassin M, Brook RH. Consensus methods: characteristics and guidelines for use. Am J Public Health. 1984;74(9):979–83.
34. Fretheim A, Schunemann HJ, Oxman AD. Improving the use of research evidence in guideline development: 5. Group processes. Health Res Policy Syst. 2006;4:17.
35. Woolf SH. Practice guidelines, a new reality in medicine. II. Methods of developing guidelines. Arch Intern Med. 1992;152(5):946–52.
36. Institute of Medicine (US) Committee on Standards for Developing Trustworthy Clinical Practice Guidelines. Current Best Practices and Standards for Development of Trustworthy CPGs: Part II, Traversing the Process. In Graham R, Mancher M, Miller Wolman D, et al., editors. Clinical Practice Guidelines We Can Trust. Washington, DC: The National Academies Press; 2011. p. 109–44.
37. Freeman AC, Sweeney K. Why general practitioners do not implement evidence: qualitative study. BMJ. 2001;323(7321):1100–2.
38. Shiffman RN, Dixon J, Brandt C, Essaihi A, Hsiao A, Michel G, et al. The GuideLine Implementability appraisal (GLIA): development of an instrument to identify obstacles to guideline implementation. BMC Med Inform Decis Mak. 2005;5:23.
39. Grol R, Grimshaw J. From best evidence to best practice: effective implementation of change in patients' care. Lancet. 2003;362(9391):1225–30.
40. Atkins D, Best D, Briss PA, Eccles M, Falck-Ytter Y, Flottorp S, et al. Grading quality of evidence and strength of recommendations. BMJ. 2004;328(7454):1490.
41. Guyatt GH, Oxman AD, Vist GE, Kunz R, Falck-Ytter Y, Alonso-Coello P, et al. GRADE: an emerging consensus on rating quality of evidence and strength of recommendations. BMJ. 2008;336(7650):924–6.
42. Schunemann HJ, Jaeschke R, Cook DJ, Bria WF, El-Solh AA, Ernst A, et al. An official ATS statement: grading the quality of evidence and strength of recommendations in ATS guidelines and recommendations. Am J Respir Crit Care Med. 2006;174(5):605–14.
43. Guyatt GH, Oxman AD, Kunz R, Vist GE, Falck-Ytter Y, Schunemann HJ, et al. What is "quality of evidence" and why is it important to clinicians? BMJ. 2008;336(7651):995–8.

44. Guyatt GH, Oxman AD, Kunz R, Falck-Ytter Y, Vist GE, Liberati A, et al. Going from evidence to recommendations. BMJ. 2008;336(7652):1049–51.
45. Schunemann HJ, Oxman AD, Brozek J, Glasziou P, Jaeschke R, Vist GE, et al. Grading quality of evidence and strength of recommendations for diagnostic tests and strategies. BMJ. 2008;336(7653):1106–10.
46. Guyatt GH, Oxman AD, Kunz R, Jaeschke R, Helfand M, Liberati A, et al. Incorporating considerations of resources use into grading recommendations. BMJ. 2008;336(7654):1170–3.
47. Jaeschke R, Guyatt GH, Dellinger P, Schunemann H, Levy MM, Kunz R, et al. Use of GRADE grid to reach decisions on clinical practice guidelines when consensus is elusive. BMJ. 2008;337:a744.
48. Ansari MT, Tsertsvadze A, Moher D. Grading quality of evidence and strength of recommendations: a perspective. PLoS Med. 2009;6(9):e1000151.
49. Harris RP, Helfand M, Woolf SH, Lohr KN, Mulrow CD, Teutsch SM, et al. Current methods of the US Preventive Services Task Force: a review of the process. Am J Prev Med. 2001;20(3 Suppl):21–35.
50. Kavanagh BP. The GRADE system for rating clinical guidelines. PLoS Med. 2009;6(9):e1000094.
51. van der Weijden T, Boivin A, Burgers J, Schunemann HJ, Elwyn G. Clinical practice guidelines and patient decision aids. An inevitable relationship. J Clin Epidemiol. 2012;65(6):584–9.
52. Guyatt GH, Schunemann HJ, Djulbegovic B, Akl EA. Guideline panels should not GRADE good practice statements. J Clin Epidemiol. 2015;68(5):597–600.
53. Thomas KW. Adoption of sepsis bundles in the emergency room and intensive care unit: a model for quality improvement. Crit Care Med. 2007;35(4):1210–2.
54. Levy MM, Pronovost PJ, Dellinger RP, Townsend S, Resar RK, Clemmer TP, et al. Sepsis change bundles: converting guidelines into meaningful change in behavior and clinical outcome. Crit Care Med. 2004;32(11 Suppl):S595–7.
55. Miller RR 3rd, Dong L, Nelson NC, Brown SM, Kuttler KG, Probst DR, et al. Multicenter implementation of a severe sepsis and septic shock treatment bundle. Am J Respir Crit Care Med. 2013;188(1):77–82.
56. Gao F, Melody T, Daniels DF, Giles S, Fox S. The impact of compliance with 6-hour and 24-hour sepsis bundles on hospital mortality in patients with severe sepsis: a prospective observational study. Crit Care. 2005;9(6):R764–70.
57. Ferrer R, Artigas A, Levy MM, Blanco J, Gonzalez-Diaz G, Garnacho-Montero J, et al. Improvement in process of care and outcome after a multicenter severe sepsis educational program in Spain. JAMA. 2008;299(19):2294–303.
58. Levy MM, Rhodes A, Phillips GS, Townsend SR, Schorr CA, Beale R, et al. Surviving Sepsis Campaign: association between performance metrics and outcomes in a 7.5-year study. Intensive Care Med. 2014;40(11):1623–33.
59. Khan P, Divatia JV. Severe sepsis bundles. Indian J Crit Care Med. 2010;14(1):8–13.
60. Shiramizo SC, Marra AR, Durao MS, Paes AT, Edmond MB, Pavao dos Santos OF. Decreasing mortality in severe sepsis and septic shock patients by implementing a sepsis bundle in a hospital setting. PLoS One. 2011;6(11):e26790.
61. Li ZQ, Xi XM, Luo X, Li J, Jiang L. Implementing Surviving Sepsis Campaign bundles in China: a prospective cohort study. Chin Med J. 2013;126(10):1819–25.
62. Shorr AF, Micek ST, Jackson WL Jr, Kollef MH. Economic implications of an evidence-based sepsis protocol: can we improve outcomes and lower costs? Crit Care Med. 2007;35(5):1257–62.
63. Djurkovic S, Baracaldo JC, Guerra JA, Sartorius J, Haupt MT. A survey of clinicians addressing the approach to the management of severe sepsis and septic shock in the United States. J Crit Care. 2010;25(4):658.e1–6.
64. Cabana MD, Rand CS, Powe NR, et al. Why don't physicians follow clinical practice guidelines? A framework for improvement. JAMA. 1999;282(15):1458–65.

65. Damiani E, Donati A, Serafini G, Rinaldi L, Adrario E, Pelaia P, et al. Effect of performance improvement programs on compliance with sepsis bundles and mortality: a systematic review and meta-analysis of observational studies. PLoS One. 2015;10(5):e0125827.
66. Noritomi DT, Ranzani OT, Monteiro MB, Ferreira EM, Santos SR, Leibel F, et al. Implementation of a multifaceted sepsis education program in an emerging country setting: clinical outcomes and cost-effectiveness in a long-term follow-up study. Intensive Care Med. 2014;40(2):182–91.
67. Schorr C, Odden A, Evans L, Escobar GJ, Gandhi S, Townsend S, et al. Implementation of a multicenter performance improvement program for early detection and treatment of severe sepsis in general medical-surgical wards. J Hosp Med. 2016;11(Suppl 1):S32–9.
68. Davis A, Henderson J, Langmack G. Development of an e-learning package for sepsis care. Br J Nurs. 2016;25(6):292–6.
69. Nguyen HB, Daniel-Underwood L, Van Ginkel C, Wong M, Lee D, Lucas AS, et al. An educational course including medical simulation for early goal-directed therapy and the severe sepsis resuscitation bundle: an evaluation for medical student training. Resuscitation. 2009;80(6):674–9.
70. Owen JA, Brashers VL, Littlewood KE, Wright E, Childress RM, Thomas S. Designing and evaluating an effective theory-based continuing interprofessional education program to improve sepsis care by enhancing healthcare team collaboration. J Interprof Care. 2014;28(3):212–7.
71. Sinuff T, Cook D, Giacomini M, Heyland D, Dodek P. Facilitating clinician adherence to guidelines in the intensive care unit: a multicenter, qualitative study. Crit Care Med. 2007;35(9):2083–9.
72. Corfield AR, Lees F, Zealley I, Houston G, Dickie S, Ward K, et al. Utility of a single early warning score in patients with sepsis in the emergency department. Emerg Med J. 2014;31(6):482.
73. Umscheid CA, Betesh J, VanZandbergen C, Hanish A, Tait G, Mikkelsen ME, et al. Development, implementation, and impact of an automated early warning and response system for sepsis. J Hosp Med. 2015;10(1):26–31.
74. Bayer O, Schwarzkopf D, Stumme C, Stacke A, Hartog CS, Hohenstein C, et al. An early warning scoring system to identify septic patients in the prehospital setting: the PRESEP score. Acad Emerg Med Off J Soc Acad Emerg Med. 2015;22(7):868–71.
75. Churpek MM, Snyder A, Han X, Sokol S, Pettit N, Howell MD, et al. Quick sepsis-related organ failure assessment, systemic inflammatory response syndrome, and early warning scores for detecting clinical deterioration in infected patients outside the intensive care unit. Am J Respir Crit Care Med. 2017;195(7):906–11.
76. Funk D, Sebat F, Kumar A. A systems approach to the early recognition and rapid administration of best practice therapy in sepsis and septic shock. Curr Opin Crit Care. 2009;15(4):301–7.
77. Liu VX, Morehouse JW, Marelich GP, Soule J, Russell T, Skeath M, et al. Multicenter implementation of a treatment bundle for patients with sepsis and intermediate lactate values. Am J Respir Crit Care Med. 2016;193(11):1264–70.
78. Nguyen HB, Corbett SW, Steele R, Banta J, Clark RT, Hayes SR, et al. Implementation of a bundle of quality indicators for the early management of severe sepsis and septic shock is associated with decreased mortality. Crit Care Med. 2007;35(4):1105–12.
79. Judd WR, Stephens DM, Kennedy CA. Clinical and economic impact of a quality improvement initiative to enhance early recognition and treatment of sepsis. Ann Pharmacother. 2014;48(10):1269–75.
80. Rivers E, Amponsah D, Coba V. Sepsis response teams. In: De Vita M, Hillman K, Bellomo R, editors. Book: textbook of rapid response systems. 1st ed. New York: Springer; 2011. p. 245–52.
81. Flynn JD, McConeghy KW, Flannery AH, Nestor M, Branson P, Hatton KW. Utilization of pharmacist responders as a component of a multidisciplinary sepsis bundle. Ann Pharmacother. 2014;48(9):1145–51.

8 Fluids in Sepsis

James R. Anstey, Adam M. Deane, and Rinaldo Bellomo

Despite being considered one of the cornerstones of treatment, many aspects of intravenous fluid administration to patients with sepsis remain controversial. While recent data have provided considerable insights, there remains uncertainty as to the type, rate and volume of fluid that should be administered. In addition, the appropriate balance between fluids and vasopressors to achieve adequate end-organ perfusion at various stages of the septic insult is open to debate. Nonetheless, there is increasing evidence that the volume, nature and timing of fluid given can have a significant influence upon patient outcome. Finally, the conventional paradigms regarding fluid administration and fluid bolus therapy are being increasingly challenged by newer evidence.

J. R. Anstey, M.B.B.S., F.R.A.C.P., F.C.I.C.M. (✉)
Intensive Care Unit, Royal Melbourne Hospital, Parkville, VIC, Australia
e-mail: James.Anstey@mh.org.au

A. M. Deane, M.B.B.S., Ph.D., F.R.A.C.P. (✉) · R. Bellomo, M.B.B.S., M.D., F.R.A.C.P.
Intensive Care Unit, Royal Melbourne Hospital, Parkville, VIC, Australia

University of Melbourne, Parkville, VIC, Australia

W. J. Wiersinga, C. W. Seymour (eds.), *Handbook of Sepsis*,
https://doi.org/10.1007/978-3-319-73506-1_8

8.1 Definitions

Fluid resuscitation can be defined as intravenous fluid administered because the clinician judges that there is inadequate end-organ perfusion. This is distinct from the ongoing maintenance fluids administered, intravenously or enterally, to meet ongoing patient needs. Sometimes the line between the two may blur.

8.2 Causes of Organ Dysfunction in the Septic Patient

Understanding of several key aspects of organ dysfunction of sepsis has increased markedly over the last 20 years, reflected in the updated International Consensus Definitions for Sepsis and Septic Shock published in 2016 [1].

In patients challenged by severe infection, the endogenous release of cytokines (e.g., tumour necrosis factor, interleukins, etc.), eicosanoids and other mediators activates an inflammatory cascade, and organ dysfunction may be due to both circulatory and cellular abnormalities that follow. In particular, several mechanisms of lethal cell injury have now been described (necroptosis [2], apoptosis [3], ferroptosis [4]) that are independent of perfusion and much more closely related to immunological and metabolic events. These observations make it uncertain whether organ injury in sepsis is an immune injury-dependent phenomenon or a tissue hypoxia-induced event or both.

The rationale underlying a 'fluid-liberal' approach is that organ dysfunction is mainly hypoperfusion-related and therefore reversible with fluid. A positive fluid balance when applied beyond the first 24 h has, however, been associated with worse outcomes [5, 6].

Here, we briefly revisit some of the major causes of circulatory disturbance and organ dysfunction in sepsis.

8.2.1 Circulatory Disturbances in Sepsis

Absolute volume depletion may be present due to poor intake or excess losses (e.g., from diarrhoea, vomiting). Ongoing fluid loss through capillary leakiness may exacerbate volume depletion beyond this initial stage [7].

Vasodilatation, mediated by increased production of nitric oxide by inflammatory mediators, contributes to vascular smooth muscle relaxation, producing the so-called vasoplegia of sepsis, presenting in its most extreme form as septic shock. The Third International Consensus Definition for Sepsis and Septic Shock (Sepsis-3) defined shock as a vasopressor requirement to achieve a mean arterial pressure of at least 65 mmHg, accompanied by a serum lactate level > 2 mmol/L, despite adequate fluid resuscitation [1]. It should be recognized that 'adequate' fluid resuscitation is challenging to define.

Septic myocardial depression, a cytokine-mediated phenomenon of decreased right and left ventricular contractility, impaired response to filling, and reversibility with resolution of sepsis [8], is common in patients with sepsis and septic shock [9]. In 1 series of 67 mechanically ventilated septic patients free from known previous cardiac disease, it was reported in 60% of patients within the first 3 days of admission [10]. In its most extreme form, septic myocardial depression can lead to profound coexisting cardiogenic shock.

8.2.2 Organ Dysfunction in Sepsis

Any of the above circulatory disturbances can affect end-organ perfusion and function in sepsis. They are accompanied by changes at a cellular level, which are only partly understood, likely driven by inflammatory mediators, as well as changes to the microcirculation.

Given that many clinicians use blood lactate concentrations and oliguria to guide fluid resuscitation, these two areas warrant specific discussion.

First, increased blood lactate concentrations that occur with sepsis are generally not due to cellular hypoxia from hypoperfusion [11], although this may sometimes be the case if there is significant intravascular volume depletion. Serum lactate concentration may be better viewed as a nonspecific indicator of cellular or metabolic 'stress' [12]. This is not to downplay its importance as a marker of illness severity, with increases strongly associated with mortality. However, attempts to increase the cardiac output using fluids or inotropes, simply in response to an elevated serum lactate concentration in sepsis, may not be effective in improving patient outcomes [13, 14].

Second, animal models of sepsis-induced renal dysfunction in the setting of a hyperdynamic circulation suggest that renal blood flow is actually increased rather than decreased – with oliguria and acute kidney injury developing in parallel with increased renal blood flow [15–17]. It is therefore hypothesized that redistribution of blood flow within the renal microvasculature, with efferent arteriolar vasodilatation, might explain the associated reduction in observed glomerular filtration rate [18, 19]. Accordingly, fluid boluses for oliguria, if given to augment renal blood flow, which may already be enhanced during sepsis, are logically unlikely to benefit and may well cause harm. Such an approach risks fluid accumulation and may explain the association between favourable outcomes and restrictive fluid regimens observed in several studies. For example, the recent Scandinavian CLASSIC (Conservative versus Liberal Approach to Fluid Therapy of Septic Shock in Intensive Care) trial reported that worsening of acute kidney injury occurred less frequently in septic patients who received a conservative approach to fluid management after their initial resuscitation (with fluid boluses only if there were signs of severe hypoperfusion), when compared to ongoing fluid boluses as long as the patient appeared to continue to respond to filling (odds ratio for worsening acute kidney injury 0.46, 0.23–0.92, $p = 0.03$) [20]. The signal from this feasibility study, which included 151 patients, requires further investigation.

8.3 The Fluid Bolus

Rapid administration of intravenous fluid with the aim of improving circulatory disturbances constitutes the 'fluid bolus', described around the birth of modern critical care by Max Harry Weil more than 50 years ago. Its effect can be judged; he wrote, 'by objective changes in circulation, such as blood pressure, mental alertness, urine flow, peripheral venous filling, and appearance and texture of the skin' [21]. Intravenous fluid resuscitation dates even further back—to the 1830s—when the life-restoring forces of a fluid bolus were eloquently described during the cholera epidemic [22]. Hence, its origins are from hypovolemic shock.

The rationale underlying the administration of a fluid bolus is to achieve an increase in end-organ perfusion rapidly and thereby minimize the duration of end-organ hypoperfusion. The 2016 Surviving Sepsis Campaign guidelines strongly recommend that 'in the initial resuscitation of sepsis-induced hypoperfusion, at least 30 mL/kg of IV crystalloid fluid be given within the first 3 h', though they acknowledge that the quality of evidence supporting this is low [23]. Interesting, a retrospective analysis of 49,331 patients receiving mandated emergency care for sepsis found that time to completion of a first bolus of intravenous fluids was unrelated to mortality (Fig. 8.1) (odds ratio 1.01, 95% CI 0.99–1.02), a result that requires prospective evaluation [24]. It is our opinion that administration of lesser volumes, particularly in those patients with significant coexisting illnesses such as congestive heart failure and chronic renal disease, may be prudent. In all patients, frequent reassessment of the haemodynamic status after initial resuscitation is recommended [23].

Conventional Guytonian physiology teaches that if a fluid bolus is to improve organ perfusion, it must increase the stressed volume of the circulation and thereby venous return and cardiac output [25]. If a fluid bolus is administered and patient is not a 'responder' (i.e., it does not produce a significant increase in cardiac output, which might arbitrarily be defined as >10–15% [26]), it may only produce tissue oedema, thereby exacerbating organ dysfunction. There are an increasing number of studies associating a positive fluid balance and increased mortality in sepsis [27, 28]. While this association may represent that higher severity of illness is associated

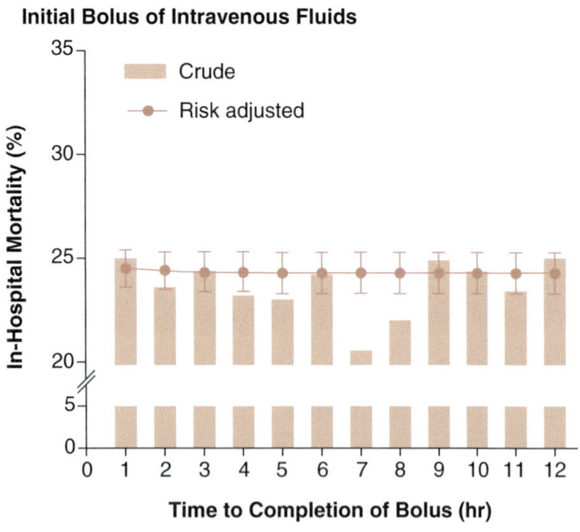

Fig. 8.1 Data from a large retrospective database of 49,331 patients looking at time to treatment and mortality during mandated emergency care for sepsis. Time to completion of the initial bolus of intravenous fluid was unrelated to risk-adjusted in-hospital mortality. Ninety-five percent confidence intervals are displayed (OR 1.01, 95% CI 0.99–1.02) [24] (With permission, New England Journal of Medicine)

with greater volumes of fluid to treat more substantial haemodynamic disturbances, an alternative explanation is that administration of less fluid—and, by extension, more vasopressor use to correct hypotension—may have merit.

A recent analysis of a large retrospective dataset of approximately 23,000 septic patients reported an association with greater mortality for those patients who received more than 5 L of fluid in the first 24 h, after adjusting for illness severity [29]. For lesser volumes, mortality appeared unaffected by volume.

In the recent FENICE study that described fluid challenge practices in 2213 patients in 46 countries, the median volume of fluid given was 500 mL (IQR 500–1000 mL), over a median time of 24 min (IQR 40–60 min) [30]. The most common indication for its administration was hypotension, present in 59% of patients [30]. Approximately half of the patients with a negative response to fluid received a further fluid bolus, the same proportion as in those who did respond. A relatively low proportion of responders, between 54.4 and 60.5% (depending on the volume and rate of administration), was also found in a recent large systematic review and meta-analysis of the fluid challenge technique [31]. This suggests that decision-making surrounding fluid boluses remains somewhat arbitrary, or at least not guided by classical teaching regarding fluid responsiveness. It has been suggested that decision-making may be driven by a clinical culture where there is a fear of not giving enough fluid, more than anything else [32].

Whether a fluid bolus is actually the best way to resuscitate a septic patient has been challenged by the observations from the landmark Fluid Expansion as Supportive Therapy (FEAST) Study [33]. This trial compared the use of fluid boluses with 5% albumin or 0.9% saline versus resuscitation without boluses, in African children with severe febrile illness and impaired perfusion. Of note, children with severe hypotension all received fluid boluses initially. These data revealed significantly greater mortality at 48 h in those patients assigned a fluid bolus: 10.6% and 10.5% mortality with albumin boluses and 0.9% saline boluses, respectively, compared with 7.3% with no bolus ($p = 0.004$). The difference in survival was apparent even after 4 h. Subsequent analysis suggested that the mechanism of death in the fluid bolus group was likely cardiovascular collapse, rather than neurological or respiratory events. This has led to the suggestion of cardiotoxicity or ischemia-reperfusion as the mechanism for these deaths [34, 35].

While these patients were generally aged between 1 and 3 years, in regions that had limited capacity for advanced supportive cardiorespiratory care that would be considered standard in many countries, and many were suffering from malaria and severe anaemia, these results are thought-provoking. To summarize, we are uncertain that the conventional approach to liberal fluid bolus therapy leads to optimal outcomes.

8.4 Indications for Fluid Administration

When considering whether to administer fluid to a patient with sepsis or septic shock, we believe that several factors may be relevant.

1. A fluid bolus (i.e., administration of fluid without any prior predictive test of responsiveness), is appropriate initially if there is evidence of hypoperfusion (e.g., delayed capillary refill, mottling, oliguria) and/or hypotension (e.g., MAP < 60 mmHg).
2. The stage of sepsis is an important consideration with regard to fluid administration. Note that an ongoing positive fluid balance beyond the early phase, particularly beyond 24 h, is associated with harm, rather than benefit [5, 6]. This remains only an association, however.
3. Dynamic predictors of fluid responsiveness (e.g. passive leg raising, pulse pressure variation) are more sensitive than static measures (e.g. central venous pressure), which are less reliable [26, 36–40].
4. An acute physiological response to fluid does not guarantee that fluid administration will lead to improved patient-centred outcomes.
5. While the optimal blood pressure is uncertain, the judicious use of vasopressors rather than persistence with large volumes of fluid should be considered.
6. Oliguria and acute kidney injury may be an epiphenomenon and are not absolute indications for further fluid.
7. Further evaluation (e.g., using echocardiogram) may have an important role when trying to understand mechanisms of shock in patients who are not responding well to initial treatment.

Predicting fluid responsiveness may be useful, particularly when deciding between ongoing fluid administration and introducing or increasing vasopressors. There are several methods to predict whether a patient will be fluid responsive. The most appropriate method used will depend on local availability, expertise, personal preference, and patient factors. Some of the more commonly employed methods are summarized in Table 8.1.

Studies incorporating fluid responsiveness as a guide to fluid resuscitation have been small and few in number, with conflicting results [41, 42]. As has been observed, such an approach may lead to cardiac output being 'maximized' rather than 'optimized', depending on the algorithm used [43]. In other words, continuing to administer fluids until a patient enters the flat part of the Frank-Starling curve may not be optimizing their haemodynamic state at all. Conversely, the potential benefit of incorporating fluid responsiveness into management would be that those unlikely to respond would be identified, thereby avoiding potentially deleterious fluid loading [41].

Moreover, when a fluid bolus is given, its actual effect may not be sustained. Knowledge about the duration of a fluid bolus' effect appears limited: a recent systematic review of the fluid challenge found that in only 5 of 85 studies was the haemodynamic effect actually assessed beyond 10 min [44]. A study of 26 postoperative patients, post general and cardiothoracic surgery, who received a 250 mL fluid bolus of Hartmann's solution over 5 min suggested that even in those patients who had an initial increase in cardiac output at 1 min as assessed by a lithium-dilution calibrated system (LiDCOplus), the haemodynamic effects had essentially dissipated after just 10 min [44]. Another study of 20 patients with predominantly

Table 8.1 Common means of predicting fluid responsiveness

Method of prediction	Underlying principle	Preconditions for use	Comments
Pulse pressure variation (PPV) Or stroke volume variation (SVV)	Cyclical changes in intrathoracic pressure with mechanical ventilation alter RV and LV preload and afterload Assess beat-to-beat variation in stroke volume as reflected by arterial pulse pressure variation (PPV) or by direct estimation of stroke volume (cardiac output monitoring device [46] or echocardiography—LVOT VTI)	PPV—arterial line SVV—continuous cardiac output monitoring device or echocardiography Patient well adapted to mechanical ventilation (often sedated, in a mandatory mode) Absence of arrhythmias	False positives if: i Arrhythmias ii Spontaneous breathing (especially if high respiratory workload) iii RV dysfunction False negatives can occur if: i Lower tidal volumes <8 mL/kg (insufficient change in cardiac preload) ii Ratio of heart rate/respiratory rate > 3.6 [26] May therefore only be used in a limited number of patients
Bilateral passive leg raise [38, 47]	Cardiac preload is transiently increased by recruiting about 200–300 mL of blood from the legs to the central circulation (a reversible fluid challenge)	May have decreased sensitivity in presence of intra-abdominal hypertension	Applicable to patients with arrhythmias and whether breathing spontaneously or mechanically ventilated [38] Assess increase in cardiac output after 1 min of leg raise by: i Change in arterial pressure ii Increase in stroke volume as measured by echocardiography (LVOT VTI) or cardiac output monitoring device Widespread applicability makes it potentially useful, with high sensitivity and specificity, though it may not be practical in all patients Avoid if intracranial hypertension
Fluid challenge (or mini-fluid challenge) [48–50]	Give small amount of fluid, e.g., 250 mL, over 5–10 min and look for change in cardiac output before committing to larger volumes (Mini-fluid challenge = 100 mL over 1 min has been more recently proposed)		No prediction before fluids are infused Allows assessment of effect prior to giving further volume May require cardiac output monitoring device or repeated echocardiography to assess effect (though an increased MAP may be a surrogate of increased CO)

(continued)

Table 8.1 (continued)

Method of prediction	Underlying principle	Preconditions for use	Comments
Echocardiography [39, 40]	Respiratory variation of the IVC and SVC can be used in mechanically ventilated patients		Respiration variation in IVC diameter (TTE) or in SVC diameter (TOE) SVC changes are more specific of the two [39], but measurement requires TOE Interpretation may be limited by significant spontaneous breathing efforts, decreased lung compliance and ventilator settings (e.g. low tidal volumes) Echocardiography also allows assessment of other important causes of shock

NB An increase in cardiac output or stroke volume of more than 10–15% in response to rapid fluid administration is a standard definition of 'fluid responsiveness' [26]
Note 1. Various definitions of fluid responsiveness exist
RV right ventricle, *LV* left ventricle, *LVOT VTI* left ventricular outflow tract velocity time integral, *TTE* transthoracic echocardiogram, *TOE* transoesophageal echocardiogram, *IVC* inferior vena cava, *SVC* superior vena cava

septic shock who received 500 mL crystalloid bolus over 30 min, after the initial resuscitation phase (greater than 6 h of vasopressor use), similarly found that cardiac output had returned to baseline within 1 h in responders [45]. While these studies focus on physiological outcomes, one might extrapolate these observations to favour vasopressor use rather than further fluid boluses beyond the early resuscitation period.

8.5 Endpoints of Initial Fluid Resuscitation

The acute physiological endpoint chosen to guide fluid administration may be clinical (e.g., blood pressure, heart rate, cognition, urine output, capillary refill, and skin temperature) or an investigation (which varies in sophistication and invasiveness, from a serum lactate to estimating changes in cardiac output and tissue perfusion). Each endpoint has various strengths and limitations and only tells part of a complex circulatory picture. For example, as mentioned above, serum lactate is a good marker of severity of illness, but is nonspecific and unreliable as a marker of organ perfusion in sepsis.

An approach known as early goal-directed therapy (EGDT), where early resuscitation of septic patients was guided by targeting central venous oxygen saturations >70%, achieved through a combination of intravenous fluids, vasopressors, inotropes, and blood transfusion, has been shown in three large RCTs from the United

States (PROCESS) [51], Australia/New Zealand (ARISE) [52] and the United Kingdom (PROMISE) [53] to not be superior to 'usual care', where treatment was guided by clinical assessment. Furthermore, EGDT led to more interventions and greater cost.

8.6 Choice of Fluid

An ideal fluid for the septic patient would be one that was inexpensive and readily available; did not accumulate, cause toxicity or metabolic derangements; and was associated with a sustained intravascular effect [54].

Crystalloids are solutions containing freely permeable ions, whereas colloids are suspensions of molecules in solution. It is important to recognize that no particular type of fluid has been proven to improve patient-centred outcomes, although starch-containing colloids have been reported to worsen some important outcomes [55, 56]. The lack of a proven superior type of fluid may explain the wide variation in fluid prescription internationally [57].

8.6.1 Colloids

Semisynthetic colloids, such as starch and gelatins, were popular due to their decreased cost when compared to albumin. Two recent landmark RCTs have compared the use of starches to crystalloid in ICU patients. The 6S Trial compared hydroxyethyl starch (130/0.42, Tetraspan) to Ringer's acetate in 798 patients admitted to the ICU with sepsis. This trial reported an increased risk of death and increased use of renal replacement therapy in patients who received starch [56]. The CHEST study compared hydroxyethyl starch (130/0.4, Voluven) with 0.9% NaCl in 6651 ICU patients. Of these, 1937 (29%) were septic. Increased renal injury and renal failure were reported in patients who received starch [55]. Gelatins, another semi-synthetic colloid, may be similarly toxic [58]. We therefore would recommend avoidance of both starches and gelatins.

An alternative colloid is albumin. In 2004, a preplanned subgroup analysis of septic patients in Australian and New Zealand SAFE study (the Saline versus Albumin Fluid Evaluation [SAFE] study), which compared 4% albumin with 0.9% saline as fluid replacement in critically ill patients, suggested that the risk of death may be lower with albumin than saline in sepsis [59]. Within the limitation of a subgroup analysis, this observation is thought-provoking, with a subsequent meta-analysis suggesting an association between the use of albumin-containing solutions in sepsis and lower mortality [60].

More recently, the results of the ALBIOS (Albumin Italian Outcome Sepsis) trial, which included 1795 patients with sepsis, who were randomized to receive daily 20% albumin aiming for an albumin concentration of 30 g/L when compared to standard care, were not superior in terms of organ failure rates—as measured by SOFA scores—or in the mortality rate [61]. However, a post hoc analysis reported a reduction in mortality in the subgroup of patients with septic shock, which requires further evaluation. While albumin appears not to be harmful in sepsis, except in traumatic brain injury patients [62], it does not have any established benefit over crystalloid.

The idea that colloids might have a dramatic volume-sparing benefit in the critically ill (as could be assumed from studies in health) was not observed in the SAFE study of 4% albumin, nor the above two starch studies, where the observed ratio of colloid to crystalloid was 1: 1.3 [55, 56, 59]. Damage to the endothelial glycocalyx layer in sepsis plays a major role in increased membrane permeability, such that the increased intravascular half-life of colloid is largely lost [63].

8.6.2 Crystalloids

Balanced crystalloid solutions (e.g., Hartmann's solution/Ringer's lactate and Plasma-Lyte) intuitively have potential benefits when compared to 0.9% NaCl, particularly as their composition is usually representative of electrolyte concentrations in humans. Other problems associated with 0.9% NaCl, including a metabolic acidosis from the chloride load, and the potential for chloride-induced nephrotoxicity, are concerns, but more likely to be problematic when the administered volume is larger. A before-after study suggested that avoidance of chloride-rich fluids might lead to decreased rates of acute kidney injury and need for renal replacement therapy [64]. However, the subsequent 'SPLIT' (Effect of a Buffered Crystalloid Solution versus Saline on Acute Kidney Injury Among Patients in the Intensive Care Unit) study failed to demonstrate any renoprotective effect from avoiding 0.9% NaCl, similar to the SALT (Balanced Crystalloids versus Saline in the Intensive Care Unit) study that also addressed this question [65, 66]. Further trials in this area are ongoing [67, 68]. Resuscitation of septic patients with hypertonic saline has an insufficient evidence basis, and as such it cannot be recommended.

The authors would currently support the use of a balanced crystalloid, or 4% (or 5%) albumin for filling in septic patients, and the avoidance of semisynthetic colloids (starch, gelatins). In the absence of any further evidence, 0.9% NaCl remains an acceptable and inexpensive alternative to balanced crystalloid solution, although it may be problematic if used in very large volumes. 4% albumin is a reasonable alternative where readily available, as long as the patient does not have a traumatic brain injury.

Conclusions

Fluid administration is a frequent intervention in septic patients, with increasing evidence that it may considerably influence the outcome. Considerations should include the patient's cumulative fluid balance, fluid responsiveness and the early use of a vasopressor to avoid excessive fluid administration beyond the initial resuscitation phase.

While there is not compelling evidence for one crystalloid over another, there is the potential that balanced crystalloids may be associated with less harm, particularly if a significant amount of fluid is given. Semisynthetic colloids (starches and gelatins) should be avoided, while 4% albumin appears safe in the absence of traumatic brain injury.

Further data are needed to determine whether fluid administered as a bolus is harmful in the adult critical care setting, to explore the optimal balance between fluids and vasopressors in the supportive phase of septic shock, and to understand whether certain crystalloids lead to better patient-centred outcomes.

References

1. Singer M, Deutschman CS, Seymour CW, Shankar-Hari M, Annane D, Bauer M, et al. The third international consensus definitions for sepsis and septic shock (Sepsis-3). JAMA. 2016;315(8):801–10.
2. Linkermann A, Stockwell BR, Krautwald S, Anders HJ. Regulated cell death and inflammation: an auto-amplification loop causes organ failure. Nat Rev Immunol. 2014;14(11): 759–67.
3. Chang KC, Unsinger J, Davis CG, Schwulst SJ, Muenzer JT, Strasser A, et al. Multiple triggers of cell death in sepsis: death receptor and mitochondrial-mediated apoptosis. FASEB J. 2007;21(3):708–19.
4. Dixon SJ, Stockwell BR. The role of iron and reactive oxygen species in cell death. Nat Chem Biol. 2014;10(1):9–17.
5. Acheampong A, Vincent JL. A positive fluid balance is an independent prognostic factor in patients with sepsis. Crit Care. 2015;19:251.
6. de Oliveira FS, Freitas FG, Ferreira EM, de Castro I, Bafi AT, de Azevedo LC, et al. Positive fluid balance as a prognostic factor for mortality and acute kidney injury in severe sepsis and septic shock. J Crit Care. 2015;30(1):97–101.
7. Siddall E, Khatri M, Radhakrishnan J. Capillary leak syndrome: etiologies, pathophysiology, and management. Kidney Int. 2017;92(1):37–46.
8. Kumar A, Haery C, Parrillo JE. Myocardial dysfunction in septic shock. Crit Care Clin. 2000;16(2):251–87.
9. Zanotti-Cavazzoni SL, Hollenberg SM. Cardiac dysfunction in severe sepsis and septic shock. Curr Opin Crit Care. 2009;15(5):392–7.
10. Vieillard-Baron A, Caille V, Charron C, Belliard G, Page B, Jardin F. Actual incidence of global left ventricular hypokinesia in adult septic shock. Crit Care Med. 2008;36(6):1701–6.
11. Garcia-Alvarez M, Marik P, Bellomo R. Stress hyperlactataemia: present understanding and controversy. Lancet Diabetes Endocrinol. 2014;2(4):339–47.
12. Garcia-Alvarez M, Marik P, Bellomo R. Sepsis-associated hyperlactatemia. Crit Care. 2014;18(5):503.
13. Bakker J, de Backer D, Hernandez G. Lactate-guided resuscitation saves lives: we are not sure. Intensive Care Med. 2016;42(3):472–4.
14. Monnet X, Delaney A, Barnato A. Lactate-guided resuscitation saves lives: no. Intensive Care Med. 2016;42(3):470–1.
15. Zafrani L, Payen D, Azoulay E, Ince C. The microcirculation of the septic kidney. Semin Nephrol. 2015;35(1):75–84.
16. Martensson J, Bellomo R. Sepsis-induced acute kidney injury. Crit Care Clin. 2015;31(4):649–60.
17. Maiden MJ, Otto S, Brealey JK, Finnis ME, Chapman MJ, Kuchel TR, et al. Structure and function of the kidney in septic shock. A prospective controlled experimental study. Am J Respir Crit Care Med. 2016;194(6):692–700.
18. Lipcsey M, Bellomo R. Septic acute kidney injury: hemodynamic syndrome, inflammatory disorder, or both? Crit Care. 2011;15(6):1008.

19. Gomez H, Ince C, De Backer D, Pickkers P, Payen D, Hotchkiss J, et al. A unified theory of sepsis-induced acute kidney injury: inflammation, microcirculatory dysfunction, bioenergetics, and the tubular cell adaptation to injury. Shock. 2014;41(1):3–11.
20. Hjortrup PB, Haase N, Bundgaard H, Thomsen SL, Winding R, Pettila V, et al. Restricting volumes of resuscitation fluid in adults with septic shock after initial management: the CLASSIC randomised, parallel-group, multicentre feasibility trial. Intensive Care Med. 2016;42(11):1695–705.
21. Weil MH, Shubin H, Rosoff L. Fluid repletion in circulatory shock: central venous pressure and other practical guides. JAMA. 1965;192:668–74.
22. Latta T. Dr Latta's cases of venous injections in cholera. Lancet. 1832;18(460):370–3.
23. Rhodes A, Evans LE, Alhazzani W, Levy MM, Antonelli M, Ferrer R, et al. Surviving Sepsis Campaign: International Guidelines for management of sepsis and septic shock: 2016. Intensive Care Med. 2017;43(3):304–77.
24. Seymour CW, Gesten F, Prescott HC, Friedrich ME, Iwashyna TJ, Phillips GS, et al. Time to treatment and mortality during mandated emergency care for sepsis. N Engl J Med. 2017;376(23):2235–44.
25. Funk DJ, Jacobsohn E, Kumar A. The role of venous return in critical illness and shock-part I: physiology. Crit Care Med. 2013;41(1):255–62.
26. Carsetti A, Cecconi M, Rhodes A. Fluid bolus therapy: monitoring and predicting fluid responsiveness. Curr Opin Crit Care. 2015;21(5):388–94.
27. Boyd JH, Forbes J, Nakada TA, Walley KR, Russell JA. Fluid resuscitation in septic shock: a positive fluid balance and elevated central venous pressure are associated with increased mortality. Crit Care Med. 2011;39(2):259–65.
28. Sadaka F, Juarez M, Naydenov S, O'Brien J. Fluid resuscitation in septic shock: the effect of increasing fluid balance on mortality. J Intensive Care Med. 2014;29(4):213–7.
29. Marik PE, Linde-Zwirble WT, Bittner EA, Sahatjian J, Hansell D. Fluid administration in severe sepsis and septic shock, patterns and outcomes: an analysis of a large national database. Intensive Care Med. 2017;43(5):625–32.
30. Cecconi M, Hofer C, Teboul JL, Pettila V, Wilkman E, Molnar Z, et al. Fluid challenges in intensive care: the FENICE study: a global inception cohort study. Intensive Care Med. 2015;41(9):1529–37.
31. Toscani L, Aya HD, Antonakaki D, Bastoni D, Watson X, Arulkumaran N, et al. What is the impact of the fluid challenge technique on diagnosis of fluid responsiveness? A systematic review and meta-analysis. Crit Care. 2017;21(1):207.
32. Perner A, Vieillard-Baron A, Bakker J. Fluid resuscitation in ICU patients: quo vadis? Intensive Care Med. 2015;41(9):1667–9.
33. Maitland K, Babiker A, Kiguli S, Molyneux E, Group FT. The FEAST trial of fluid bolus in African children with severe infection. Lancet. 2012;379(9816):613. author reply –4
34. Maitland K, George EC, Evans JA, Kiguli S, Olupot-Olupot P, Akech SO, et al. Exploring mechanisms of excess mortality with early fluid resuscitation: insights from the FEAST trial. BMC Med. 2013;11:68.
35. Myburgh J, Finfer S. Causes of death after fluid bolus resuscitation: new insights from FEAST. BMC Med. 2013;11:67.
36. Magder S. Fluid status and fluid responsiveness. Curr Opin Crit Care. 2010;16(4):289–96.
37. Marik PE, Baram M, Vahid B. Does central venous pressure predict fluid responsiveness? A systematic review of the literature and the tale of seven mares. Chest. 2008;134(1): 172–8.
38. Mesquida J, Gruartmoner G, Ferrer R. Passive leg raising for assessment of volume responsiveness: a review. Curr Opin Crit Care. 2017;23(3):237–43.
39. Vignon P, Repesse X, Begot E, Leger J, Jacob C, Bouferrache K, et al. Comparison of echocardiographic indices used to predict fluid responsiveness in ventilated patients. Am J Respir Crit Care Med. 2017;195(8):1022–32.
40. Charron C, Caille V, Jardin F, Vieillard-Baron A. Echocardiographic measurement of fluid responsiveness. Curr Opin Crit Care. 2006;12(3):249–54.

41. Richard JC, Bayle F, Bourdin G, Leray V, Debord S, Delannoy B, et al. Preload dependence indices to titrate volume expansion during septic shock: a randomized controlled trial. Crit Care. 2015;19:5.
42. See KC, Mukhopadhyay A, Lau SC, Tan SM, Lim TK, Phua J. Shock in the first 24 h of intensive care unit stay: observational study of protocol-based fluid management. Shock. 2015;43(5):456–62.
43. Saugel B, Vincent JL, Wagner JY. Personalized hemodynamic management. Curr Opin Crit Care. 2017;23(4):334–41.
44. Aya HD, Ster IC, Fletcher N, Grounds RM, Rhodes A, Cecconi M. Pharmacodynamic analysis of a fluid challenge. Crit Care Med. 2016;44(5):880–91.
45. Nunes TS, Ladeira RT, Bafi AT, de Azevedo LC, Machado FR, Freitas FG. Duration of hemodynamic effects of crystalloids in patients with circulatory shock after initial resuscitation. Ann Intensive Care. 2014;4:25.
46. Geisen M, Rhodes A, Cecconi M. Less-invasive approaches to perioperative haemodynamic optimization. Curr Opin Crit Care. 2012;18(4):377–84.
47. Boyd JH, Sirounis D. Assessment of adequacy of volume resuscitation. Curr Opin Crit Care. 2016;22(5):424–7.
48. Biais M, de Courson H, Lanchon R, Pereira B, Bardonneau G, Griton M, et al. Mini-fluid challenge of 100 ml of crystalloid predicts fluid responsiveness in the operating room. Anesthesiology. 2017;127:450–6.
49. Guinot PG, Bernard E, Deleporte K, Petiot S, Dupont H, Lorne E. Mini-fluid challenge can predict arterial pressure response to volume expansion in spontaneously breathing patients under spinal anaesthesia. Anaesth Crit Care Pain Med. 2015;34(6):333–7.
50. Marik PE. Fluid therapy in 2015 and beyond: the mini-fluid challenge and mini-fluid bolus approach. Br J Anaesth. 2015;115(3):347–9.
51. Pro CI, Yealy DM, Kellum JA, Huang DT, Barnato AE, Weissfeld LA, et al. A randomized trial of protocol-based care for early septic shock. N Engl J Med. 2014;370(18):1683–93.
52. Investigators A, Group ACT, Peake SL, Delaney A, Bailey M, Bellomo R, et al. Goal-directed resuscitation for patients with early septic shock. N Engl J Med. 2014;371(16):1496–506.
53. Mouncey PR, Osborn TM, Power GS, Harrison DA, Sadique MZ, Grieve RD, et al. Trial of early, goal-directed resuscitation for septic shock. N Engl J Med. 2015;372(14):1301–11.
54. Myburgh JA, Mythen MG. Resuscitation fluids. N Engl J Med. 2013;369(25):2462–3.
55. Myburgh JA, Finfer S, Bellomo R, Billot L, Cass A, Gattas D, et al. Hydroxyethyl starch or saline for fluid resuscitation in intensive care. N Engl J Med. 2012;367(20):1901–11.
56. Perner A, Haase N, Guttormsen AB, Tenhunen J, Klemenzson G, Aneman A, et al. Hydroxyethyl starch 130/0.42 versus Ringer's acetate in severe sepsis. N Engl J Med. 2012;367(2):124–34.
57. Hammond NE, Taylor C, Finfer S, Machado FR, An Y, Billot L, et al. Patterns of intravenous fluid resuscitation use in adult intensive care patients between 2007 and 2014: an international cross-sectional study. PLoS One. 2017;12(5):e0176292.
58. Pisano A, Landoni G, Bellomo R. The risk of infusing gelatin? Die-hard misconceptions and forgotten (or ignored) truths. Minerva Anestesiol. 2016;82(10):1107–14.
59. Finfer S, Bellomo R, Boyce N, French J, Myburgh J, Norton R, et al. A comparison of albumin and saline for fluid resuscitation in the intensive care unit. N Engl J Med. 2004;350(22):2247–56.
60. Delaney AP, Dan A, McCaffrey J, Finfer S. The role of albumin as a resuscitation fluid for patients with sepsis: a systematic review and meta-analysis. Crit Care Med. 2011;39(2):386–91.
61. Caironi P, Tognoni G, Masson S, Fumagalli R, Pesenti A, Romero M, et al. Albumin replacement in patients with severe sepsis or septic shock. N Engl J Med. 2014;370(15):1412–21.
62. Myburgh J, Investigators SS, Australian, New Zealand Intensive Care Society Clinical Trials G, Australian Red Cross Blood S, George Institute for International H, et al. Saline or albumin for fluid resuscitation in patients with traumatic brain injury. N Engl J Med. 2007;357(9):874–84.
63. Lee WL, Slutsky AS. Sepsis and endothelial permeability. N Engl J Med. 2010;363(7):689–91.
64. Yunos NM, Bellomo R, Hegarty C, Story D, Ho L, Bailey M. Association between a chloride-liberal vs chloride-restrictive intravenous fluid administration strategy and kidney injury in critically ill adults. JAMA. 2012;308(15):1566–72.

65. Young P, Bailey M, Beasley R, Henderson S, Mackle D, McArthur C, et al. Effect of a buffered crystalloid solution vs saline on acute kidney injury among patients in the intensive care unit: the SPLIT randomized clinical trial. JAMA. 2015;314(16):1701–10.
66. Semler MW, Wanderer JP, Ehrenfeld JM, Stollings JL, Self WH, Siew ED, et al. Balanced crystalloids versus saline in the intensive care unit. The SALT randomized trial. Am J Respir Crit Care Med. 2017;195(10):1362–72.
67. Zampieri FG, Azevedo LCP, Correa TD, Falavigna M, Machado FR, Assuncao MSC, et al. Study protocol for the balanced solution versus saline in intensive care study (BaSICS): a factorial randomised trial. Crit Care Resusc. 2017;19(2):175–82.
68. Semler MW, Self WH, Wang L, Byrne DW, Wanderer JP, Ehrenfeld JM, et al. Balanced crystalloids versus saline in the intensive care unit: study protocol for a cluster-randomized, multiple-crossover trial. Trials. 2017;18(1):129.

9 Vasopressors in Sepsis

Julian Arias Ortiz and Daniel De Backer

Septic shock is the most severe form of sepsis in which profound circulatory, cellular, and metabolic abnormalities occur [1, 2]. It is clinically identified by persistent arterial hypotension despite optimal fluid resuscitation requiring vasopressor agents and associated with signs of altered tissue perfusion (altered skin perfusion, oliguria, altered mental state) and confirmed by elevated blood lactate levels reflecting abnormal oxygen metabolism [3]. The hemodynamic alterations of septic shock are characterized by impaired endothelial function resulting in profound alterations in vascular tone leading to arterial and venular dilation, associated with severe hypotension, hypovolemia (volume loss due to impaired endothelial barrier function and increased permeability and volume redistribution related to dilation of venous reservoir), and impaired blood flow distribution between organs and within organs (microcirculatory level). In addition, myocardial depression frequently occurs. In most cases myocardial depression has minimal impact on cardiac output and tissue perfusion, but in some cases it may result in an inadequate cardiac output. These hemodynamic alterations are typical of those of distributive shock [4].

Vasopressors are administered to correct hypotension, aiming at restoring tissue perfusion. In this chapter we will review the indications for vasopressor use, the target blood pressure, the hemodynamic and other effects of vasopressors, and the different types of vasopressors.

J. A. Ortiz, M.D.
Surgical Intensive Care Unit, Calderon Guardia Hospital, Universidad de Costa Rica, San José, Costa Rica
e-mail: julian.ariasortiz@gmail.com

D. De Backer, M.D., Ph.D. (✉)
Department of Intensive Care, CHIREC Hospitals, Université Libre de Bruxelles, Brussels, Belgium
e-mail: ddebacke@ulb.ac.be

W. J. Wiersinga, C. W. Seymour (eds.), *Handbook of Sepsis*,
https://doi.org/10.1007/978-3-319-73506-1_9

9.1 Indications and Goals

9.1.1 Hypotension May Contribute to Impaired Organ and Tissue Perfusion

Septic shock is characterized by a decreased vascular tone leading to hypotension and worsening of tissue perfusion. Several mechanisms contribute to the decreased vascular tone and include either activation of guanylate cyclase, leading to vasodilation, or impaired sensitivity to vasoconstrictive substances such as catecholamines, vasopressin, and angiotensin (Fig. 9.1) [5]. Among the mediators implicated in vasodilation, nitric oxide (NO) through the activation of inducible nitric oxide synthase (iNOS) and vasodilatory prostaglandins may play a key role. The decreased sensitivity to catecholamines, vasopressin, and angiotensin is related both to a reduction in the number of the respective receptors and to uncoupling of the receptor from its intracellular effectors [6–8]. Interestingly, the desensitization can vary according to the receptor type, between patients, as well as over time, which may have implications for selection of the vasopressor agents. A patient failing to respond to one agent may respond to an agent from another class. In addition, relative adrenal insufficiency may also contribute in some cases [9].

Hypotension is generally considered as systolic arterial pressure <90 mmHg or a mean arterial pressure (MAP)<65 mmHg [1, 2]. While one may naively consider

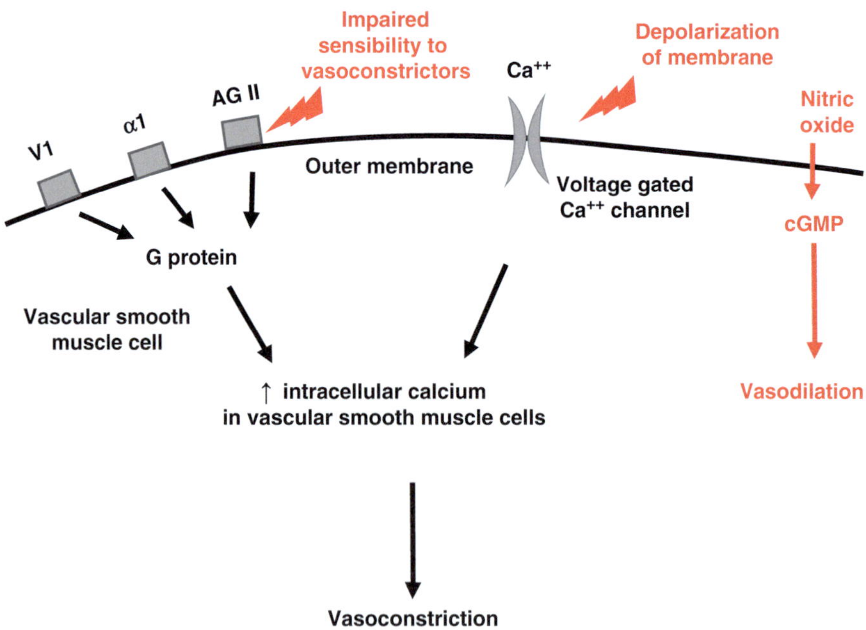

Fig. 9.1 Mechanisms leading to arteriolar contraction

that hypotension should not be an issue as long as blood flow is preserved, hypotension is the driving pressure of the different organs. In septic pigs, maintaining MAP 50–60 was associated with a higher degree of impairment in renal function compared to 75–85 mmHg, even though there were no differences in cardiac output [10]. In patients with septic shock, correction of severe hypotension is associated with improvement in creatinine clearance and lactate [11].

Profound and persistent hypotension represents an independent risk of death [12, 13]. Even non-sustained hypotension (<60 min) is associated with poor outcome and should not be neglected [14].

9.1.2 Specificities of Some Organs (Kidney, Brain, etc.)

The principal autoregulatory mechanisms that control the regional blood flow distribution and perfusion of the microcirculation are the global autonomic control, global and local pressure-flow relations, and local autoregulatory control (via neuroendocrine, paracrine, and mechanosensory pathways). Normally different vascular beds have different pressure-flow relations (regional P/Q) [15], and they also have different O_2 extraction capacities (regional VO_2/DO_2) [16]. These mechanisms adapt the locoregional tissue oxygen transport to metabolic needs. Alteration of these processes in sepsis is mainly due to a decreased adrenergic responsiveness and a pathologic imbalance between local vasoconstrictor and vasodilatory mediators (NO, endothelin, thromboxane A_2, etc.) leading to blood flow heterogeneity within organs, with a consequent dissociation between blood flow and metabolic demand.

Endothelial dysfunction in sepsis induces changes in blood flow distribution between the different organs. These variably affect the different vascular beds. The mesenteric circulation is typically altered as a result of increased sympathetic tone and renin-angiotensin activation inducing vasoconstriction of the mesenteric territory, whereas downregulation of endothelial nitric oxide synthase (eNOS) can decrease the endothelium-dependent vasodilation. In humans, hepatic flow generally increases in parallel with cardiac output, but hepatic venous saturation (Sho_2) can decrease [17]. Renal blood flow is generally increased in hyperkinetic models but the repartition between medullar and cortical flow is altered probably largely because of an increased release of NO. As mentioned above, hypotension is associated with development of AKI [18]. Cerebral blood flow is typically preserved, even in hypokinetic models. However, autoregulation of cerebral perfusion can be altered in sepsis [19], and cerebral blood flow may be dependent on blood pressure at MAP levels between 65 and 85 mmHg and can even be affected by changes in cardiac output [20]. Autopsy findings and nuclear magnetic resonance studies suggest ischemic lesions may occur in patients with septic shock [21]. These data suggest that preservation of perfusion pressure is particularly important in sepsis, but that the level of the ideal perfusion pressure for a given individual is difficult to predict.

9.1.3 Implications for the Microcirculation

The microcirculation is responsible for the fine tuning of distribution of flow at the organ level. The generalized endothelial dysfunction of sepsis has been associated with severe microcirculatory alterations in sepsis. these are characterized by capillary rarefaction and heterogeneity of perfusion, with no-flow capillaries in close viscinity to well perfused capillaries [22, 23].

The effects of vasopressors on microvascular perfusion are not straightforward. On the one hand, vasopressors vasoconstrict precapillary sphincters and venous outflow, which may impair microvascular perfusion. On the other hand, correction of hypotension may restore the driving pressure of capillaries. Accordingly, the effects of vasopressors on the microcirculation are expected to be highly variable and depend on patient condition.

9.2 Timing of Introduction

Vasopressor therapy is used to counteract life-threatening hypotension. It is important to consider introduce a vasopressor early in the resuscitation phase of septic shock (salvage phase [4]), even when hypovolemia has not been completely resolved.

Early initiation of vasopressors may be associated with several beneficial effects in septic shock. By restoring vascular tone in capacitance veins, norepinephrine increases cardiac preload. This results in an increase in cardiac output in preload-dependent patients and reduces the degree of preload dependency [24]. This could help to limit the positive fluid balance and prevent harmful fluid overload. Administration of norepinephrine with restoration of the MAP also improves the microcirculation, recruiting microvessels, and improving tissue oxygenation [25].

Early correction of hypotension is probably associated with improved outcome. Both duration and degree of hypotension have been associated with increased mortality in septic shock patients [12, 13] so that it sounds attractive to rapidly correct hypotension. While it is difficult to conduct randomized trials delaying introduction of vasopressor therapy, observational trials have shown that delay in correcting severe hypotension is associated with an increased mortality rate [26]. Altogether these data suggest that hypotension should be corrected without delay.

9.3 Target of Arterial Pressure

Targeting a MAP of 65–70 mmHg is considered as a good initial goal [27]. Observational trials showed that a MAP below 65 mmHg was associated with an increased mortality rate in septic shock patients. Interestingly, these trials failed to show differences in outcome between 65 and 70 mmHg and higher values. In an experimental model of sepsis, conflicting results have been observed: targeting a MAP of 50–60 mmHg was associated with an increased incidence of acute kidney injury (AKI) compared to a higher MAP of 75–85 mmHg, but it didn't translate into a survival benefit maybe because targeting the higher MAP level was also associated with a more positive fluid balance and greater vasopressor load [10]. Vasopressors cause vasoconstriction, and excessive vasoconstriction can cause two main problems: (1) it can alter the microcirculation and interfere with the mechanisms regulating the distribution of blood flow in the periphery, and (2) vasoconstriction can increase afterload and result in impaired right and left ventricular function. In addition, vasopressor agents are associated with their intrinsic side effects (i.e., arrhythmias with adrenergic agents, impaired splanchnic perfusion with vasopressin) which are dose dependent, and reaching higher MAP levels requires higher doses of vasopressors.

Limited size interventional trials evaluated the effects of different MAP levels on various indices of tissue perfusion and renal function in patients with septic shock [28, 29]. Overall these trials were unable to show a significant benefit for a higher MAP level but demonstrated an important individual response. In a trial randomizing 776 patients with septic shock to a higher (80–85 mmHg) or a lower (65–70 mmHg) MAP, no differences in mortality at 28 or 90 days between the two groups [30]. However the higher MAP target was associated with an improved kidney function and less requirement than the low MAP target. This potential beneficial effect was mitigated by an increase in the incidence of arrhythmias and in myocardial infarction.

Even though increasing MAP to higher values than 65 mmHg could be beneficial in some patients, it can also be associated with harmful effects. For each patient a balance needs to be made between achieving an adequate arterial pressure and limiting adverse effects associated with fluid and vasopressor administration.

It is very difficult to identify patients who may benefit from a higher MAP value. Some factors like age and history of hypertension suggest that a higher MAP value may be desired, but even in these cases a high individual variability has still been observed. One of the key problems in defining "optimal" arterial pressure at the individual level is that global measures of perfusion (cardiac output, central or mixed venous oxygen saturation) do not always reflect what occurs at the tissue level, both in terms of regional perfusion (i.e., renal perfusion) and microvascular perfusion. One may thus consider to use surrogates of organ or microvascular perfusion (i.e., urine output, lactate, venoarterial difference in PCO2) and perform a MAP challenge during which the changes in these variables are evaluated. In case of absence of improvement at higher MAP target, it is probably wiser to come back to the 65 mmHg target.

So after achieving an initial value of at least 65 mmHg, the MAP level should be adjusted taking into account various indices of tissue perfusion including mental state, skin perfusion (mottling and capillary refill time), urine output, lactate levels, and venoarterial PCO_2 gradients.

9.4 Which Vasopressor

Different classes of vasopressor agents may be considered. It should be noted that even though alpha-adrenergic agents, vasopressin, and angiotensin stimulate different receptors (Fig. 9.1), the underlying mechanism leading to constriction is identical: after activation of the surface receptor, the increase in phospholipase C and

Table 9.1 Main effects of vasopressors

Agent	Receptor stimulation	Effect
Adrenergic	Alpha-adrenergic	Vasopressor effect
	Beta-adrenergic	+ Inotropic, splanchnic, and microvascular perfusions /–/ Tachycardia and arrhythmias, metabolic
	Dopaminergic	+ Splanchnic and renal perfusions (Questionnable in critically ill patients) /–/ Tachycardia and arrhythmias, immunologic, impact on pituitary axis
Vasopressin	V1	Vasopressor effect, improved glomerular filtration rate, decreased permeability, inhibition of KATP channels
	V2	Anti-diuresis, platelet aggregation
	V3	ACTH release
	Octreotide receptor	Vasodilation
Angiotensin II	Angiotensin	+ Vasopressor effect
		/–/ Antidiuretic effect (ADH release)

+ positive effect, /–/ negative effect

Table 9.2 Stimulation of the different adrenergic receptors

	Alpha	Beta	Dopaminergic
Dopamine	++	++	+
Norepinephrine	++++	+	/–/
Epinephrine	++++	++++	/–/
Phenylephrine	++++	/–/	/–/

protein kinase C leads to mobilization of calcium stores and entry of calcium in the cell which induce vasoconstriction. The different response to these agents arises because of the density and localization of the different receptors (density varies in the different vascular beds, resulting in difference in regional perfusions), downregulation of these receptors in sepsis (the downregulation of adrenergic, vasopressin, and angiotensin II varies individually), and the associated stimulation of other receptors (i.e., beta-adrenergic, dopaminergic, vasopressin 2 and 3, etc.) with its own hemodynamic and metabolic consequences (Table 9.1).

It should be noted that all vasopressor agents carry the risk to impair cardiac function: the septic heart is very sensitive to an increase in afterload; restoring blood pressure may hence unmask sepsis-associated myocardial depression and compromise cardiac output and hence tissue perfusion.

9.4.1 Adrenergic Agents

Adrenergic agonists are the first-line vasopressors because of their rapid onset of action, high potency, and short half-life, which allows easy dose titration.

Each vasopressor (dopamine, norepinephrine, phenylephrine, and epinephrine) has specific hemodynamic, metabolic, immunomodulating effects (Table 9.2). While norepinephrine, phenylephrine, and epinephrine have similar vasopressor effects (a similar increase in blood pressure is achieved by administering a similar dose of these agents), dopamine is less potent. The other effects depend on the additional stimulation of beta-adrenergic and/or dopaminergic receptors. Stimulation of each type of adrenergic receptors has pros and cons. For example, α-adrenergic stimulation will increase vascular tone and blood pressure, but it could increase the afterload to the left and right ventricle, potentially decreasing cardiac output and regional blood flows, especially in the hepatosplanchnic region; for these reasons, phenylephrine (pure alpha-adrenergic agent) is rarely indicated. At the other extreme, beta-adrenergic stimulation can increase regional blood flows by increasing cardiac output, but also increases the risk of myocardial ischemia, promotes arrhythmias, and is associated with immunodepression and metabolic effects (hyperglycemia, hyperlactatemia). Epinephrine has a combined alpha- and beta-adrenergic effect. As the dose of the agent is driven by the response in arterial pressure (and thus the alpha-adrenergic effect), epinephrine at low doses has minimal metabolic effect and increases tissue perfusion, while at higher doses this agent is associated with strong metabolic effects. At high doses, epinephrine decreased splanchnic blood flow and increased blood lactate levels compared to norepinephrine in septic shock patients [31]. Epinephrine is also with tachycardia and an increased incidence of arrhythmia. In a randomized controlled trial comparing norepinephrine and epinephrine in patients with septic shock, epinephrine was associated with arrhythmic and metabolic effects that resulted in withdrawal of 13% of patients from the study, but there were no differences in the achievement in hemodynamic targets [32]. It is difficult to determine the impact of these effects on mortality as it was evaluated only in one underpowered randomized study which showed a nonsignificant increase in day 28 mortality with epinephrine compared to norepinephrine [33].

Dopamine was initially considered as having a beneficial combination of alpha-, beta-, and dopaminergic effects. However it became rapidly obvious that the potentially beneficial effects of dopaminergic stimulation on splanchnic and renal perfusion are blunted in patients with shock, while the negative impact on heart rate and pituitary axis are still observed. As a result, dopamine is associated with tachycardia and an increased incidence of arrhythmias [34]. More importantly, dopamine is associated with an increased risk of death compared to norepinephrine (relative risk: 1.1 (1.01–1.20); $p = 0.035$) [35]. Hence, dopamine is no longer recommended for the treatment of patients with septic shock.

Norepinephrine has predominantly α-adrenergic properties, but its modest β-adrenergic effect helps to maintain cardiac output. Its administration generally results in a clinically significant increase in mean arterial pressure, with little change in heart rate or cardiac output. The usual dose is 0.1–2.0 mcg/kg min.

Given its favorable head-to-head comparisons with other adrenergic vasopressors, norepinephrine is considered as the vasopressor of choice in septic shock patients [36]. Epinephrine may at best be considered as a second-line agent for severe cases [36]. The authors consider that if norepinephrine is unable to increase

MAP to the desired target, it is better to use vasopressin or angiotensin which are acting on alternative receptors than to give an additional alpha-adrenergic agent with potentially more adverse effects.

9.4.2 Non-adrenergic Agents

In cases of septic shock not responding satisfactorily to norepinephrine, adding another vasopressor with a different mechanism of action may be considered. Non-adrenergic vasopressors can be considered either as an alternative to adrenergic agents in order to limit their potential adverse effects (arrhythmias and metabolic effects) or as additional agents in case of limited response to alpha-adrenergic agents. Both vasopressin and angiotensin II can be considered for this purpose.

9.4.2.1 Vasopressin

Vasopressin and its analog terlipressin exert their effects by way of vascular $V1_a$ receptors and renal tubular V2 receptors. $V1_a$ receptor stimulation leads to arterial vasoconstriction and V2 stimulation increases renal free water reabsorption. Terlipressin has higher affinity for vascular receptors than vasopressin as assessed by a higher $V1_a$/V2 ratio compared with vasopressin (2.2 vs. 1, respectively). While the vasopressor effect is related to V1 receptor stimulation, stimulation of the other vasopressin receptors can generate other less desired effects (Table 9.1). At high doses vasopressin impairs splanchnic perfusion and can lead to gut and liver ischemia.

Vasopressin has emerged as an adjunct to catecholamines for patients who have severe septic shock. The rationale for its use is the relative vasopressin deficiency, described in septic shock especially when not responding to norepinephrine, but vasopressin receptor desensitization should also be considered. Administration of vasopressin usually increases vascular tone and blood pressure, helping to reduce the need for the use of adrenergic vasopressors. Of note, vasopressin may decrease blood flow in the heart, kidneys, and intestine, so it should be administered only in patients with a high level of cardiac output.

In the Vasopressin and Septic Shock Trial (VASST), the investigators found that the addition of low-dose vasopressin to norepinephrine in the treatment of patients with septic shock was safe, spared norepinephrine infusion and may have been associated with a survival benefit for patients receiving limited doses of norepinephrine [26]. The VANISH trial evaluated the impact of early vasopressin use versus norepinephrine on kidney failure in patients with septic shock; the early use of vasopressin did not improve the number of kidney failure-free days [37]. More importantly, this study failed to confirm the hypothesis that less severe patients may benefit from vasopressin compared to norepinephrine, as survival rates were identical with the two agents.

Altogether, these trials demonstrated that (1) a low-dose vasopressin can be used to spare doses of norepinephrine or to help to restore blood pressure in patients with limited response to norepinephrine; (2) a low-dose vasopressin is safe and associated with minimal adverse effects; (3) a low-dose vasopressin has neutral effects on mortality compared to norepinephrine and can thus be used as a safe alternative/adjunct to this agent.

The current recommendations suggest adding vasopressin to norepinephrine as a second-line vasopressor, with the intent of raising mean arterial pressure to target and/or to decrease norepinephrine dosage [36]. Vasopressin should not be used at doses higher than 0.03–0.04 U per minute.

Terlipressin, an analog of vasopressin, has a duration of action of several hours, as compared with minutes for vasopressin. For this reason, it does not offer an advantage over vasopressin in the ICU. The ideal dose of terlipressin remains to be determined.

New V1 derivatives (selepressin, etc.) are currently under investigation in humans and have shown promising effects in experimental conditions.

9.4.2.2 Angiotensin

Angiotensin II is a strong vasoconstrictive peptide which may help to restore blood pressure in cases of septic shock not responding to norepinephrine. In sepsis, a decreased angiotensin II sensitivity has also been reported. Nevertheless, experimental studies have shown that angiotensin II administration can help to maintain blood pressure with minimal metabolic effects. In a recent trial, angiotensin II was shown to increase blood pressure and to spare norepinephrine doses [38]. Interestingly, administration of angiotensin II was associated with a trend toward a decrease mortality at day 28 (46 vs. 54%, $p = 0.12$) which may justify conduction of further trials to ensure the safety and effectiveness of this agent. At this stage and in the absence of large-scale trials evaluating the effects of angiotensin II on outcome, it is probably premature to use this promising agent outside clinical research.

9.4.2.3 Nitric Oxide (NO) Inhibitors

Nitric oxide plays a pivotal role in the development of vasodilatation during septic shock. In the healthy state, nitric oxide is continuously produced at low concentrations by a calcium-dependent nitric oxide synthase (NOS1 and NOS3, cNOS) from the substrate L-arginine. This enzyme resides in the vascular endothelial cells and plays an important role in the control of normal vascular tone. Endotoxin and cytokines released during the host response to infection induce a calcium-independent NOS (NOS2, iNOS). Induction of iNOS can result in the sustained production of nitric oxide for a prolonged period of time (up to 10 h), despite the presence of negative feedback mechanisms. The increased production of nitric oxide has been associated with hypotension, decreased responsiveness to vasoconstrictors, and development of multiple organ dysfunction. Inhibiting the production of nitric oxide or modulating its effects was thought to be beneficial in patients with septic shock. Several agents had been used as NOS inhibitors in sepsis, such as methylarginine (L-NMMA) and nitroarginine (L-NNA). The study done by Lopez et al., a multiple-center, randomized, placebo-controlled trial, using a nonselective nitric oxide synthase inhibitor (L-NMMA) in septic shock patients, showed a detrimental effect with an increase in mortality [39]. Accordingly, the administration of nonselective NOS inhibitors is currently not recommended in septic shock patients.

Methylene blue inhibits guanylate cyclase and hence modulates the effects of nitric oxide. Limited size clinical trials have shown that this compound can effectively increase blood pressure without detrimental effects on cardiac function [40], but large-scales trials are required to ensure safety and effectiveness of this agent.

9.4.2.4 Steroids

Corticosteroids have been investigated for more than 60 years in the management of patients with septic shock. Yet their use in practice still remains controversial. While so-called low-dose hydrocortisone may help to restore responsiveness to vasoconstrictive substances and shorten shock duration, their impact on outcome remains controversial. Current guidelines suggest adding IV hydrocortisone to treat septic shock patients if adequate fluid resuscitation and vasopressor therapy are unable to restore hemodynamic stability. The recommended hydrocortisone dose is 200 mg per day, eventually as a continuous infusion to improve glycemic control, and it is suggested by the Surviving Sepsis Campaign as a weak recommendation, with low quality of evidence [27]. Two ongoing large-scale double-blind randomized trials will provide new information in close future and may clarify these controversies on the use of hydrocortisone in septic shock.

Conclusions

Prompt correction of hypotension seems desirable as both severity and duration of hypotension are associated with a poor outcome. Norepinephrine, an alpha-adrenergic agent, is considered as first-line vasopressor agent. When the patient fails to respond to norepinephrine, alternative agents acting on different receptors should be considered as second-line agents rather than adding another adrenergic agent. Vasopressin at low dose is an excellent second-line agent. The role of angiotensin II requires further investigations.

References

1. Singer M, Deutschman CS, Seymour CW, Shankar-Hari M, Annane D, Bauer M, et al. The third international consensus definitions for sepsis and septic shock (Sepsis-3). JAMA. 2016;315(8):801–10.
2. Cecconi M, De Backer D, Antonelli M, Beale RJ, Bakker J, Hofer C, et al. Consensus on circulatory shock and hemodynamic monitoring. Task force of the European Society of Intensive Care Medicine. Intensive Care Med. 2014;40(12):1795–815.
3. Shankar-Hari M, Phillips GS, Levy ML, Seymour CW, Liu VX, Deutschman CS, et al. Developing a new definition and assessing new clinical criteria for septic shock: for the Third International Consensus definitions for sepsis and septic shock (Sepsis-3). JAMA. 2016;315(8):775–87.
4. Vincent JL, De Backer D. Circulatory shock. N Engl J Med. 2013;369(18):1726–34.
5. De BD, Scolletta S. Clinical management of the cardiovascular failure in sepsis. Curr Vasc Pharmacol. 2013;11(2):222–42.
6. Bucher M, Kees F, Taeger K, Kurtz A. Cytokines down-regulate alpha1-adrenergic receptor expression during endotoxemia. Crit Care Med. 2003;31(2):566–71.

7. Bucher M, Hobbhahn J, Kurtz A. Nitric oxide-dependent down-regulation of angiotensin II type 2 receptors during experimental sepsis. Crit Care Med. 2001;29(9):1750–5.
8. Bucher M, Hobbhahn J, Taeger K, Kurtz A. Cytokine-mediated downregulation of vasopressin V(1A) receptors during acute endotoxemia in rats. Am J Physiol Regul Integr Comp Physiol. 2002;282(4):R979–84.
9. Annane D, Bellissant E, Sebille V, Lesieur O, Mathieu B, Raphael JC, et al. Impaired pressor sensitivity to noradrenaline in septic shock patients with and without impaired adrenal function reserve. Br J Clin Pharmacol. 1998;46:589–97.
10. Correa TD, Vuda M, Takala J, Djafarzadeh S, Silva E, Jakob SM. Increasing mean arterial blood pressure in sepsis: effects on fluid balance, vasopressor load and renal function. Crit Care. 2013;17(1):R21.
11. Albanese J, Leone M, Garnier F, Bourgoin A, Antonini F, Martin C. Renal effects of norepinephrine in septic and nonseptic patients. Chest. 2004;126(2):534–9.
12. Dunser MW, Takala J, Ulmer H, Mayr VD, Luckner G, Jochberger S, et al. Arterial blood pressure during early sepsis and outcome. Intensive Care Med. 2009;35(7):1225–33.
13. Varpula M, Tallgren M, Saukkonen K, Voipio-Pulkki LM, Pettila V. Hemodynamic variables related to outcome in septic shock. Intensive Care Med. 2005;31(8):1066–71.
14. Marchick MR, Kline JA, Jones AE. The significance of non-sustained hypotension in emergency department patients with sepsis. Intensive Care Med. 2009;35(7):1261–4.
15. Magder SA. The highs and lows of blood pressure: toward meaningful clinical targets in patients with shock. Crit Care Med. 2014;42(5):1241–51.
16. Schlichtig R, Kramer DJ, Pinsky MR. Flow redistribution during progressive hemorrhage is a determinent of critical O2 delivery. J Appl Physiol. 1991;70:169–78.
17. De Backer D, Creteur J, Noordally O, Smail N, Gulbis B, Vincent JL. Does hepato-splanchnic VO2/DO2 dependency exist in critically ill septic patients? Am J Respir Crit Care Med. 1998;157:1219–25.
18. Izawa J, Kitamura T, Iwami T, Uchino S, Takinami M, Kellum JA, et al. Early-phase cumulative hypotension duration and severe-stage progression in oliguric acute kidney injury with and without sepsis: an observational study. Crit Care. 2016;20(1):405.
19. Taccone FS, Castanares-Zapatero D, Peres-Bota D, Vincent JL, Berre' J, Melot C. Cerebral autoregulation is influenced by carbon dioxide levels in patients with septic shock. Neurocrit Care. 2010;12(1):35–42.
20. Berre J, De Backer D, Moraine JJ, Melot C, Kahn RJ, Vincent JL. Dobutamine increases cerebral blood flow velocity and jugular bulb hemoglobin saturation. Crit Care Med. 1997;25:392–8.
21. Sharshar T, Gray F, Lorin dG, Hopkinson NS, Ross E, Dorandeu A, et al. Apoptosis of neurons in cardiovascular autonomic centres triggered by inducible nitric oxide synthase after death from septic shock. Lancet. 2003;362(9398):1799–805.
22. De Backer D, Creteur J, Preiser JC, Dubois MJ, Vincent JL. Microvascular blood flow is altered in patients with sepsis. Am J Respir Crit Care Med. 2002;166:98–04.
23. De Backer D, Donadello K, Sakr Y, Ospina-Tascon GA, Salgado DR, Scolletta S, et al. Microcirculatory alterations in patients with severe sepsis: impact of time of assessment and relationship with outcome. Crit Care Med 2013;41(3):791–9.
24. Monnet X, Jabot J, Maizel J, Richard C, Teboul JL. Norepinephrine increases cardiac preload and reduces preload dependency assessed by passive leg raising in septic shock patients. Crit Care Med. 2011;39(4):689–94.
25. Georger JF, Hamzaoui O, Chaari A, Maizel J, Richard C, Teboul JL. Restoring arterial pressure with norepinephrine improves muscle tissue oxygenation assessed by near-infrared spectroscopy in severely hypotensive septic patients. Intensive Care Med. 2010;36:1882–9.
26. Bai X, Yu W, Ji W, Lin Z, Tan S, Duan K, et al. Early versus delayed administration of norepinephrine in patients with septic shock. Crit Care. 2014;18(5):532.
27. Rhodes A, Evans LE, Alhazzani W, Levy MM, Antonelli M, Ferrer R, et al. Surviving sepsis campaign: international guidelines for management of sepsis and septic shock: 2016. Intensive Care Med, 2017;43(3):304–77.

28. Thooft A, Favory R, Salgado DR, Taccone FS, Donadello K, De Backer D, et al. Effects of changes in arterial pressure on organ perfusion during septic shock. Crit Care. 2011;15:R222.
29. Deruddre S, Cheisson G, Mazoit JX, Vicaut E, Benhamou D, Duranteau J. Renal arterial resistance in septic shock: effects of increasing mean arterial pressure with norepinephrine on the renal resistive index assessed with Doppler ultrasonography. Intensive Care Med. 2007;33(9):1557–62.
30. Asfar P, Meziani F, Hamel JF, Grelon F, Megarbane B, Anguel N, et al. High versus low blood-pressure target in patients with septic shock. N Engl J Med. 2014;370(17):1583–93.
31. De Backer D, Creteur J, Silva E, Vincent JL. Effects of dopamine, norepinephrine, and epinephrine on the splanchnic circulation in septic shock: which is best? Crit Care Med. 2003;31:1659–67.
32. Myburgh JA, Higgins A, Jovanovska A, Lipman J, Ramakrishnan N, Santamaria J. A comparison of epinephrine and norepinephrine in critically ill patients. Intensive Care Med. 2008;34(12):2226–34.
33. Annane D, Vignon P, Renault A, Bollaert PE, Charpentier C, Martin C, et al. Norepinephrine plus dobutamine versus epinephrine alone for management of septic shock: a randomised trial. Lancet. 2007;370(9588):676–84.
34. De Backer D, Biston P, Devriendt J, Madl C, Chochrad D, Aldecoa C, et al. Comparison of dopamine and norepinephrine in the treatment of shock. N Engl J Med. 2010;362(9):779–89.
35. De Backer D, Aldecoa C, Njimi H, Vincent J-L. Dopamine versus norepinephrine in the treatment of septic shock: a metaanalysis. Crit Care Med. 2012;40:725–30.
36. Russell JA, Walley KR, Singer J, Gordon AC, Hebert PC, Cooper DJ, et al. Vasopressin versus norepinephrine infusion in patients with septic shock. N Engl J Med. 2008;358(9):877–87.
37. Gordon AC, Mason AJ, Thirunavukkarasu N, Perkins GD, Cecconi M, Cepkova M, et al. Effect of early vasopressin vs norepinephrine on kidney failure in patients with septic shock: the VANISH randomized clinical trial. JAMA. 2016;316(5):509–18.
38. Khanna A, English SW, Wang XS, Ham K, Tumlin J, Szerlip H, et al. Angiotensin II for the treatment of vasodilatory shock. N Engl J Med. 2017;377(5):419–30.
39. Lopez A, Lorente JA, Steingrub J, Bakker J, McLuckie A, Willatts S, et al. Multiple-center, randomized, placebo-controlled, double-blind study of the nitric oxide synthase inhibitor 546C88: effect on survival in patients with septic shock. Crit Care Med. 2004;32:21–30.
40. Myburgh JA, Webb RK, Worthley LIG. The P50 is reduced in critically ill patients. Intensive Care Med. 1991;17:355–8.

Management of Multiorgan Failure in Sepsis

10

Ithan D. Peltan and Samuel M. Brown

10.1 The History of Multiorgan Failure

Organ dysfunction resulting from a maladaptive host response to infection defines the sepsis syndrome [1]. For many patients, the simultaneous or sequential failure of multiple organ systems triggered by the infection poses a greater threat to life and health than the primary infection.

The emergence of multiorgan failure (MOF) as a recognized syndrome complicating multiple acute illnesses paralleled the rise of the modern intensive care unit (ICU) in the 1970s [2, 3]. Advances in the early care of medical and surgical disease combined with the development of methods to support failing organs—including particularly vasopressors, hemodialysis, closed chest cardiac massage, and positive pressure ventilation—unmasked MOF in many patients [4]. In other words, MOF represented a new state of biological existence made possible by the ICU: patients who would once have been dead were now alive, albeit in a state of profound organ dysfunction.

MOF has been commonly defined as "altered organ function in an acutely ill patient such that homeostasis cannot be maintained without intervention" [5]. MOF is also defined as failure or significant dysfunction of two or more organ systems [6]. Some advocate substituting "multiple organ dysfunction syndrome" (MODS) for MOF because impaired organ homeostasis exists on a continuum and to emphasize the need to interrupt progression of dysfunction to failure [5, 6]. In current usage, however, MOF/MODS commonly refer to severe single organ failure *or* milder dysfunction affecting multiple organs. Sepsis III added another twist, since the term sepsis itself now incorporates MOF [1]. Regardless of definition, the MOF *concept* is robust, with good construct and predictive validity [7] (Box 10.1). For clarity, we use here "sepsis-associated MOF" rather than the more ambiguous term "sepsis."

I. D. Peltan, M.D., M.Sc. · S. M. Brown, M.D., M.S. (✉)
Intermountain Medical Center, Murray, UT, USA

University of Utah School of Medicine, Salt Lake City, UT, USA
e-mail: samuel.brown@hsc.utah.edu

W. J. Wiersinga, C. W. Seymour (eds.), *Handbook of Sepsis*,
https://doi.org/10.1007/978-3-319-73506-1_10

Box 10.1: Terminology Applied to Multiorgan Failure
Multiple organ or multiorgan failure
Multiple systems failure
Progressive system(s) failure
Sequential system(s) failure
Acute organ system failure
Multiple system(s) organ failure
Remote organ failure
Multiple organ dysfunction syndrome
Organ dysfunction in the ICU

10.2 MOF Criteria and Scoring Systems

While MOF may be easy to recognize clinically, explicit diagnostic criteria were necessary for research. Multiple scores exist [8], with most rating pulmonary, cardiovascular, and renal function and many also rating neurologic, hepatic, and hematologic function (Table 10.1). Scoring systems mainly describe the extent of organ dysfunction rather than predict patient outcomes [9]. Nevertheless, and regardless of the specific criteria, the number of organ failures predicts mortality [10, 11].

The three most widely used sepsis-associated MOF scores all evaluate the same six organ systems: the Multiple Organ Dysfunction Score (MODS), the Logistic Organ

Table 10.1 Organ systems included in selected multiorgan failure criteria and scores

	CV	Pulm	Renal	Neuro	GI	Heme	Hepatic	Other system(s)
Baue [2]	•	•	•	•	•	•	•	Pancreas/ endocrine
Goris et al. [15]	•	•	•	•	•	•	•	
Fry et al. [16]		•	•		•		•	
Stevens [17]	•	•	•	•	•	•	•	
Knauss et al. [18]	•	•	•	•		•		
Caricco et al. [19]	•	•	•	•		•	•	Metabolic, general
Marshall et al. [20]	•	•	•	•		•	•	Metabolic, immunologic
Hébert et al. [10]	•	•	•	•	•	•	•	
Kollef [21]	•	•	•	•	•	•	•	
Fagon et al. [22]	•	•	•	•		•	•	Infection
Moore et al. [23]	•	•	•				•	
Marshall et al. [6]	•	•	•	•		•	•	
Le Gall et al. [12]	•	•	•	•		•	•	
Vincent et al. [13]	•	•	•	•		•	•	
Levy et al. [24]	•	•	•	•	•	•	•	Metabolic
Howell et al. [25]	•	•	•			•		

Abbreviations: *CV* cardiovascular, *GI* gastrointestinal, *Heme* hematologic, *Neuro* neurologic, *Pulm* pulmonary

Table 10.2 Sequential Organ Failure Assessment score[a]

SOFA score	1	2	3	4
Respiration PaO_2/FiO_2, mmHg	<400	<300	<200 ——— with respiratory support ———	<100
Coagulation Platelets × $10^3/mm^3$	<150	<100	<50	<20
Liver Bilirubin, mg/dL (μmol/L)	1.2–1.9 (20–32)	2.0–5.9 (33–101)	6.0–11.9 (102–204)	>12.0 (<204)
Cardiovascular Hypotension	MAP <70 mmHg	Dopamine ≤5 or dobutamine (any dose)	Dopamine >5 or epinephrine ≤0.1 or norepinephrine ≤0.1	Dopamine >15 or epinephrine >0.1 or norepinephrine >0.1
Central nervous system Glasgow Coma Score	13–14	10–12	6–9	<6
Renal Creatinine, mg/dL (μmol/L) or urine output	1.2–1.9 (110–170)	2.0–3.4 (171–299)	3.5–4.9 (300–440) or <500 mL/day	>5.0 (>440) or <200 mL/day

Dysfunction System (LODS) score, and the Sequential Organ Failure Assessment (SOFA) score (Table 10.2) [6, 12, 13]. Despite its informal development, the SOFA score's simplicity and (admittedly modest) predictive validation [11, 14] led to its broad adoption, including its incorporation into the Sepsis III definitions [1, 11].

Sepsis III also introduced the qSOFA, a simplified SOFA score measuring only pulmonary, cardiovascular, and neurologic function [11]. External validations of the qSOFA have been mixed, dependent on the care setting, clinical outcome, and model priorities [26, 27].

10.3 Epidemiology

10.3.1 Incidence

The incidence of sepsis-associated MOF depends on the criteria employed and population investigated [28]. In infected patients admitted to French EDs, 34% had a SOFA ≥2 [26]. In a cohort of 184,000 ICU patients with suspected infection, 90% had a SOFA ≥2 [27]. In a multinational study ($N = 8353$), 34% of patients in the ICU at least 24 h had infection on ICU admission, and 50% had MOF [29].

10.3.2 Genetics

Evidence points to a heritable risk of death from infection not attributable to the risk of acquiring infection. Among adoptees, early death from infection is increased by a factor of six if the biological—but not the adoptive—parent died early from infection [30]. If the adoptee died from infection, biological siblings' risk of death from infection was dramatically higher (HR 9.36, 95% CI 2.94–29.8) [31]. Similarly, familial risk of influenza mortality appears independent of viral factors or shared environment [32]. Because MOF is the usual mode by which acute infection causes death, these findings indicate the risk of MOF from infection has a genetic component. Despite methodological limitations and the challenges posed by sepsis's heterogeneity [33], polymorphisms related to TLR4, TNF, and IL-1 have been linked to organ failure development and trajectory [34].

10.3.3 Natural History and Outcomes

The distribution of septic organ failures depends on the care setting, diagnostic criteria, and case identification methods. In a Spanish ICU cohort ($N = 2619$), most patients (56%) had 2–3 organ failures at the time of sepsis diagnosis [35]. Pulmonary failure was most common (75%), followed by cardiovascular (59%) and renal (40%). Early descriptions emphasized a characteristic sequence of organ failures, beginning with respiratory and progressing to hepatic, neurologic, and cardiac failure [2, 4, 36], but later studies deemphasized this concept. Regardless, MOF is the most common cause of death in sepsis: among 1201 deaths in five sepsis trials, death from MOF (43%) was more common than cardiovascular collapse (23%) or refractory hypoxemia (13%) [37].

10.4 Pathophysiology and Heterogeneity of Sepsis-Associated MOF

The pathophysiology of sepsis-associated MOF involves multiple overlapping pathways influenced by the physiologic insult and both fixed (e.g., genetic) and variable (e.g., nutritional status) host characteristics. Sepsis may initiate a self-sustaining organ failure cascade such that removal of the inciting infectious stimulus does not lead to MOF resolution. Relevant pathways include microvascular hypoperfusion, direct cell injury, inflammation, and cell hibernation/stunning [38]. Cross talk between organ systems—crucial to MOF propagation—is mediated by hormones, cytokines, perfusion irregularities, oxygenation, and production, release, or accumulation of toxins.

No pathway in isolation dominates the progression from infection to MOF. Sepsis-associated MOF is itself an amalgam of multiple phenotypes (clinical) and endotypes (biological), each of which may have a different prognosis and optimal management [39]. A multicenter study of 2533 septic patients employing a form of neural networks identified four phenotypes: (a) minimal MOF, (b) predominant hepatic dysfunction, (c) shock with hypoxemia and altered mental status, and (d) shock with isolated renal dysfunction [40]. Clusters were not synonymous with sepsis etiology, preexisting conditions, or sepsis severity but nevertheless predicted distinct mortality patterns. Meanwhile, the leukocyte transcriptome displays two distinct "sepsis response signatures," one of which is characterized by immune tolerance, T cell "exhaustion," and higher mortality [41].

Importantly, the host response to infection behaves as a complex nonlinear system [42]. Infection's progression to MOF is determined by a dynamic network of high-dimensional interactions. Such complexity may explain why treatments of sepsis-associated MOF targeting a single plausible pathophysiologic mechanism have been almost uniformly unsuccessful in clinical trials [43]. Absent a simple linear chain from infection to MOF, therapeutic failure may result from the targeted pathway's insufficiency for organ failure development or progression, its inactivity at the time of treatment, or unpredictable effects of the therapeutic perturbation on other pathways [44].

10.5 MOF Prevention and Treatment

10.5.1 Global Sepsis Treatments

Dozens of pharmacologic agents targeting pathophysiological mechanisms of MOF have been tested in clinical trials. So far, none have clear efficacy, even when restricted to biomarker-identified subgroups. Sepsis treatments targeting immunomodulation are discussed in detail in Chap. 13.

10.5.2 High-Quality Supportive Care

Sepsis care defies easy protocolization [45]. Outcome optimization requires individualized management in addition to early, appropriate antibiotics and, when applicable, source control [46, 47]. While antibiotic management is discussed elsewhere, we emphasize that delayed antibiotic administration is associated with worse MOF [48, 49].

ICUs exist largely to treat or prevent MOF progression. However, which patients benefit from ICU admission is unclear. While treatment guidelines for community-acquired pneumonia direct location of care, such guidance is lacking for other infections. Validated pneumonia risk scores explicitly [50] favor outpatient management for some pneumonia patients despite sepsis-qualifying organ dysfunction. Even when both infection and organ failure are diagnosed, at least 2% of sepsis patients are discharged home [51]. Additional research on triage for sepsis patients is indicated.

Septic inpatients merit careful attention to prevention of complications. Components of optimal care likely include:

- Deep vein thrombosis prophylaxis [52]
- Removal of invasive catheters as soon as they are unnecessary [53]

- Measures to prevent ventilator-associated pneumonia, though some interventions are recently in question [54]
- Attention to the patient as a person, including engaging patients and families in care [55, 56]

10.5.3 Treatments Targeting Specific Organ Systems

While ICU interventions may aid restoration of "normal" organ physiology, such interventions can also reverse an adaptive response to infection, damage the target organ more than they help it, or trigger adverse effects in distant organs via organ cross talk [57]. As a result, many—though not all—evidence-based approaches to sepsis-induced MOF reflect *deadoption* of harmful or useless interventions.

10.5.3.1 Pulmonary System

The quintessence of sepsis-associated pulmonary failure, the acute respiratory distress syndrome (ARDS), is defined by the onset of hypoxemia ($PaO_2/FIO_2 \leq 300$ mmHg despite at least 5 cmH_20 positive end expiratory pressure [PEEP]) and bilateral airspace opacities not fully explained by left atrial hypertension within 1 week of a known insult [58]. Infection is by far the most common cause of ARDS [59].

Lung-protective ventilation (LPV) is the standard of care for ARDS. LPV involves administration of small tidal volumes, PEEP titration in parallel with FIO_2, and maintaining plateau pressure <30 cmH_2O to reduce progressive ventilator-induced lung injury. The ARMA trial demonstrated that low (6–8 mL/kg ideal body weight [IBW]) versus traditional (10–12 mL/kg IBW) tidal volumes improved survival and resolution of pulmonary organ failure [60]. LPV should be begun on intubation, as higher initial tidal volumes early in treatment are associated with increased mortality [61].

"Open lung" strategies—which escalate PEEP before FIO_2 to maintain target PaO_2—likely benefit patients with a PaO_2/FIO_2 ration ≤200 mmHg [62]. Recently, the ART study ($N = 1010$) reported increased mortality in patients randomized to an open-lung strategy, but overly aggressive recruitment maneuvers and high overall mortality appear to limit these findings' generalizability [63]. Approximately two-thirds of patients with sepsis-associated ARDS exhibit a subtype associated with an inflammatory cytokine profile, prolonged MOF, higher mortality, and improved outcomes with an open-lung strategy [64]. The effect of restrictive versus liberal fluid management may also vary across ARDS subtypes [65].

Prone positioning improves ventilation of dependent lung units and likely improves ARDS outcomes [66]. The most recent and influential trial of proning studied 466 patients with at least moderate ARDS, demonstrating lower mortality (16% vs. 33%, $p < 0.001$) with proning [67]. Many clinicians and investigators feel that equipoise has been lost on the question of proning for at least moderate ARDS [68].

Neuromuscular blockade (NMB) is the only pharmacologic therapy that currently has reasonable evidence for efficacy in ARDS. In 340 ARDS patients randomized to a 48-hour infusion of cisatracurium or placebo, the NMB group had 32% lower 90-day adjusted mortality [69]. Efficacy appeared greatest in patients with baseline $PaO_2/FIO_2 \leq 120$ mmHg. Due to generalizability concerns related to protocolized deep sedation of control patients, a large, multicenter study comparing NMB to standard care (i.e., light sedation and early mobilization where possible) for severe ARDS is underway [70].

The timing of intubation may also be important. Noninvasive ventilation (NIV) to "protect" the patient from intubation and mechanical ventilation with NIV may adversely influence outcomes [59, 71]. Whether this reflects distinct ARDS dynamics or NIV-related "self-inflicted lung injury" [72] from high tidal-volume respiration cannot be determined from observational data.

Numerous other ventilator-related interventions have failed investigation for routine application in ARDS. Importantly, almost no data inform "rescue" therapy for the rare ARDS patient with refractory hypoxemia. Failed therapies include high-frequency oscillatory ventilation (which may even increase mortality versus LPV) [73] and inhaled pulmonary vasodilators [74, 75]. Recent multi-society consensus guidelines recommend against routine HFOV use [76]. While extracorporeal life support (ECLS) allows radically lung-protective ventilation while preserving life in severe ARDS, the evidence supporting its routine use for ARDS is poor, including observational data from the H1N1 influenza pandemic [77] and a methodologically limited trial that suggested referral to an ECLS-capable center improved outcomes [78–80]. Randomized trials currently underway should improve the ECLS evidence base in the next few years.

Many opportunities to improve ARDS outcomes involve increasing utilization of proven therapies. Nearly 15 years after publication of ARMA, the LUNG-SAFE study of 3022 ARDS patients from 50 countries found that only 60% were clinically diagnosed with ARDS and 35% received tidal volumes >8 mL/kg IBW [59]. Among patients with severe ARDS, only 38% received neuromuscular blockade, and 16% underwent prone positioning. Further improvements in pulmonary organ failure will likely require implementation science approaches to investigate why evidence-based therapies are not applied, the reasons disproven therapies continue to be utilized, and methods to aid evidence-based adoption and deadoption of therapies [81].

ARDS Prevention

Most (though not all) experts see ARDS prevention as a worthwhile goal [82, 83]. Early application of LPV in at-risk patients likely reduces progression to ARDS [84]. In contrast to older studies (in the pre-LPV era) in which IV steroids did not prevent ARDS [85, 86], a meta-analysis suggested IV corticosteroids may reduce ARDS development in patients presenting with severe community-acquired pneumonia [87]. To date, no other pharmacologic therapies have proven effective for ARDS prevention [83]. Early administration of aspirin for patients at risk for ARDS (including 78% with suspected sepsis), for instance, recently failed to reduce ARDS incidence in a notably underpowered trial [88]. Agents of potential future interest include inhaled corticosteroids and β-agonists, vitamin D, vitamin C, and inhibitors of the renin-angiotensin-aldosterone axis [89].

Oxygenation Goals

Tissue dysoxia is common in MOF, making oxygen supplementation an attractive therapy. Given the biology of hemoglobin, however, hyperoxia does little to increase oxygen delivery and may increase formation of reactive oxygen species. High FIO_2 is also toxic to the lung, worsens ventilation/perfusion matching, and is associated with worse outcomes in multiple other critical syndromes [90].

Two recent studies suggest harm from higher oxygenation targets in sepsis-associated MOF. A trial of FIO_2 1.0 versus FIO_2 titrated to SpO_2 88–95% in 442 intubated patients with septic shock was stopped early for possible harm from hyperoxia (28-day mortality 45% vs. 35%, $p = 0.12$) [91]. A single-center trial ($N = 480$), stopped early for slow enrollment, also suggested lower mortality and improved MOF among patients randomized to SpO_2 94–98% versus 97–100% [92].

10.5.3.2 Cardiovascular System

Cardiovascular failure is common in sepsis-associated MOF. Current MOF scores measure distributive shock, which is associated with worse prognosis [93] and is covered in Chap. 9. Here, we consider other forms of sepsis-associated cardiac dysfunction.

Myocardial Dysfunction

Left ventricular (LV) systolic and diastolic dysfunction affects as many as 60–70% of sepsis patients, depending on the criteria used and population studied [94]. Whereas depressed LV ejection fraction does not clearly portend poor prognosis and often normalizes over time, the link to increased mortality is stronger for LV strain and diastolic dysfunction. Toxicity from adrenergic overstimulation (both endogenous and exogenous) may be more important than inflammatory cytokines as a cause of microvascular dysfunction generally and cardiomyocyte toxicity specifically [95].

Inotropic support for septic cardiomyopathy has a long history but poor supporting evidence. Adrenergic agonism for inotropic support targeted to $ScvO_2 > 70\%$ was enshrined in early goal-directed therapy (EGDT) [96], but enthusiasm has waned since EGDT failed validation in subsequent trials [45]. The non-adrenergic inotrope, levosimendan, is a calcium-sensitizing agent also tested in septic shock. In a trial of 516 septic shock patients, treatment with levosimendan may have worsened MOF compared to placebo [97].

Although seemingly counterintuitive, analogous to the benefits of reducing adrenergic tone in systolic heart failure, β-blockade may improve septic shock outcomes by reducing ventricular work, interrupting adrenergic cardiomyocyte toxicity, and improving diastolic and endovascular function [98, 99]. Infusion of the short-acting β-blocker esmolol appears safe in septic shock. However, while one randomized trial of esmolol suggested benefit, its interpretation is limited by a lack of placebo control, extremely high control group mortality, and heavy reliance on levosimendan [100]. Trials are therefore underway to clarify this agent's role in septic shock.

Cardiac Dysrhythmias

Almost a third of sepsis patients experience new-onset atrial fibrillation [101]. Incident atrial fibrillation is associated with worse outcomes, including mortality, although causation is unclear. Optimal treatment is also unclear, as observational data suggesting improved outcomes with β-blocker treatment rather than digoxin or amiodarone suffer from confounding by indication [102].

10.5.3.3 Renal System

Up to 50% of ICU patients suffer acute kidney injury (AKI), with sepsis the most common cause [103]. AKI is the most common element of sepsis-associated MOF, and AKI in sepsis confers higher mortality [104]. Prevention and treatment of sepsis-associated AKI are therefore a high priority.

Dopamine Receptor Agonists

Though low-dose dopamine (≤5 μg/kg/min) increases renal blood flow and urine output, dopamine infusion is ineffective for AKI prevention or treatment [105]. While data are more encouraging for the D1 receptor agonist fenoldopam, its application in sepsis remains unclear and may be limited by its prominent antihypertensive effect [106].

Renal Replacement Therapy

Management of sepsis-associated AKI is largely expectant until renal replacement therapy (RRT) is begun. The timing, mode, and intensity (or dose) of RRT are all important questions.

- Mode: While continuous RRT (CRRT) has fewer hemodynamic consequences than intermittent hemodialysis (HD), randomized trials have not shown a benefit for CRRT over HD [107]. Hemofiltration using polymyxin B cartridges also has not shown efficacy in randomized trials [108].
- Timing: In one trial, initiating RRT at onset of KDIGO stage III AKI rather than waiting for traditional indications for RRT showed no mortality benefit, but only 51% of delayed RRT strategy subjects eventually received RRT [109]. By contrast, in a trial comparing RRT initiation at KDIGO stage II versus stage III (or any traditional RRT indication), 90% of delayed RRT patients received RRT, and the early-initiation strategy reduced 90-day mortality (39% vs. 55%, $p = 0.03$) and improved renal recovery [110]. Interpretation of this study is challenging, as the delayed-treatment arm does not represent standard care in the United States.
- Dose: In multicenter trials enrolling general ICU populations (49–63% sepsis), increased intensity RRT did not improve outcomes [111, 112].

10.5.3.4 Hematologic System

Hematologic dysfunction in sepsis patients may manifest as disseminated intravascular coagulation (DIC), venous thromboembolism (VTE), or anemia due to bone marrow suppression or bleeding.

Thrombotic Pathways

The coagulation system aids the fight against infection but can also contribute to the dysregulated host response (Fig. 10.1) [113]. Multiple anticoagulant agents have been tested in sepsis without durable evidence of efficacy.

Activated Protein C

Activated protein C (APC) was the only targeted agent approved to treat sepsis in the United States. In complex with protein S, APC deactivates clotting factors V and VIII and exhibits anti-inflammatory properties [114]. The original large APC study, PROWESS, was stopped early for efficacy for 28-day mortality (25% vs 31%, $p = 0.005$) [115]. Post hoc analyses suggested the observed benefit began only after protocol/agent modification midway through the trial and was restricted to more severely ill patients [116]. Regulatory approval thus limited APC's indication to sepsis patients with an APACHE II score ≥ 25 and mandated additional trials, which yielded null results in less severely ill adults and in children [117, 118]. Ultimately, PROWESS-SHOCK randomized 1697 septic shock patients without evidence of APC benefit [119]. The manufacturer subsequently withdrew APC from the market.

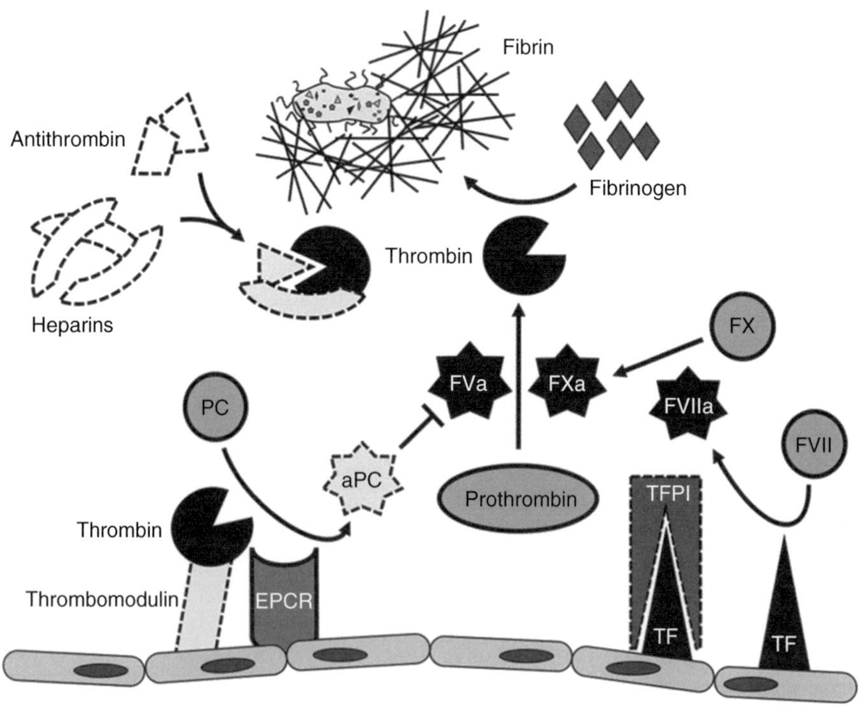

Fig. 10.1 Thrombotic pathways involved in sepsis and associated candidate anticoagulant treatment targets. Dotted lines indicate endogenous anticoagulants evaluated as treatment targets for sepsis. Abbreviations: *a* activated, *EPCR* endothelial protein C receptor, *FV* factor V, *FX* factor X, *FVII* factor VII, *PC* protein C, *TF* tissue factor, *TFPI* tissue factor pathway inhibitor

Other Anticoagulants

- Antithrombin is a circulating anticoagulant that binds and inactivates thrombin and other procoagulants. Treatment of sepsis patients with exogenous antithrombin increased bleeding but did not improve mortality [120, 121].
- Thrombomodulin is an endothelial membrane-bound protein that activates protein C from its zymogen after binding thrombin. A phase II trial ($N = 741$) of thrombomodulin treatment in sepsis suggested nonsignificant improvement in mortality, especially in sicker patients with overt DIC [122]. A phase III study in this population is underway [123].
- Tissue factor pathway inhibitor (TFPI) binds to and inhibits tissue factor, a key initiator of sepsis-related coagulation. Trials in pneumonia and general sepsis showed no benefit with exogenous TFPI treatment, and the sepsis trial demonstrated increased bleeding [124, 125].
- Heparinoids act by binding antithrombin and increasing its efficiency and activity. A meta-analysis of trials testing heparin versus a comparator suggested borderline significant mortality reduction with heparin (RR 0.88, 95% CI 0.77–1.00, $p = 0.05$) [126], but analysis was dominated by a study in which prophylactic heparin was withdrawn in control patients. Based on current evidence, chemoprophylaxis for venous thromboembolism is reasonable, but higher doses are not supported by the data.

Anemia and Transfusions

Hemoglobin levels in sepsis patients commonly start low and fall further due to inflammatory bone marrow suppression, serial phlebotomy, and invasive procedures [127]. Furthermore, derangements common in sepsis—including acidemia and fever—impair hemoglobin's oxygen affinity and may reduce erythrocytes' oxygen transport efficiency. Transfusion to target hemoglobin >10 g/dL in sepsis was once common based on the physiology of oxygen delivery and a single-center trial of protocolized resuscitation [96], but benefit was not borne out in large trials [45]. Transfusion to maintain hemoglobin >7 g/dL appears prudent in sepsis-associated MOF.

10.5.3.5 Endocrine System and Metabolism

The endocrine system in sepsis is discussed in detail in Chap. 5. Here, we highlight data on vitamins, micronutrients, and modulators of mitochondrial metabolism as sepsis treatments.

- Vitamin D: Besides regulating calcium levels, vitamin D exerts pleiotropic effects on the innate immune system and lung function. A massive dose of vitamin D may reduce hospital mortality in critically ill patients with baseline vitamin D $\leq$ 12 ng/dL [128]. A large trial of high-dose vitamin D in patients at risk for ARDS (commonly due to sepsis) is underway [129].
- Nitric oxide (NO) inhibition: Increased NO production in sepsis may contribute to distributive shock and tissue damage from reactive oxygen species. Unfortunately, therapies attempting to reduce NO production or scavenge NO have proven harmful [130, 131].

- Thiamine: Thiamine, an important cofactor for mitochondrial respiration and antioxidant production, is often low in septic patients [132]. A single-center trial of thiamine in septic shock showed no benefit overall but may have reduced mortality among the third of patients with thiamine deficiency [133].
- Selenium: Selenium is an essential trace nutrient integrated into enzymes with important antioxidant roles that is depleted in sepsis [134]. A large RCT including 1089 patients with severe sepsis or septic shock found no difference in mortality with sodium selenite supplementation [135].
- Vitamin C: A small, single-center, observational study suggested improved survival and MOF in sepsis patients treated with a cocktail of high-dose vitamin C, thiamine, and hydrocortisone [136]. These and related hypothesis-generating observations have created equipoise for randomized trials of vitamin C-based cocktails in sepsis.

10.5.3.6 Gastrointestinal System

Although it has not figured in standard scoring systems, gut failure—manifested by "ileus" (feeding intolerance, bowel distension, absent bowel sounds, vomiting, or high gastric residuals), gastrointestinal bleeding, and diarrhea—may portend worse prognosis among ICU patients [137]. Disturbances in the gut's barrier functions, increased virulence of the gut microbiome, and post-antibiotic abrogation of the gut microbiome's ability to promote immune autoregulation may play a role in the development and progression of MOF [138]. Both selective gastrointestinal decontamination and replenishment of the nonpathogenic microbiome with probiotics have shown positive effects [139, 140]. Treatment of persistent sepsis-associated MOF with fecal microbiota transplant (after eradication of the inciting infection) is an intriguing concept that needs further evaluation [141, 142].

Though an element of the SOFA score and other MOF scores, the implications of sepsis-associated cholestasis are poorly understood [143]. Management is conservative. Frank hepatic failure is rare as a result of sepsis-associated MOF and should raise concern for an alternative diagnosis.

10.5.3.7 Nervous System

Sepsis-associated encephalopathy (SAE) is a distressingly common manifestation of sepsis-associated MOF and likely represents a mix of MOF and iatrogenic effects from medications. Patients with SAE may manifest impairment ranging from mild cognitive slowing to coma. Patients with SAE are at risk for long-term cognitive impairment and other adverse outcomes [144]. Treatments for SAE are not yet evidence-based. Strategies to minimize sedation and increase early mobility may be helpful [145, 146]. Early evidence of utility of N-acetyl cysteine (NAC) in chronic cognitive impairment may suggest the need for further study of NAC in SAE.

Beyond cognitive impairment, sepsis survivors commonly suffer serious psychological disability, including post-traumatic stress disorder, anxiety, and depression. Whether these outcomes are directly related to SAE or the psychological experience of immobilization and life support therapies is not yet known.

10.6 Organ Failure as an Outcome

The need for efficiency in critical care trials, especially at and before phase 2, has motivated interest in surrogate and/or composite outcomes. For sepsis, MOF may be an attractive target for such surrogate outcomes. The best-known composite outcome in critical care research is ventilator-free days (the VFD score). The VFD score combines a primary outcome (mortality) and a proposed surrogate outcome (duration of mechanical ventilation) into a single composite [147]. This unitless score—reflecting probability of death and duration of ventilation among survivors—has been widely used in ARDS trials. More generally, organ failure trajectory represents an attractive surrogate outcome (including as a constituent of a composite outcome) in sepsis trials because it is the most common final cause of death for this syndrome. In fact, in a recent meta-analysis of randomized trials, the effect of a treatment on SOFA trajectory—but not the MODS severity measured by the SOFA score measured at a fixed point in time—was strongly correlated with the observed effect of the tested treatment on mortality [148]. Challenges to routine application of organ-failure-free days as a surrogate outcome, however, include persistent criteria variation and limited validation to date of the outcome's statistical properties.

Conclusion

MOF is a syndrome enabled by the modern ICU, which made survival possible after previously fatal physiologic insults such as overwhelming infection or serious trauma. Currently, prevention and management of sepsis-associated MOF focus on integrated, supportive care and avoidance of toxic therapies. The most familiar organ systems affected by MOF, the lung and kidney, have reasonable treatments, including non-injurious mechanical ventilation and renal replacement therapy, even as controversies persist. Expanding implementation of proven therapies and deadoption of disproven treatments would likely improve sepsis outcomes. The complex, nonlinear nature of MOF and the number of endotypes underlying this syndrome have hampered the development of specific therapies even as mortality has improved overall. While speedy assessment of sepsis endotypes is likely to aid therapeutic targeting in the future, reliable evidence may require new study designs and alternative outcome targets.

References

1. Singer M, Deutschman CS, Seymour CW, et al. The third international consensus definitions for sepsis and septic shock (Sepsis-3). JAMA. 2016;315:801–10.
2. Baue AE. Multiple, progressive, or sequential systems failure: a syndrome of the 1970s. Arch Surg. 1975;110:779–81.
3. Shoemaker WC. Editorial: multiple injuries and multiple organ failure. Crit Care Med. 1973;1:157.
4. Eiseman B, Beart R, Norton L. Multiple organ failure. Surg Gynecol Obstet. 1977;144:323–6.

5. Bone RC, Balk RA, Cerra FB, et al. Definitions for sepsis and organ failure and guidelines for the use of innovative therapies in sepsis. Chest. 1992;101:1644–55.
6. Marshall JC, Cook DJ, Christou NV, Bernard GR, Sprung CL, Sibbald WJ. Multiple organ dysfunction score: a reliable descriptor of a complex clinical outcome. Crit Care Med. 1995;23:1638–52.
7. Seymour CW, Coopersmith CM, Deutschman CS, et al. Application of a framework to assess the usefulness of alternative sepsis criteria. Crit Care Med. 2016;44:e122–30.
8. Baue AE. MOF, MODS, and SIRS: what is in a name or an acronym? Shock. 2006;26: 438–49.
9. Vincent J-L, Moreno R. Clinical review: scoring systems in the critically ill. Crit Care. 2010;14:207.
10. Hébert PC, Drummond AJ, Singer J, Bernard GR, Russell JA. A simple multiple system organ failure scoring system predicts mortality of patients who have sepsis syndrome. Chest. 1993;104:230–5.
11. Seymour CW, Liu VX, Iwashyna TJ, et al. Assessment of clinical criteria for sepsis: for the third international consensus definitions for sepsis and septic shock (Sepsis-3). JAMA. 2016;315:762–74.
12. Le Gall JR, Klar J, Lemeshow S, et al. The logistic organ dysfunction system: a new way to assess organ dysfunction in the intensive care unit. JAMA. 1996;276(10):802–10.
13. Vincent J-L, Moreno R, Takala J, et al. The SOFA (Sepsis-related Organ Failure Assessment) score to describe organ dysfunction/failure. Intensive Care Med. 1996;22:707–10.
14. Peres Bota D, Melot C, Lopes Ferreira F, Nguyen B-V, Vincent J-L. The Multiple Organ Dysfunction Score (MODS) versus the Sequential Organ Failure Assessment (SOFA) score in outcome prediction. Intensive Care Med. 2002;28:1619–24.
15. Goris RJ, te Boekhorst TP, Nuytinck JK, Gimbrère JS. Multiple-organ failure: generalized autodestructive inflammation? Arch Surg. 1985;120:1109–15.
16. Fry DE, Pearlstein L, Fulton RL, Polk HC. Multiple system organ failure: the role of uncontrolled infection. Arch Surg. 1980;115:136–40.
17. Stevens LE. Gauging the severity of surgical sepsis. Arch Surg. 1983;118:1190–2.
18. Knaus WA, Draper EA, Wagner DP, Zimmerman JE. Prognosis in acute organ-system failure. Ann Surg. 1985;202:685–93.
19. Carrico CJ, Meakins JL, Marshall JC, Fry D, Maier RV. Multiple-organ-failure syndrome. Arch Surg. 1986;121:196–208.
20. Marshall JC, Christou NV, Horn R, Meakins JL. The microbiology of multiple organ failure. The proximal gastrointestinal tract as an occult reservoir of pathogens. Arch Surg. 1988;123:309–15.
21. Kollef MH. Ventilator-associated pneumonia: a multivariate analysis. JAMA. 1993;270:1965–70.
22. Fagon JY, Chastre J, Novara A, Medioni P, Gibert C. Characterization of intensive care unit patients using a model based on the presence or absence of organ dysfunctions and/or infection: the ODIN model. Intensive Care Med. 1993;19:137–44.
23. Moore FA, Sauaia A, Moore EE, Haenel JB, Burch JM, Lezotte DC. Postinjury multiple organ failure: a bimodal phenomenon. J Trauma. 1996;40:501–10. discussion 510–2.
24. Levy MM, Fink MP, Marshall JC, et al. 2001 SCCM/ESICM/ACCP/ATS/SIS international sepsis definitions conference. Crit Care Med. 2003;31:1250–6.
25. Howell MD, Talmor D, Schuetz P, Hunziker S, Jones AE, Shapiro NI. Proof of principle: the predisposition, infection, response, organ failure sepsis staging system. Crit Care Med. 2011;39:322–7.
26. Freund Y, Lemachatti N, Krastinova E, et al. Prognostic accuracy of Sepsis-3 criteria for in-hospital mortality among patients with suspected infection presenting to the emergency department. JAMA. 2017;317:301–8.
27. Raith EP, Udy AA, Bailey M, et al. Prognostic accuracy of the SOFA score, SIRS criteria, and qSOFA score for in-hospital mortality among adults with suspected infection admitted to the intensive care unit. JAMA. 2017;317:290–300.

28. Sauaia A, Moore EE, Johnson JL, Ciesla DJ, Biffl WL, Banerjee A. Validation of post-injury multiple organ failure scores. Shock. 2009;31:438–47.
29. Alberti C, Brun-Buisson C, Chevret S, et al. Systemic inflammatory response and progression to severe sepsis in critically ill infected patients. Am J Respir Crit Care Med. 2005; 171:461–8.
30. Sørensen TI, Nielsen GG, Andersen PK, Teasdale TW. Genetic and environmental influences on premature death in adult adoptees. N Engl J Med. 1988;318:727–32.
31. Petersen L, Andersen PK, Sørensen TIA. Genetic influences on incidence and case-fatality of infectious disease. PLoS One. 2010;5:e10603.
32. Albright FS, Orlando P, Pavia AT, Jackson GG, Cannon Albright LA. Evidence for a heritable predisposition to death due to influenza. J Infect Dis. 2008;197:18–24.
33. Clark MF, Baudouin SVA. Systematic review of the quality of genetic association studies in human sepsis. Intensive Care Med. 2006;32:1706–12.
34. Sutherland AM, Walley KR. Bench-to-bedside review: association of genetic variation with sepsis. Crit Care. 2009;13:210.
35. Blanco J, Muriel-Bombín A, Sagredo V, et al. Incidence, organ dysfunction and mortality in severe sepsis: a Spanish multicentre study. Crit Care. 2008;12:R158.
36. Tilney NL, Bailey GL, Morgan AP. Sequential system failure after rupture of abdominal aortic aneurysms: an unsolved problem in postoperative care. Ann Surg. 1973;178:117–22.
37. Vincent J-L, Nelson DR, Williams MDI. Worsening multiple organ failure the cause of death in patients with severe sepsis? Crit Care Med. 2011;39:1050–5.
38. Graetz TJ, Hotchkiss RS. Sepsis: preventing organ failure in sepsis–the search continues. Nat Rev Nephrol. 2017;13:5–6.
39. Prescott HC, Calfee CS, Thompson BT, Angus DC, Liu VX. Toward smarter lumping and smarter splitting: rethinking strategies for sepsis and acute respiratory distress syndrome clinical trial design. Am J Respir Crit Care Med. 2016;194:147–55.
40. Knox DB, Lanspa MJ, Kuttler KG, Brewer SC, Brown SM. Phenotypic clusters within sepsis-associated multiple organ dysfunction syndrome. Intensive Care Med. 2015;41:814–22.
41. Davenport EE, Burnham KL, Radhakrishnan J, et al. Genomic landscape of the individual host response and outcomes in sepsis: a prospective cohort study. Lancet Respir Med. 2016;4:259–71.
42. Seely AJ, Christou NV. Multiple organ dysfunction syndrome: exploring the paradigm of complex nonlinear systems. Crit Care Med. 2000;28:2193–200.
43. Vincent J-L. We should abandon randomized controlled trials in the intensive care unit. Crit Care Med. 2010;38:S534–8.
44. Carlet J, Cohen J, Calandra T, Opal SM, Masur H. Sepsis: time to reconsider the concept. Crit Care Med. 2008;36:964–6.
45. Investigators PRISM, Rowan KM, Angus DC, et al. Early, goal-directed therapy for septic shock—a patient-level meta-analysis. N Engl J Med. 2017;376:2223–34.
46. Kalil AC, Johnson DW, Lisco SJ, Sun J. Early goal-directed therapy for sepsis: a novel solution for discordant survival outcomes in clinical trials. Crit Care Med. 2017;45:607–14.
47. Seymour CW, Gesten F, Prescott HC, et al. Time to treatment and mortality during mandated emergency care for sepsis. N Engl J Med. 2017;376:2235–44.
48. Whiles BB, Deis AS, Simpson SQ. Increased time to initial antimicrobial administration is associated with progression to septic shock in severe sepsis patients. Crit Care Med. 2017;45:623–9.
49. Leisman D, Huang V, Zhou Q, et al. Delayed second dose antibiotics for patients admitted from the emergency department with sepsis: prevalence, risk factors, and outcomes. Crit Care Med. 2017;45:956–65.
50. Mandell LA, Wunderink RG, Anzueto A, et al. Infectious diseases society of America/American thoracic society consensus guidelines on the management of community-acquired pneumonia in adults. Clin Infect Dis. 2007;44(suppl 2):S27–72.
51. Strehlow MC, Emond SD, Shapiro NI, Pelletier AJ, Camargo CA. National study of emergency department visits for sepsis, 1992 to 2001. Ann Emerg Med. 2006;48:326–31.

52. Kahn SR, Lim W, Dunn AS, et al. Prevention of VTE in nonsurgical patients: antithrombotic therapy and prevention of thrombosis, 9th ed: American college of chest physicians evidence-based clinical practice guidelines. Chest. 2012;141:e195S–226S.
53. Pronovost P, Needham D, Berenholtz S, et al. An intervention to decrease catheter-related bloodstream infections in the ICU. N Engl J Med. 2006;355:2725–32.
54. Klompas M. What is new in the prevention of nosocomial pneumonia in the ICU? Curr Opin Crit Care. 2017;23(5):378–84.
55. Brown SM. Through the valley of shadows: living wills, intensive care, and making medicine human. Oxford: Oxford University Press; 2016.
56. Brown SM, Rozenblum R, Aboumatar H, et al. Defining patient and family engagement in the intensive care unit. Am J Respir Crit Care Med. 2015;191:358–60.
57. Quílez ME, López-Aguilar J, Blanch L. Organ crosstalk during acute lung injury, acute respiratory distress syndrome, and mechanical ventilation. Curr Opin Crit Care. 2012;18:23–8.
58. Ranieri VM, Rubenfeld GD, ARDS Definition Task Force, et al. Acute respiratory distress syndrome: the Berlin definition. JAMA. 2012;307:2526–33.
59. Bellani G, Laffey JG, Pham T, et al. Epidemiology, patterns of care, and mortality for patients with acute respiratory distress syndrome in intensive care units in 50 countries. JAMA. 2016;315:788–800.
60. The Acute Respiratory Distress Syndrome Network. Ventilation with lower tidal volumes as compared with traditional tidal volumes for acute lung injury and the acute respiratory distress syndrome. N Engl J Med. 2000;342:1301–8.
61. Needham DM, Yang T, Dinglas VD, et al. Timing of low tidal volume ventilation and intensive care unit mortality in acute respiratory distress syndrome: prospective cohort study. Am J Respir Crit Care Med. 2015;191:177–85.
62. Briel M, Meade M, Mercat A, et al. Higher vs lower positive end-expiratory pressure in patients with acute lung injury and acute respiratory distress syndrome: systematic review and meta-analysis. JAMA. 2010;303:865–73.
63. Cavalcanti AB, Suzumura ÉA, Writing Group for the Alveolar Recruitment for Acute Respiratory Distress Syndrome Trial (ART) Investigators, et al. Effect of lung recruitment and titrated positive end-expiratory pressure (PEEP) vs low PEEP on mortality in patients with acute respiratory distress syndrome: a randomized clinical trial. JAMA. 2017;318:1335–45.
64. Calfee CS, Delucchi K, Parsons PE, et al. Subphenotypes in acute respiratory distress syndrome: latent class analysis of data from two randomised controlled trials. Lancet Respir Med. 2014;2:611–20.
65. Famous KR, Delucchi K, Ware LB, et al. Acute respiratory distress syndrome subphenotypes respond differently to randomized fluid management strategy. Am J Respir Crit Care Med. 2017;195:331–8.
66. Munshi L, Del Sorbo L, Adhikari NKJ, et al. Prone position for acute respiratory distress syndrome: a systematic review and meta-analysis. Ann Am Thorac Soc. 2017;14:S280–8.
67. Guérin C, Reignier J, Richard J-C, et al. Prone positioning in severe acute respiratory distress syndrome. N Engl J Med. 2013;368:2159–68.
68. Fan E, Cheek F, Chlan L, et al. An official American Thoracic Society clinical practice guideline: the diagnosis of intensive care unit-acquired weakness in adults. Am J Respir Crit Care Med. 2014;190:1437–46.
69. Papazian L, Forel J-M, Gacouin A, et al. Neuromuscular blockers in early acute respiratory distress syndrome. N Engl J Med. 2010;363:1107–16.
70. Reevaluation of systemic early neuromuscular blockade (ROSE). ClinicalTrials.gov. 2015.:NCT02509078. https://clinicaltrials.gov/ct2/show/NCT02509078. Accessed 6 Aug 2017.
71. Frat J-P, Thille AW, Mercat A, et al. High-flow oxygen through nasal cannula in acute hypoxemic respiratory failure. N Engl J Med. 2015;372:2185–96.
72. Brochard L, Slutsky A, Pesenti A. Mechanical ventilation to minimize progression of lung injury in acute respiratory failure. Am J Respir Crit Care Med. 2017;195:438–42.

73. Young D, Lamb SE, Shah S, et al. High-frequency oscillation for acute respiratory distress syndrome. N Engl J Med. 2013;368:806–13.
74. Taylor RW, Zimmerman JL, Dellinger RP, et al. Low-dose inhaled nitric oxide in patients with acute lung injury: a randomized controlled trial. JAMA. 2004;291:1603–9.
75. Gebistorf F, Karam O, Wetterslev J, Afshari A. Inhaled nitric oxide for acute respiratory distress syndrome (ARDS) in children and adults. Cochrane Database Syst Rev. 2016;6:CD002787.
76. Fan E, Del Sorbo L, Goligher EC, et al. An official American Thoracic Society/European Society of Intensive Care Medicine/Society of Critical Care Medicine clinical practice guideline: mechanical ventilation in adult patients with acute respiratory distress syndrome. Am J Respir Crit Care Med. 2017;195:1253–63.
77. Davies A, Jones D, Australia and New Zealand Extracorporeal Membrane Oxygenation (ANZ ECMO) Influenza Investigators, et al. Extracorporeal membrane oxygenation for 2009 influenza A (H1N1) acute respiratory distress syndrome. JAMA. 2009;302:1888–95.
78. Zapol WM, Snider MT, Hill JD, et al. Extracorporeal membrane oxygenation in severe acute respiratory failure: a randomized prospective study. JAMA. 1979;242:2193–6.
79. Morris AH, Wallace CJ, Menlove RL, et al. Randomized clinical trial of pressure-controlled inverse ratio ventilation and extracorporeal CO2 removal for adult respiratory distress syndrome. Am J Respir Crit Care Med. 1994;149:295–305.
80. Peek GJ, Mugford M, Tiruvoipati R, et al. Efficacy and economic assessment of conventional ventilatory support versus extracorporeal membrane oxygenation for severe adult respiratory failure (CESAR): a multicentre randomised controlled trial. Lancet. 2009;374: 1351–63.
81. Weiss CH, Krishnan JA, Au DH, et al. An official American Thoracic Society research statement: implementation science in pulmonary, critical care, and sleep medicine. Am J Respir Crit Care Med. 2016;194:1015–25.
82. Rubenfeld GD. Who cares about preventing acute respiratory distress syndrome? Am J Respir Crit Care Med. 2015;191:255–60.
83. Beitler JR, Schoenfeld DA, Thompson BT, Preventing ARDS. progress, promise, and pitfalls. Chest. 2014;146:1102–13.
84. Serpa Neto A, Cardoso SO, Manetta JA, et al. Association between use of lung-protective ventilation with lower tidal volumes and clinical outcomes among patients without acute respiratory distress syndrome: a meta-analysis. JAMA. 2012;308:1651–9.
85. Luce JM, Montgomery AB, Marks JD, Turner J, Metz CA, Murray JF. Ineffectiveness of high-dose methylprednisolone in preventing parenchymal lung injury and improving mortality in patients with septic shock. Am Rev Respir Dis. 1988;138:62–8.
86. Weigelt JA, Norcross JF, Borman KR, Snyder WH. Early steroid therapy for respiratory failure. Arch Surg. 1985;120:536–40.
87. Wan Y-D, Sun T-W, Liu Z-Q, Zhang S-G, Wang L-X, Kan Q-C. Efficacy and safety of corticosteroids for community-acquired pneumonia: a systematic review and meta-analysis. Chest. 2016;149:209–19.
88. Kor DJ, Carter RE, Park PK, et al. Effect of aspirin on development of ards in at-risk patients presenting to the emergency department: the LIPS-A randomized clinical trial. JAMA. 2016;315:2406–14.
89. Levitt JE, Matthay MA. Clinical review: early treatment of acute lung injury–paradigm shift toward prevention and treatment prior to respiratory failure. Crit Care. 2012;16:223.
90. Damiani E, Adrario E, Girardis M, et al. Arterial hyperoxia and mortality in critically ill patients: a systematic review and meta-analysis. Crit Care. 2014;18:711.
91. Asfar P, Schortgen F, Boisramé-Helms J, et al. Hyperoxia and hypertonic saline in patients with septic shock (HYPERS2S): a two-by-two factorial, multicentre, randomised, clinical trial. Lancet Respir Med. 2017;5:180–90.
92. Girardis M, Busani S, Damiani E, et al. Effect of conservative vs conventional oxygen therapy on mortality among patients in an intensive care unit: the OXYGEN-ICU randomized clinical trial. JAMA. 2016;316:1583–9.

93. Shankar-Hari M, Phillips GS, Levy ML, et al. Developing a new definition and assessing new clinical criteria for septic shock: for the third international consensus definitions for sepsis and septic shock (Sepsis-3). JAMA. 2016;315:775–87.
94. Beesley SJ, Weber G, Sarge T, et al. Septic cardiomyopathy. Crit Care Med. https://doi.org/10.1097/CCM.0000000000002851.
95. Landesberg G, Levin PD, Gilon D, et al. Myocardial dysfunction in severe sepsis and septic shock: no correlation with inflammatory cytokines in real-life clinical setting. Chest. 2015;148:93–102.
96. Rivers E, Nguyen B, Havstad S, et al. Early goal-directed therapy in the treatment of severe sepsis and septic shock. N Engl J Med. 2001;345:1368–77.
97. Gordon AC, Perkins GD, Singer M, et al. Levosimendan for the prevention of acute organ dysfunction in sepsis. N Engl J Med. 2016;375:1638–48.
98. Lechat P, Packer M, Chalon S, Cucherat M, Arab T, Boissel JP. Clinical effects of beta-adrenergic blockade in chronic heart failure: a meta-analysis of double-blind, placebo-controlled, randomized trials. Circulation. 1998;98:1184–91.
99. Reuter DA, Russell JA, Mekontso Dessap A. Beta-blockers in septic shock to optimize hemodynamics? Yes. Intensive Care Med. 2016;42:1607–9.
100. Morelli A, Ertmer C, Westphal M, et al. Effect of heart rate control with esmolol on hemodynamic and clinical outcomes in patients with septic shock: a randomized clinical trial. JAMA. 2013;310:1683–91.
101. Walkey AJ, Hammill BG, Curtis LH, Benjamin EJ. Long-term outcomes following development of new-onset atrial fibrillation during sepsis. Chest. 2014;146:1187–95.
102. Walkey AJ, Evans SR, Winter MR, Benjamin EJ. Practice patterns and outcomes of treatments for atrial fibrillation during sepsis: a propensity-matched cohort study. Chest. 2016;149:74–83.
103. Hoste EAJ, Bagshaw SM, Bellomo R, et al. Epidemiology of acute kidney injury in critically ill patients: the multinational AKI-EPI study. Intensive Care Med. 2015;41:1411–23.
104. Poukkanen M, Vaara ST, Pettila V, et al. Acute kidney injury in patients with severe sepsis in Finnish intensive care units. Acta Anaesthesiol Scand. 2013;57:863–72.
105. Friedrich JO, Adhikari N, Herridge MS, Beyene J. Meta-analysis: low-dose dopamine increases urine output but does not prevent renal dysfunction or death. Ann Intern Med. 2005;142:510–24.
106. Landoni G, Biondi-Zoccai GGL, Tumlin JA, et al. Beneficial impact of fenoldopam in critically ill patients with or at risk for acute renal failure: a meta-analysis of randomized clinical trials. Am J Kidney Dis. 2007;49:56–68.
107. Vinsonneau C, Camus C, Combes A, et al. Continuous venovenous haemodiafiltration versus intermittent haemodialysis for acute renal failure in patients with multiple-organ dysfunction syndrome: a multicentre randomised trial. Lancet. 2006;368:379–85.
108. Payen DM, Guilhot J, Launey Y, et al. Early use of polymyxin B hemoperfusion in patients with septic shock due to peritonitis: a multicenter randomized control trial. Intensive Care Med. 2015;41:975–84.
109. Gaudry S, Hajage D, Schortgen F, et al. Initiation strategies for renal-replacement therapy in the intensive care unit. N Engl J Med. 2016;375:122–33.
110. Zarbock A, Kellum JA, Schmidt C, et al. Effect of early vs delayed initiation of renal replacement therapy on mortality in critically ill patients with acute kidney injury: the ELAIN randomized clinical trial. JAMA. 2016;315:2190–9.
111. Palevsky PM, Zhang JH, VA/NIH Acute Renal Failure Trial Network, et al. Intensity of renal support in critically ill patients with acute kidney injury. N Engl J Med. 2008;359:7–20.
112. Bellomo R, Cass A, RENAL Replacement Therapy Study Investigators, et al. Intensity of continuous renal-replacement therapy in critically ill patients. N Engl J Med. 2009;361:1627–38.
113. Fourrier F. Severe sepsis, coagulation, and fibrinolysis: dead end or one way? Crit Care Med. 2012;40:2704–8.
114. Levi M, van der Poll T. Recombinant human activated protein C: current insights into its mechanism of action. Crit Care. 2007;11(Suppl 5):S3.

115. Bernard GR, Vincent J-L, Laterre PF, et al. Efficacy and safety of recombinant human activated protein C for severe sepsis. N Engl J Med. 2001;344:699–709.
116. Warren HS, Suffredini AF, Eichacker PQ, Munford RS. Risks and benefits of activated protein C treatment for severe sepsis. N Engl J Med. 2002;347:1027–30.
117. Abraham E, Laterre P-F, Garg R, et al. Drotrecogin alfa (activated) for adults with severe sepsis and a low risk of death. N Engl J Med. 2005;353:1332–41.
118. Nadel S, Goldstein B, Williams MD, et al. Drotrecogin alfa (activated) in children with severe sepsis: a multicentre phase III randomised controlled trial. Lancet. 2007;369:836–43.
119. Ranieri VM, Thompson BT, Barie PS, et al. Drotrecogin alfa (activated) in adults with septic shock. N Engl J Med. 2012;366:2055–64.
120. Warren BL, Eid A, Singer P, et al. High-dose antithrombin III in severe sepsis: a randomized controlled trial. JAMA. 2001;286:1869–78.
121. Hoffmann JN, Wiedermann CJ, Juers M, et al. Benefit/risk profile of high-dose antithrombin in patients with severe sepsis treated with and without concomitant heparin. Thromb Haemost. 2006;95(5):850–6.
122. Vincent J-L, Ramesh MK, Ernest D, et al. A randomized, double-blind, placebo-controlled, Phase 2b study to evaluate the safety and efficacy of recombinant human soluble thrombomodulin, ART-123, in patients with sepsis and suspected disseminated intravascular coagulation. Crit Care Med. 2013;41:2069–79.
123. Phase 3 Safety and Efficacy Study of ART-123 in Subjects With Severe Sepsis and Coagulopathy. ClinicalTrials.gov. 2012. https://clinicaltrials.gov/ct2/show/NCT01598831. Accessed 28 Oct 2017.
124. Abraham E, Reinhart K, Opal S, et al. Efficacy and safety of tifacogin (recombinant tissue factor pathway inhibitor) in severe sepsis: a randomized controlled trial. JAMA. 2003;290:238–47.
125. Wunderink RG, Laterre P-F, François B, et al. Recombinant tissue factor pathway inhibitor in severe community-acquired pneumonia: a randomized trial. Am J Respir Crit Care Med. 2011;183:1561–8.
126. Zarychanski R, Abou-Setta AM, Kanji S, et al. The efficacy and safety of heparin in patients with sepsis: a systematic review and metaanalysis. Crit Care Med. 2015;43:511–8.
127. Goyette RE, Key NS, Ely EW. Hematologic changes in sepsis and their therapeutic implications. Semin Respir Crit Care Med. 2004;25:645–59.
128. Amrein K, Schnedl C, Holl A, et al. Effect of high-dose vitamin D3 on hospital length of stay in critically ill patients with vitamin D deficiency: the VITdAL-ICU randomized clinical trial. JAMA. 2014;312:1520–30.
129. Vitamin D to improve outcomes by leveraging early treatment (VIOLET). ClinicalTrials.gov. 2017.:NCT03096314. https://clinicaltrials.gov/ct2/show/NCT03096314. Accessed 5 Aug 2017.
130. López A, Lorente JA, Steingrub J, et al. Multiple-center, randomized, placebo-controlled, double-blind study of the nitric oxide synthase inhibitor 546C88: effect on survival in patients with septic shock. Crit Care Med. 2004;32:21–30.
131. Vincent J-L, Privalle CT, Singer M, et al. Multicenter, randomized, placebo-controlled phase III study of pyridoxalated hemoglobin polyoxyethylene in distributive shock (PHOENIX). Crit Care Med. 2015;43:57–64.
132. Donnino MW, Carney E, Cocchi MN, et al. Thiamine deficiency in critically ill patients with sepsis. J Crit Care. 2010;25:576–81.
133. Donnino MW, Andersen LW, Chase M, et al. Randomized, double-blind, placebo-controlled trial of thiamine as a metabolic resuscitator in septic shock: a pilot study. Crit Care Med. 2016;44:360–7.
134. Sakr Y, Reinhart K, Bloos F, et al. Time course and relationship between plasma selenium concentrations, systemic inflammatory response, sepsis, and multiorgan failure. Br J Anaesth. 2007;98:775–84.
135. Bloos F, Trips E, Nierhaus A, et al. Effect of sodium selenite administration and procalcitonin-guided therapy on mortality in patients with severe sepsis or septic shock: a randomized clinical trial. JAMA Intern Med. 2016;176:1266–76.

136. Marik PE, Khangoora V, Rivera R, Hooper MH, Catravas J. Hydrocortisone, Vitamin C, and thiamine for the treatment of severe sepsis and septic shock: a retrospective before-after study. Chest. 2017;151:1229–38.
137. Reintam Blaser A, Poeze M, Malbrain MLNG, et al. Gastrointestinal symptoms during the first week of intensive care are associated with poor outcome: a prospective multicentre study. Intensive Care Med. 2013;39:899–909.
138. Klingensmith NJ, Coopersmith CM. The gut as the motor of multiple organ dysfunction in critical illness. Crit Care Clin. 2016;32:203–12.
139. Price R, MacLennan G, Glen J, SuDDICU Collaboration. Selective digestive or oropharyngeal decontamination and topical oropharyngeal chlorhexidine for prevention of death in general intensive care: systematic review and network meta-analysis. BMJ. 2014;348:g2197.
140. Manzanares W, Lemieux M, Langlois PL, Wischmeyer PE. Probiotic and synbiotic therapy in critical illness: a systematic review and meta-analysis. Crit Care. 2016;20:1–19.
141. Wei Y, Yang J, Wang J, et al. Successful treatment with fecal microbiota transplantation in patients with multiple organ dysfunction syndrome and diarrhea following severe sepsis. Crit Care. 2016;20:332.
142. Klingensmith NJ, Coopersmith CM. Fecal microbiota transplantation for multiple organ dysfunction syndrome. Crit Care. 2016;20:398.
143. Jenniskens M, Langouche L, Vanwijngaerden Y-M, Mesotten D, Van den Berghe G. Cholestatic liver (dys)function during sepsis and other critical illnesses. Intensive Care Med. 2016;42:16–27.
144. Pandharipande PP, Girard TD, Jackson JC, et al. Long-term cognitive impairment after critical illness. N Engl J Med. 2013;369:1306–16.
145. Barr J, Fraser GL, Puntillo K, et al. Clinical practice guidelines for the management of pain, agitation, and delirium in adult patients in the intensive care unit. Crit Care Med. 2013;41:263–306.
146. Schweickert WD, Pohlman MC, Pohlman AS, et al. Early physical and occupational therapy in mechanically ventilated, critically ill patients: a randomised controlled trial. Lancet. 2009;373:1874–82.
147. Schoenfeld DA, Bernard GR, Network ARDS. Statistical evaluation of ventilator-free days as an efficacy measure in clinical trials of treatments for acute respiratory distress syndrome. Crit Care Med. 2002;30:1772–7.
148. de Grooth H-J, Geenen IL, Girbes AR, Vincent J-L, Parienti J-J, Oudemans-van Straaten HM. SOFA and mortality endpoints in randomized controlled trials: a systematic review and meta-regression analysis. Crit Care. 2017;21:38.

Sepsis Management: Importance of the Pathogen

11

Russell J. McCulloh and Steven M. Opal

11.1 Introduction

11.1.1 Do Identity and Nature of the Causative Pathogen Really Matter in Sepsis?

Sepsis is now defined as "life-threatening organ dysfunction caused by a dysregulated host response to infection" [1]. This definition appropriately focuses upon the deleterious and dysregulated host response as the principal pathophysiologic event in sepsis. However, this definition seems to imply that while infection might be the initiating factor causing sepsis, pathogens play little or no role to the generation of the potentially fatal sequence of events underway in septic patients. With some highly pathogenic organisms, the causative microorganism can directly damage host tissues and play an active role in the pathogenesis of sepsis.

Does the treating physician really need to know the precise identity of the causative organism and its virulence properties to effectively resuscitate and prevent irreversible damage to organ systems in septic patients? Probably not, but ignoring the contribution of the pathogen to the ongoing microcirculatory tissue perfusion abnormalities and organ dysfunction would be unwise. Perhaps the most enduring, lifesaving intervention in numerous sepsis clinical studies is the urgent administration of appropriate antimicrobial agents [1–4]. Choosing the right initial antibiotic(s)

R. J. McCulloh, M.D.
Infectious Diseases, University of Missouri-Kansas City, Kansas City, MO, USA

Ocean State Clinical Coordinating Center of Rhode Island Hospital, Providence, RI, USA

S. M. Opal, M.D. (✉)
Ocean State Clinical Coordinating Center of Rhode Island Hospital, Providence, RI, USA

Infectious Disease Division, Alpert Medical School of Brown University,
Providence, RI, USA
e-mail: Steven_Opal@brown.edu

W. J. Wiersinga, C. W. Seymour (eds.), *Handbook of Sepsis*,
https://doi.org/10.1007/978-3-319-73506-1_11

requires some knowledge of the likely pathogens responsible for sepsis, even if the final identity of the actual microorganism in the microbiology laboratory might take many hours or days to precisely define. Broad-spectrum antibiotics covering the most likely pathogens are usually employed to assure a reasonable chance that the offending microorganism(s) is effectively treated. Rapid molecular diagnostics to identify the causative microorganism and determine its antimicrobial susceptibility profile in sepsis management are greatly needed in tailoring antimicrobial agents to the identified pathogen [5]. Knowing the pathogen causing sepsis in individual patients can also help direct diagnostic efforts to identify the site of origin of infection (e.g., *Streptococcus pyogenes*—skin and soft tissue sites, *Bacteroides fragilis*—anaerobic abscesses in the abdomen). Additionally, finding the pathogen and beginning specific therapy in an expeditious fashion can limit ongoing microbial growth, toxin production, and organ injury by controlling total microbial biomass (i.e., bacterial load) within the host before potentially lethal pathogen levels have accumulated [6].

11.2 Microbial Features That Contribute to Pathogenicity

Microbial invasion of the human host across the epithelial barriers to infection is an uncommon event and only occurs with a highly virulent pathogen, a significant break in the integumental barrier, or a major defect in innate or acquired immune defenses. This chapter will focus upon the special characteristics needed to permit a microbial invader to successfully cross physical barriers, evade host defenses, and disseminate within the host.

Capable pathogens must possess an array of virulence properties to invade and to replicate at a greater rate than the impressive capacity of the human host to clear microorganisms from the systemic circulation [7, 8]. If a pathogen has succeeded in finding a breach in the physical barriers to infection, the microorganism immediately finds itself in an unhospitable environment and is under attack from innate host defenses. Antimicrobial peptides, oxidant stress, heat stress, severe iron limitation, complement opsonic and lytic activity, pathogen-associated pattern recognition receptor binding, opsonophagocytic antibodies, and phagocytosis and killing by innate immune cells of the myeloid lineage, neutrophils, dendritic cells, and monocyte/macrophage cells await the opportunity to eliminate pathogens.

The most immediate threat to invading pathogens as they enter the plasma compartment is likely complement itself [9, 10]. Complement (C′) fixation by either the alternate C′ system or the mannose-binding lectin pathway can rapidly kill gram-negative bacteria within a few minutes by the assembly of the C′-mediated membrane attack complex. Gram-positive bacteria are also susceptible to C′-mediated, pattern recognition, opsonization, and lysis within phagocytic cells. If the host has previously been exposed to this specific pathogen, immunologic memory in terms of pre-existing, specific antibodies will bind, fix complement, and rapidly kill bacteria, fungi, and viruses by the classical C′ pathway. The terminal membrane attack complex (C5b-C9) creates pores through the outer and inner membranes of gram-negative organisms and rapidly lyses the bacterium. With the exception of bacteremia associated with infected intravascular catheters, essentially all bacterial strains that cause bloodstream infection express "serum resistance," the capacity to prevent rapid lysis from circulation C′ components. Most urinary and intestinal strains of *E. coli* and other enteric bacteria do not have the capacity to avoid C′-mediated lysis. Only certain virulent subsets of gram-negative bacilli and cocci can prevent lysis from C′ and disseminate in the bloodstream [9–11].

Prevention of complement clearance by bacteria is generally accomplished by one of three mechanisms: (1) covering the bacterial outer membrane with anticomplement factors, (2) steric inhibition of C′ components from reaching the inner membrane via synthesis of excessively long and complex O′-specific side chains of the lipopolysaccharide (LPS) outer membrane (see Fig. 11.1), or (3) synthesis of secretion of specific, thick exocapsular polysaccharide coats that shield bacteria of complement attack [10]. Bacterial expression of binding sites for specific complement inhibitors (such as factor H) is found in some gram-negative and gram-positive bacterial pathogens. The synthesis of excessively long and complex O′-specific side chains of the lipopolysaccharide (LPS) outer membrane is a characteristic of gram-negative bacilli and gram-negative cocci (see Fig. 11.1). Exocapsules are anti-C′ defenses commonly employed by both gram-positive and gram-negative pathogens [10, 11].

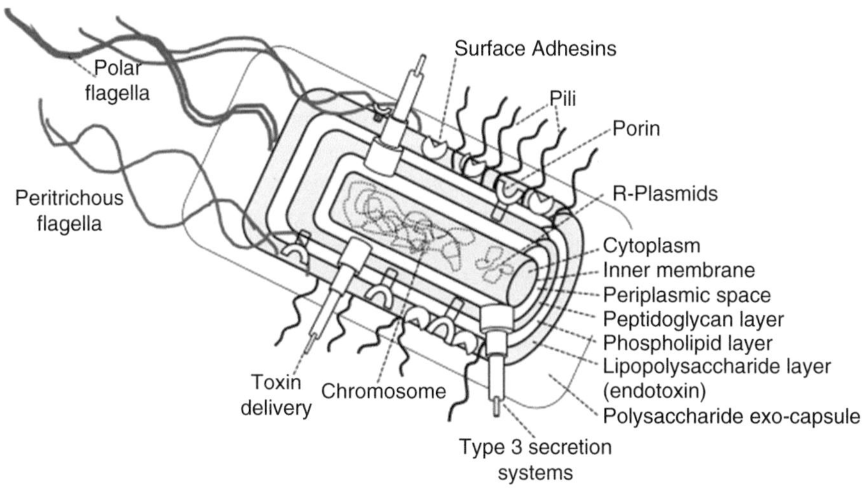

Fig. 11.1 Basic morphology of a gram-negative bacillus. Bacteria are 0.5–5 μm, unicellular organisms that have a simple di-phospholipid inner membrane and a complex, multilayer outer membrane. The chromosome is usually a single, covalently closed DNA molecule without histones or a nuclear membrane. Separate, autonomously replicating, extrachromosomal DNA elements known as plasmids are frequent sites for antibiotic resistance genes. Plasmids can transmit resistance genes horizontally to other bacteria. Bacteria communicate with each other by quorum sensing systems to act like a team of pathogens in biofilm formation and during microbial invasion. Motile bacteria use either polar flagella (e.g., *Pseudomonas aeruginosa*) or multiple peritrichous flagella (enteric bacilli) for locomotion. Secretion of exotoxins and extracellular enzymes is accomplished by multicomponent secretion systems

When adequately opsonized bacteria are detected in the bloodstream, they are rapidly and efficiently removed from the circulation by the liver. The liver is a huge organ (about 1500 g in an adult human), and its endothelial surface receives about 25% of the total cardiac output. Hepatic sinusoids are heavily invested with Kupffer cells which avidly bind bacteria and kill invading organisms, assisted by neutrophils from within the liver microcirculation [7, 8]. Splenic sinusoids are the most capable sites for removing poorly opsonized bacteria in the early stages of bloodstream infection. This accounts for the well-known risk of sudden and at times devastating systemic infections following splenectomy or with congenital or acquired splenic hypofunction (e.g., sickle cell disease and other hemoglobinopathies, congenital asplenia, graft-versus-host disease, etc.) [12].

11.3 Microbial Virulence, Genomic Regions of Diversity, Pathogenicity Islands, and Integrons

Pathogenic microorganisms express an array of virulence factors allowing them to invade, avoid host defenses, cause disease, and replicate fast to outcompete antimicrobial clearance mechanisms of the host innate and adaptive immune systems. Comparative genomic analyses find that many gram-positive and gram-negative pathogens often arrange their chromosomes with a common set of core genes intrinsic to each bacterial species and discrete regions where virulence genes are clustered. The core genomic components consist of essential gene products for normal cell homeostasis, metabolic and structural genes, and gene products for transcription, translation, and replication. Interspersed among the core genome are regions of diversity (RDs) and are recognized by tightly compacted regions of invasion genes, toxins, adhesins, and anti-phagocytic or anticomplement elements. These 10–100 kb RDs are part of the "flexible gene pool" distinguishable from more stable core regions which make up the rest of the pathogen chromosome. Importantly, RD sequences significantly differ in their guanine-cytosine (G + C) ratio and/or different codon usage pattern from core regions, suggesting that these genes have been relatively recently inherited by horizontal transfer of DNA from other bacterial species [13–15]. They are also referred to as "pathogenicity islands," "genomic islands," or "mobile genetic elements (MGEs)" to emphasize their recent and extrinsic genetic acquisition along the bacterial chromosome. These regions also feature accumulations of toxin genes originally derived from lysogenic bacteriophage remnants and other mobile genetic elements such as insertion sequences and transposons [15]. Bacterial genomes retain core regions but are surprisingly mobile and tolerate variability and chromosomal rearrangements within the flexible gene pool found in genomic islands.

This genomic plasticity provides microorganisms an evolutionary advantage in a rapidly changing and often toxic environment as seen in an ICU where patients often receive multiple antibacterial agents during their hospital stay. This variability in genomic islands allows for rapid recombination events and inheritance of large sequences of DNA from related species, involving many functional genes, all at the same time. This property allows bacteria to rapidly adapt to environmental changes, a process referred to as "evolution by quantum leaps" [16]. This capability has confounded efforts to eliminate bacterial pathogens by modern antimicrobial chemotherapeutic agents and fosters the evolution of multiple drug-resistant (MDR) bacterial pathogens.

Another evolutionary advantage for bacteria is the facility to readily acquire and sample exogenous DNA for potentially advantageous genes such as those mediating antibiotic resistance. Such a genetic system is in widespread use, particularly in enteric bacterial species, and known as integrons [13, 17]. Integrons are often located on bacterial chromosomes and are especially common on accessory extra-chromosomal genetic elements known as plasmids (Fig. 11.1). Integrons feature an integrase enzyme that allows transient DNA strand cleavage and uptake of new sequences derived from foreign DNA that has entered the cell from the environment. These new sequences are strategically placed to attachment sites and linked together with other adjacent DNA sequences as a series of inserted cassettes. A high-frequency promoter site exists at the 5′ end of integrons, thereby facilitating efficient transcription and translation of the newly acquired DNA cassette.

If this newly acquired DNA happens to encode a gene for an antibiotic resistance mechanism, this genetic event provides the host bacterium with an enormous survival advantage in a hospital setting filled with patients receiving an array of antibiotics. Integrons are commonplace within the genomes or plasmids of MDR pathogens. A cluster of different resistance genes to various classes of antibiotics can be found lined up one after another as integron gene cassettes. If such integrons are located on transferable plasmids, multiple resistance genes can spread rapidly as a single conjugal event by an integron-bearing plasmid that transfers MDR genes to susceptible recipient bacteria. Resistance plasmids carrying integrons and transposable elements are regularly shared among bacteria, even across species and genera barriers, aiding to the rapid evolution of MDR pathogens. This capacity is highly favored and adds to the fitness of microorganisms in a world awash in antibiotics. As a recent example, investigation of a newly discovered gene for colistin resistance (*mcr-3*) in China was found on a self-conjugating plasmid encoding 18 other antibiotic resistance genes [18]. The flexible gene pool of antibiotic resistance genes is often found on plasmids which can be readily gained or lost independent from the core genes predominately found along the bacterial chromosome [15]. These plasmid-derived resistance genes are disposable to bacteria in an antibiotic-free environment when no longer needed. Such plasmids become an unnecessary metabolic burden by wasting DNA substrates for replication if the resistance genes are no longer needed to protect the bacterial host from antibiotics. Bacteria can rapidly reacquire resistance genes through continuous horizontal transfer of R plasmids in antibiotic-rich locations such as the hospital wards.

11.4 Common Bacterial Pathogens That Cause Sepsis

An overview of the current types of bacterial pathogens felt to be responsible for causing sepsis in recent sepsis trials is provided in Table 11.1 [19–32]. This summary includes over 11,000 patients from 14 recent trials in which only slightly over half ($n = 6105$) had an identifiable, causative pathogen defined as the probable or definite pathogen responsible for sepsis by the treating physician. Presumably early

Table 11.1 Frequency of pathogen types causing sepsis in recent interventional trials

Gram-positive pathogens	Total $n = 2701$ (% of gram-positive bacteria)	Gram-negative pathogens	Total $n = 3404$ (% of gram-negative bacteria)
Streptococcus pneumoniae	890 (32.9%)	*Escherichia coli*	1460 (42.3%)
Staphylococcus aureus	849 (31.4%)	*Klebsiella* spp.	491 (14.4%)
Enterococcus spp.	326 (12.1%)	*Pseudomonas aeruginosa*	329 (9.7%)
Streptococcus pyogenes (Group A streptococci)	158 (5.8%)	*Enterobacter* spp.	327 (9.6%)
Coagulase-negative staphylococci	120 (4.4%)	*Bacteroides* spp.	301 (8.8%)
Streptococcus agalactiae (Group B streptococci)	98 (3.6%)	*Haemophilus influenzae*	270 (7.9%)
Other gram-positive bacteria including: *Clostridium*, *Corynebacterium*, *Listeria*, *Lactobacillus*, *Propionibacterium* spp. anaerobic streptococci, other gram-positive anaerobes	260 (9.6%)	Other gram-negative bacteria including: *Serratia*, *Proteus*, *Acinetobacter*, *Legionella*, *Citrobacter*, *Mycoplasma*, *Chlamydophila*, *Fusobacterium*, *Neisseria* spp., other gram-negative anaerobes	226 (6.6%)

Distribution summary of microorganisms determined by the clinical investigators to be the probable or definite causative pathogen or co-pathogen in patients with sepsis. These data were derived from large sepsis intervention studies conducted over the past 20 years (Refs. [18–31]). These studies included a total of 11,848 patients in which a definite or probable pathogen was determined in 6105 of these patients (51.5%). A total of 44.2% were gram-positive bacteria, and 55.8% were gram-negative bacterial pathogens. *Candida* spp. accounted for an additional 209 infections in these studies (1.7% of total septic population in this summary)

antimicrobial therapy stymied attempts to culture the causative pathogen in almost one half the septic population. Hopefully, non-culture dependent, genomic methodologies will allow us to identify more thoroughly the precise etiologic agent responsible as the cause of sepsis and septic shock [33].

Within the patients with identifiable causative bacterial organisms, gram-negative bacteria slightly outnumbered gram-positive bacteria (55.8% vs. 44.2%), while fungal organisms (also exclusively *Candida* species) accounted for a small (1.7% of total septic population in this summary) but important group of patients with an excessively high mortality. Only about one third of septic patients from these interventional sepsis trials had positive blood cultures thought to represent the causative microorganism. Again, non-culture, PCR-based diagnostic systems might be more useful to detect bloodstream pathogens no longer cultivatable as a result of empiric antibiotic therapy [32, 33].

11.5 Bacterial Communication Systems

A wide variety of pathogenic bacterial pathogens communicate with each other via small molecule signaling molecules and specific receptors (see Table 11.2). These signaling networks are called quorum sensing systems as they inform individual

Table 11.2 Quorum sensing systems in bacterial communities and their role in pathogenesis

Quorum sensing type	Bacterial species using this system	Basic signaling molecules	Primary functions
Autoinducer 1 (AI-1)	*Vibrio* spp., *Pseudomonas aeruginosa*, other gram-negative bacilli	Acyl homoserine lactones of different length freely diffuse across membranes to recipient receptors to activate target operons	Increasing concentrations of bacteria reaches threshold of AI-1 and activates expression of virulence genes for dissemination
Oligopeptide autoinducing peptides (AIP)	*S. aureus* and other gram-positive bacteria	Cyclic short peptides are transported outside the cell wall and bound to surface sensor histidine kinases which phosphorylate transcription factors	Transcription of the *agr* locus activates virulence genes (alpha toxin, proteases, superantigens) in *S. aureus* while limiting biofilm formation
Autoinducer 2 (AI-2)	*P. aeruginosa*, *Vibrio* spp. enteric gram-negative pathogens, EHEC	Complex small molecule signaling structures derived from SAM-mediated furanone-borate ring formations. AI-2 is secreted by specific transporters	*V. cholerae* expresses virulence factors (cholera toxin, mucinases, biofilm formation at low concentration) and shuts off virulence during diarrhea phase to disseminate
Autoinducer 3 (AI-3)	Enteric bacteria, EHEC	Catechol-like molecules, epinephrine, and norepinephrine require adrenergic receptors to signal between cells	Full expression of *E. coli* attachment and effacing lesions in colon during bloody diarrhea and hemolytic uremic syndrome

AI autoinducer, *AIP* autoinducer peptides, *agr* accessory gene regulator, *SAM* *S*-adenosylmethionine, *EHEC* enterohemorrhagic *Escherichia coli* (see Refs. [34–36])

bacteria about the quantity and density of highly related strains of bacteria within their immediate vicinity [34]. Once a critical threshold of related bacteria reach a predesignated quorum, the population density level changes the transcriptional profiles of the microbial pathogens in a specific manner. Usually when low population densities are present, this signals the bacteria to remain inactive and not express virulence factors in an attempt to avoid detection by the recognition by the vertebrate host. However, when large concentrations of similar organisms have accumulated, the necessary quorum has been assembled to turn on virulence genes and attack the host [35]. Quorum sensing plays a role in directing bacterial populations in many cooperative behaviors such as formation of complex, stable biofilms, sporulation, toxin production, secretion delivery systems, and dissemination with fully activated invasion genes. Some bacteria do not make quorum sensing effector molecules but still express receptors for other bacterial signaling molecules, perhaps "listening" to what other competing bacteria might be up to nearby.

An impressive array of chemical signals are involved in quorum sensing [34–36]. Gram-negative bacteria primarily rely upon homoserine lactone signals, while most gram-positive bacteria utilize short cyclical peptide signaling molecules. The signaling receptor systems are highly reminiscent of receptor signaling in eukaryotes with an extracellular receptor linked to an intracellular kinase molecule that phosphorylates transcriptional activators to change bacterial expression of growth, virulence, bacterial defenses and toxin secretion. Experimentally, natural and synthetic inhibitors of quorum sensing have been discovered and offered some level of protection in some experimental animal studies. Whether type of intervention could be successfully deployed in human infections or not remains an open question worth further investigation [36].

11.6 Selected Traits of the Common Bloodstream Gram-Negative Pathogens Causing Sepsis

11.6.1 *Escherichia coli*

E. coli remains the most common gram-negative bacillus causing severe sepsis or septic shock in numerous clinical studies in sepsis over the past 20 years [19–33]. A highly selected subset of *E. coli* clones are capable of causing bloodstream infections [9, 10, 37]. These virulent clones that are capable of bloodstream invasion are called extraintestinal pathogenic *E. coli* (exPEC) [38]. Using molecular typing systems from single-nucleotide polymorphism pyrosequencing to whole genome sequencing, a multi-locus sequence type (MLST) can now be generated to define relatedness of *E. coli* bacterial clones at the chromosomal level [39].

Recent surveys of blood isolates of *E. coli* in the North America and several European countries reveal that over half of these strains belong to only three, highly adapted, sequence types known as ST131, ST73, and ST69 [38, 40, 41]. Typically blood isolates of *E. coli* are more likely to carry an array of virulence factors (protection against complement and neutrophil killing, adhesins, toxin production, iron acquisition systems, attachment fimbriae, etc.) than commensal *E. coli* isolates cultured from the gastrointestinal or urinary tract [40–43]. Serum and neutrophil phagocytosis resistance were found in the majority of blood isolates. These virulence traits were less prevalent when the bacteremic strain of *E. coli* was isolated from patients with intravenous catheters or patients with nosocomial infections or with severely immunocompromised states [41, 43, 44].

The emerging role of *E. coli* ST131 (serotype O25b:H4) as a dominant cause of extraintestinal bloodstream infection is a disturbing development highlighting the interplay between fitness, virulence, and antibiotic selection pressures existing in the environment and within the patient residing in and outside the hospital setting [45–47]. This strain of bacteria contains an impressive array of virulence factors in its genome and expresses a large number of antibiotic resistance genes, usually encoded on R plasmids, to commonly employ antimicrobial compounds. The majority of isolates within this clone carries an extended spectrum beta-lactamase $bla_{CTX\text{-}M\text{-}15,}$ along with two or more DNA gyrase mutations resulting in high-level fluoroquinolone resistance. Most strains also feature resistance genes to trimethoprim-sulfamethoxazole and even a number of aminoglycosides.

The end result is that a patient admitted with an apparently uncomplicated *E. coli* urinary tract infection, treated with a seemingly appropriate antibiotic regimen with a third-generation cephalosporin or ciprofloxacin, might become increasingly ill over the first 8 h into hospital admission from an as yet untreated systemic infection from this MDR pathogen. While awaiting the culture and susceptibility test results, the astute clinician might detect a failure to respond to the original antibiotic choice and decide to add an aminoglycoside or trimethoprim-sulfamethoxazole. This patient would still not be receiving an effective antibiotic for another 12–36 h while awaiting the susceptibility results. Delayed effective antibiotic therapy during bacteremic sepsis is well known to be associated with poor outcomes in treating sepsis [1–4]. Treatment with carbapenems or extended spectrum beta-lactams with beta-lactamase inhibitors would work against most stains of *E. coli* ST131, but such agents are usually and appropriately reserved for difficult to treat nosocomially acquired infections. Regrettably, clone ST131 is now being isolated from the environment and commercial food products, even organically grown chickens supposedly not exposed to antibiotics [46].

Another adverse trend in the epidemiology of *E. coli* ST131 is the increasing prevalence of bloodstream infections with this virulent, MDR pathogen in elderly patients exposed to multiple courses of antibiotics during prolonged hospitalizations. The modest fitness cost to *E. coli* ST131 from the metabolic burden needed to maintain multiple resistance genes on R plasmids might be worth it in a hospital environment where repeated courses of antibiotics are administered over time [47–50]. Rapid molecular detection and resistance testing will be needed to correctly detect and treat this emerging microbial threat [47].

11.6.2 *Klebsiella pneumoniae*

This resourceful and often recalcitrant nosocomial pathogen is the second most common, gram-negative bacterial pathogen causing sepsis in recent clinical trials (Table 11.1). Human infections with *Klebsiella* spp. are becoming more frequent, more virulent, more antibiotic resistant, and more widely disseminated than in previous decades [51, 52]. The epidemiology of K. *pneumoniae* is changing with more virulent, community-acquired infections in previously healthy people and more pronounced dissemination of multiple resistance genes within nosocomial infections worldwide [51–54]. A cluster of highly virulent clones of *K. pneumoniae* expressing hypermucovicosity exo-polysaccharides have been identified in invasive infection community acquired in Taiwan, other regions in Southeast Asia, and South Africa for the past three decades. These infections are associated with primary pyogenic liver abscesses, bloodstream infections, and occasional complications of septic endophthalmitis and meningitis. These acute infections are usually community acquired and are often found in previously healthy persons or diabetic patients [53]. They are caused by hyper-viscous, heavily mucoid strains of *K. pneumoniae* primarily belonging to serotype K1 or K2 (favored sequence types ST23, ST25, 65, and 231). Their virulence is attributed to heavy capsular polysaccharide production, iron acquisition siderophores, and perhaps other virulence factors [52, 53, 55]. These infections are now spreading and are now reported in several European countries along with reports from the North America and Australia [56–59].

Another separate yet emerging threat with *K. pneumoniae* within the hospital environment is the dissemination of favored clones of *Klebsiella* spp. (such as ST258) which possess a remarkable proclivity to rapidly evolve by the horizontal spread of antibiotic resistance genes including carbapenemases (KPCs). These clones rapidly adapt to new antibiotic threats by the spread of antibiotic resistance genes by plasmids and transposable elements from other *Klebsiella* spp. or even other genera of bacteria (including New Delhi metallo-beta-lactamase-1 [NDM-1], oxacillinase-48 [oxa-48], and others) [51, 52]. Fortunately, the highly invasive liver abscess-forming, community-acquired strains have not yet acquired many resistance genes with MDR nosocomial strains of *K. pneumoniae*. This eventuality might only be a matter of time and bear careful monitoring.

11.6.3 *Pseudomonas aeruginosa*

The third most frequently recognized gram-negative bacterial pathogen causing sepsis in recent large clinical trials is *Pseudomonas aeruginosa* (see Table 11.1). Other than their similar appearance on routine Gram stain, *P. aeruginosa* shares little in common with *E. coli*, *K. pneumoniae*, or the other enteric bacterial species. Enteric bacteria are part of the normal resident microbiota of humans throughout life. *Pseudomonas aeruginosa*, on the other hand, primarily resides in freshwater and soil environments and are only accidental, opportunistic pathogens of humans [60]. The large pangenome content of *P. aeruginosa* differs markedly from enteric bacteria, and sharing of resistance genes and virulence genes is relatively uncommon. Horizontal gene transfer does occur between *Pseudomonas* spp. and other bacteria, and genomic pathogenicity islands are identifiable in the chromosomes and plasmids of these organisms. They communicate with each other through quorum sensing systems (see Table 11.2) but usually only communicate with quorum sensing molecules recognized between other members of their own species [34, 36].

P. aeruginosa is notorious among microbiologists and clinicians for its remarkable ability to intrinsically resist the actions of many common antibiotics. Moreover, *Pseudomonas* spp. possess the distressing capacity to become more resistant to antibiotics, to which they were initially susceptible, during the actual treatment period itself. Intrinsic and rapidly developing resistance to antibiotics in this species is accomplished primarily by point mutations altering the permeability characteristics of their cell wall porin genes (e.g., *opr*D), the derepression of existing resistance genes by accumulation of mutations in regulatory genes, and upregulation of the actions of multiple efflux pumps [50, 60]. They can also acquire and express resistance genes from conjugal transfer of R plasmids from related bacterial species. MDR strains and even XDR (extreme drug resistance) strains are becoming more prevalent over time in *P. aeruginosa* and exist in specific, high-risk clones such as sequence types ST111, ST175, and ST235 [60].

In addition to intrinsic and acquired antibiotic resistance development, *P. aeruginosa* has the potential capability for high-level virulence expression during dissemination of pathogens into a compromised host. This capacity is related to two major factors: (1) expression of PAMPs (pathogen-associated molecular patterns) and (2) expression and secretion of a myriad of highly potent exotoxins. PAMPs of *P. aeruginosa* include cell wall lipopolysaccharide (toll-like receptor TLR-4) TLR2 agonists (e.g., lipopeptides, peptidoglycans) and TLR5 agonists (polar flagella). When these PAMPs are released systemically, they activate innate immune cell signaling and procoagulant activity inducing septic shock [4, 5]. A second critical factor in disease pathogenesis from *Pseudomonas aeruginosa* is its synthesis and secretory release of multiple, highly injurious, exotoxins.

These exotoxins are delivered to the microenvironment surrounding the organism by a series of ingenious, energy-requiring, nanomachine structures known as bacterial secretion systems (types 1–7 SS) [61]. Other common gram-negative bacteria also employ toxin secretion systems, but *P. aeruginosa* is perhaps the most proficient bacterial pathogen at creating these toxin delivery systems to injure host cells. By electron microscopy these secretion systems appear like syringe structures that pass from the bacterial inner membrane through the outer membrane of the bacterium. This is usually a one-stage event, although two-step secretion systems exist (T2SS and T5SS). The toxin or protease can be released to the extracellular space or directly into the cytoplasm of host cells thereby delivering a fatal blow to the patient's cells without warning or immune recognition (e.g., type 3 SS). The characteristics of the seven currently identified secretion systems of bacteria are described in more detail in Table 11.3 and diagrammatically shown in Fig. 11.1.

P. aeruginosa possesses at least five of the secretion systems known to bacteriologists at present [61]. The type 1 SS is used to deliver proteases, cytotoxins, iron acquisition, and heme-binding proteins to the extracellular environment during infection to acquire iron and damage cells during infection. Type 2 SS is used to deliver the highly injurious protease elastase, a series of phospholipases and phosphatases, and the critically important exotoxin A, the two component ADP-ribosylating, lethal inhibitor of human cell transcription into the microenvironment surrounding *P. aeruginosa* [61]. The type 3 secretion system directly delivers four important toxins into human cells including the cytoskeletal inhibitor of phagocytosis ExoS, the cytotoxins exoU and exoT, and the adenylate cyclase inhibitor of phagocytosis, exoY, to impair innate immune cell defenses against invasive infection [62].

The type 4 secretion system is widely used by many gram-negative bacteria for DNA exchange during bacterial transformation and conjugation but does not appear to be expressed or found in the genome of *P. aeruginosa* [63, 64]. Type 5 secretion systems are used by *P. aeruginosa* for the release of inflammatory proteases and to deliver substrates necessary for fimbria assembly on the bacterial outer membrane [61]. The type 6 system deploys the cellular toxin hemolysin-coregulated protein to the extracellular space for *P. aeruginosa* [65–68]. The recently described type 7 system is important in the pathogenesis of mycobacterial infections, but no homologues of this system have been identified in *Pseudomonas* spp. [69, 70].

Table 11.3 Bacterial secretion systems and their role in toxin delivery and virulence

Secretion system type	Bacterial species using this system	Basic structure	Primary functions
TISS	*Pseudomonas aeruginosa*, other gram-negative bacilli	Forms a 12-stranded beta-barrel OMP, powered by an ABC transporter	Delivers alkaline proteases to OM surface and heme-binding protein to acquire iron, hemolysins, cytotoxins
TIISS	Widely expressed in gram-negative bacteria	Two-phase transport system to cross the IM and then the OM	Secretion of lytic enzymes, proteases, elastase, and A/B exoA in *P. aeruginosa*, lipases, phospholipases, phosphatases
TIIISS	*P. aeruginosa*, *Vibrio* spp. enteric gram-negative pathogens	Needle structure that delivers toxins directly into cytosol of eukaryotic cells	ExoS interferes with cytoskeleton impairs phagocytosis, exoU and ExoT are cytotoxic, exoY adenylate cyclase, impairs phagocytosis, TIIISS is recognized by the inflammasome
TIVSS	Enteric bacteria, *Legionella*, *Neisseria*, *and Brucella* spp.	Pilus like, form mating bridge for transformation, conjugation, cytotoxin delivery	Intracellular toxin delivery into human cells, DNA transfer, impair phago-lysosome fusion for intracellular survival for *Legionella*, *Brucella* spp.
TVSS	*Pseudomonas*, other gram-negatives	Two-phase transport system to cross the IM and then the OM	Exports materials for fimbriae synthesis, also delivers a protease that activates NF*k*B via PAR-1
TVISS	*Pseudomonas* spp., other gram-negative bacteria	Bacteriophage-like tubular structure, punctures host cells, and other bacteria	Can deliver toxins to human cells, primary role is eliminating competitors within bacterial communities (wounds, airways, GI tract)
TVIISS	*Mycobacterium* spp. and some gram-positive bacteria	Tubular structure extending through IM and mycolic acid containing layer	Secretes the virulence factors ESAT-6 and CFP-10 into extracellular space, which can impair and kill macrophages
Sec	Gram-negative and gram-positive bacteria	Three-part system: protein targeting, motor protein, IM channel SecYEG translocase	Transports unfolded (SecA) or folded proteins (SecB) across IM. Common mechanism for transporting proteins across IM (CM for gram positives)
SecA2	*L. monocytogenes*, *C. difficile*, MTB, *S. aureus*, some *Streptococcus spp.*	Smaller proteins missing the helical wing domain found in other secretases	Cell wall adhesion delivery, hemolysins (including pneumolysin), facilitate biofilm formation
Tat	*P. aeruginosa*, *E. coli*, MTB, gram-positive	2–3 subunits (TatA, B, C) form IM spanning channel	Transports various proteins across IM (CM for gram positives)
Sortase	Most gram-positive organisms	Cysteine transpeptidase with transmembrane domain	Anchors surface proteins to cell wall, including protein A, clumping factors A and B, fibronectin-binding protein

OMP outer membrane pore; *ABC* adenosine triphosphate-binding cassette; *OM* outer membrane; *IM* inner membrane (see Fig. 11.1); *MTB Mycobacterium tuberculosis*; *CM* cytoplasmic membrane; A/B binary toxins with an active domain (A) and a binding domain (B), exo-exotoxin; exoA in *P. aeruginosa* uses the B subunit to bind to cell membranes and an A component to ADP-ribosylate elongation factor 2, inhibiting eukaryotic protein synthesis which kills cells; NF*k*B nuclear factor kappa B cell is a transcriptional factor for activation of acute phase proteins by innate immune cells; *PAR-1* protease-activated receptor 1 activates human cells to secret cytokines and inflammatory mediators; *ESAT-6* early secreted antigenic target of 6 kDa; *CFP-10*, culture filtrate protein of 10 kDa (see Refs. [61–70, 145])

Armed with this formidable array of toxins, and a series of complex secretion systems to deliver these toxins, it comes as no surprise that multidrug-resistant *P. aeruginosa* infections are feared pathogens in immunocompromised patients. Considerable efforts are now underway to come up with new ways to deal effectively with this microorganism by vaccine strategies, monoclonal antibodies, quorum sensing inhibitors, and a spectrum of other novel therapeutic approaches against *P. aeruginosa* [50, 60, 61].

11.7 Selected Traits of the Common Bloodstream Gram-Positive Pathogens Causing Sepsis

11.7.1 *Staphylococcus aureus*

Staphylococcus aureus is one of the most common gram-positive pathogens causing severe sepsis, particularly among hospitalized patients [71–73]. *S. aureus* is by far the most virulent species of the genus *Staphylococcus*, due partly to its ability to acquire and integrate virulence-conferring genetic elements [74]. These mobile genetic elements (MGEs), which include plasmids, transposons, prophages (genes inserted by bacteriophages), and pathogenicity islands, can contain an immense array of virulence factors and antimicrobial resistance genes. Additionally, *S. aureus* possesses a sophisticated network of regulatory mechanisms that allow differential gene expression of toxins, surface proteins, and capsular polysaccharides depending upon external environmental stressors [75].

Like many gram-positive cocci, many clinically relevant *S. aureus* isolates produce a polysaccharide capsule, of which at least 13 serotypes have been identified [76]. Serotypes 5 and 8 appear to be most prevalent in human infection, although the reasons for this finding remain uncertain [77, 78]. Encapsulation, as in other organisms, protects the organism from opsonophagocytosis, although it may reduce adhesion to endothelial cell surfaces and may alter virulence in vivo. Conjugate capsular polysaccharide vaccines have been developed and trialed for serotypes 5 and 8, but no trial to date has met its predetermined successful end points [79].

Several surface proteins expressed on *S. aureus* may play a role in pathogenesis. Adhesins recognize mammalian extracellular matrix molecules and serve a critical role in bacterial colonization [80]. Coagulase binds to host prothrombin, forming staphylothrombin, which catalyzes the formation of fibrin from fibrinogen. This function cloaks *S. aureus* from immune system detection and facilitates intravascular infection. Clumping factors A and B facilitate this activity and also play a role in intravascular and skin surface adhesion and clustering of free-floating bacteria in plasma [81]. Protein A (an adhesin) both plays a powerful role in immune activation/sepsis and binds the Fc portion of human immunoglobulin, facilitating immune system evasion [82].

S. aureus elaborates many proteins to facilitate nutrient acquisition and tissue invasion and plays a powerful role in pathogenesis due to infection. Several hemolysins, most notably α-hemolysin, induce erythrocyte hemolysis and can also cause skin necrosis, cytokine release, and shock [83]. Isolates expressing γ-hemolysin (sometimes called γ-leucocidin) may cause necrotizing skin infections. Several toxins, including γ-hemolysin and Panton-Valentine leucocidin (PVL), are bicomponent, secreted toxins that polymerize on host cell surfaces, forming pores in the cytoplasmic membranes of specific host cell types [84]. For example, PVL forms from the combination of the proteins lukS-PV and lukF-PV. These toxins are also part of a group of secreted proteins called invasins, which also include matrix metalloprotease, hyaluronidase, and phospholipase C. As a group, these proteins facilitate tissue invasion and release of nutrients vital to continued growth and survival.

Finally, *S. aureus* can elaborate several toxins which can cause "toxin-mediated" diseases. Staphylococcal scalded skin syndrome (SSSS) is mediated by exfoliative toxins A and B (ETA and ETB) which cleave glycoprotein desmoglein 1, thus allowing the organism to more effectively spread beneath the stratum corneum [85]. Staphylococcal enterotoxin A (SEA) is part of a family of enterotoxins that can cause food poisoning, and some have been studied as potential biological weapons [86]. Staphylococcal enterotoxins B and C (SEB and SEC) and toxic shock syndrome toxin 1 (TSST-1) are the most common causes of staphylococcal toxic shock syndrome (TSS) and will be discussed with other superantigens, below.

Antimicrobial resistance in *S. aureus* is derived from acquisition of genes both from other, often less pathogenic, species and from other *S. aureus* isolates [87–89]. Resistance to penicillin rapidly emerged after its introduction in the 1940s through the elaboration of a beta-lactamase, and strains producing modified penicillin-binding proteins, conferring resistance to beta-lactamase-resistant penicillins (e.g., oxacillin, nafcillin) followed decades later. In recent decades *S. aureus* species with resistance to vancomycin have emerged, apparently through the transfer of plasmids from enterococci [87, 88]. Biofilm production, which is regulated at least in part via quorum sensing and nutrient availability, also protects *S. aureus* from antimicrobial activity. Bacteria deep within biofilms tend to be dormant and therefore less susceptible to antimicrobials, and concentrations of antimicrobials achieved within biofilms may be significantly lower than in surrounding tissues or intravascularly.

11.7.2 *Streptococcus pneumoniae*

The most commonly reported gram-positive bacterial pathogen causing severe sepsis or septic shock in most intervention trials, particularly among patients with community-onset sepsis, is *Streptococcus pneumoniae* [19–31]. A common colonizer of the nasopharynx of healthy individuals, *S. pneumoniae* can cause focal-invasive disease due to contiguous spread that progresses to bacteremia, meningitis, and sepsis. The most prominent virulence factor of pneumococci is its polysaccharide capsule, of which at least 90 distinct types within 45 serogroups have been identified [90]. Invasive pneumococcal disease (IPD) most commonly follows colonization with a new serotype. Specific serotypes (notably 1, 2, 7F, 9, 14, 16) are most likely to cause IPD, many of which are now included in the 13-serotype pneumococcal conjugate vaccine. Vaccination has resulted in decreases in IPD of up to 80% in some populations [91]. Non-encapsulated *S. pneumoniae* isolates may create biofilms and are associated with higher rates of antimicrobial resistance than their encapsulated counterparts [92].

Other virulence factors expressed by *S. pneumoniae* can include adhesins CbpA and phosphorylcholine that promote myocardial adhesion and invasion via interactions with vascular endothelial surface receptors [93]. Pneumolysin, a cholesterol-dependent pore-forming toxin that can lyse a variety of cell types, promotes tissue invasion/damage and is secreted via the accessory Sec system [94]. Other virulence factors facilitate immune evasion by preventing complement-mediated attach (elongation factor Tu [Tuf]) and promoting biofilm formation (polyamine transporter [potABCD]) [95, 96].

11.7.3 *Streptococcus pyogenes*

Streptococcus pyogenes (group A streptococci, GAS) causes severe disease through a combination of three main mechanisms: immune-mediated inflammation, release of toxins, and suppuration/pus formation [97]. A primary virulence factor of GAS is the M surface protein, which is anchored to the surface in a manner similar to that of the sortase gene in *S. aureus* [98]. M protein, along with fibronectin, facilitates adherence and internalization into host epithelial cells [99]. Pili, which are assembled and inserted into the cell wall by sortases, facilitate attachment and adhesion to tonsillar epithelium, a primary location for initial colonization [100].

Once colonization is established, several factors facilitate tissue invasion. Streptococcal pyrogenic exotoxin B (SpeB), a cysteine protease, degrades complement proteins, immunoglobulins, and cytokines, thus inhibiting host responses to invasive infection [101–103]. M proteins bind complement and the Fc portion of immunoglobulins and, when released from the cell surface, form complexes with fibrinogen that induces neutrophil activation and capillary leakage and potentiates the development of septic shock [104]. Additionally, M protein, in concert with streptokinase, binds host plasminogen and activates it to plasmin, creating a proteolytic-coated bacterial cell surface that facilitates tissue invasion [105].

GAS also secretes a variety of proteins that serve as potent toxins to a variety of cell types. Streptolysins S and O (SLS and SLO) induce cell lysis through pore formation and facilitate tissue invasion [106, 107]. At lower concentrations SLO inhibits neutrophil phagocytosis and oxidative burst activity [108]. The hyperinvasive GAS clone M1T1 also elaborates a powerful serum inhibitor of complement (SIC), promoting innate immune evasion and Sda1, a phage-encoded protein that prevents toll-like receptor recognition resulting in decreased cytokine response and macrophage bactericidal activity [109, 110]. Several superantigens are also elaborated by GAS, including SpeA and SpeC, which are discussed below.

11.7.4 *Streptococcus agalactiae*

Streptococcus agalactiae (group B streptococcus, GBS) is the most common cause of neonatal sepsis in the developed world and a common cause of skin and soft tissue infection leading to sepsis in adults, particularly in diabetic or medically debilitated patients [111, 112]. A normal component of the intestinal microbiome in up to 20% of patients, GBS, is often considered a "pathobiont," a potentially pathogenic colonizing species that usually coexists with the host but is capable of causing invasive and/or severe disease [113]. Similar to GAS, virulence factors critical to establishing invasive infection include adhesion, invasion, and immune evasion. Fibrinogen-binding protein FbsA promotes adhesion, while FbsB mediates tissue invasion [114]. Pili facilitate both adhesion to epithelial cell surfaces and translocation across the blood-brain barrier [115, 116]. The hypervirulent clonal complex ST-17 of serotype III GBS expresses an adhesin (HvgA) that facilitates colonization and tissue invasion and has a tropism for meninges [117].

Tissue invasion is facilitated by both surface proteins (notably alpha C proteins) and beta-hemolysins [118, 119]. Of previous diagnostic relevance, the co-hemolysin CAMP factor may facilitate invasion and survival but likely plays a more minor role in the development of severe systemic infection [120]. Capsular polysaccharides prevent opsonophagocytosis and have been studied as potential vaccine targets [121]. Streptococcal C5a peptidase of GBS (SCPB) inhibits the complement response, and factors H and BibA (GBS immunogenic bacterial adhesin) inhibit complement binding [122, 123].

Unlike GAS, the severe systemic inflammatory response of GBS infection, particularly in neonates, is not due to secreted toxins but to dysregulated immune responses to cell wall and intracellular components. Bacterial lipopeptides induce tumor necrosis factor (TNF) formation and release via interactions with toll-like receptor 2 (TLR2) [124]. Intracellular recognition of GBS DNA occurs in a TLR-independent fashion and results in type I interferon formation [125]. Finally, RNA is recognized via a TLR7 pathway in dendritic cells and via the NOD-like receptor family pyrin domain containing three (NLRP3) inflammasomes resulting in macrophage and dendritic cell activation [126]. This resulting activation of innate immune system cells is exacerbated in young infants by immature/poor opsonophagocytosis and intracytoplasmic killing that allows GBS to persist in the host and Th2-dominated adaptive immune responses that further contribute to a hyperinflammatory state, resulting in the rapid development of fulminant sepsis [113].

11.8 Superantigens

S. aureus, GAS, and some strains of other beta-hemolytic streptococci secrete proteins from a family of virulence factors called superantigens [127]. Superantigens are non-glycosylated low-molecular-weight exoproteins that undergo N-terminal cleavage and secretion through the Sec pathway. This family of exoproteins includes 24 different superantigens among *S. aureus* and 11 serologically distinct proteins among GAS. For *S. aureus*, the most commonly recognized superantigens clinically include TSST-1 and staphylococcal exotoxins; among GAS streptococcal pyrogenic exotoxins (SPEs), streptococcal superantigen (SSA), and streptococcal mitogenic exotoxin Z_n ($SMEZ_n$) are most commonly discussed [128]. Superantigens non-specifically cross-bridge T-cell receptors and major histocompatibility complex class II (MHC II) molecules on antigen-presenting cells, thus inducing T-cell proliferation and APC activation [129]. Superantigens stimulate up to 50% of T cells (as compared to the typical 1 in 10,000 ratio of other conventional processed antigens), inducing a runaway immune response often termed a "cytokine storm." During this process LPS clearance (an ongoing imperative due to endogenous intestinal flora) drops precipitously, and the lethality of circulating LPS increases by 10^6-fold [130].

Several clinical syndromes result from host exposure to superantigens, with variation due in part to host factors, site of infection, and specific superantigen. Staphylococcal TSS due to TSST-1 was first commonly reported among menstruating women, where growth of *S. aureus* on intravaginal tampons resulted in TSST-1 elaboration and the development of illness [131]. Symptoms of TSS in these cases include high fever, hypotension, erythematous rash (erythroderma), and multiorgan dysfunction or failure. Diarrhea and/or vomiting are also common symptoms early in disease, a common feature among shock syndromes due to other superantigens. Importantly, for staphylococcal TSS, toxin is often elaborated by bacteria that are extrinsic to the circulation, making it possible for staphylococcal TSS to occur as a complication of nearly any infection due to *S. aureus*. Some staphylococcal superantigens (particularly SEs) also produce an intense response when ingested, resulting in episodes of severe retching, vomiting, and diarrhea every 15–30 min for up to 48 h, an illness termed staphylococcal food poisoning. Streptococcal TSS has most often been described in association with skin and soft tissue infections (a classic example being post varicella infection in childhood) and is most commonly seen in conjunction with bacteremia [132]. Necrotizing fasciitis is commonly complicated by streptococcal TSS, and failure to achieve prompt source control (which may require extensive tissue resection or amputation) greatly increases the risk of mortality.

Treating sepsis complicated by TSS or milder forms of cytokine storming due to superantigens requires prompt source identification and control and antibiotic administration. Clindamycin use as part of antibiotic therapy regimens in TSS can reduce superantigen production, which can improve symptom course and clinical outcome [133]. Reducing circulating superantigen concentrations has been demonstrated through administration of intravenous immune globulin (IVIG) which has been shown to reduce fatality among patients with streptococcal TSS [134]. Monoclonal antibodies to certain superantigens have been proposed, but no preparation has made it to market. Studies of active immunization strategies are also underway but remain in early stages [135].

11.9 Virulence Traits of *Candida* Species Causing Sepsis

Of the many species of fungi capable of causing invasive disease and sepsis in humans, *Candida* species are by far most prominent. *Candida* species have been attributed as the cause of up to 7% of cases of septic shock in some reports [136]. The most common species causing infection include *C. albicans*, *C. glabrata*, *C. krusei*, *C. parapsilosis*, and *C. tropicalis* [137]. More recently, the multidrug-resistant species *C. auris* (first identified from cultures of the ear of a patient in Japan) has emerged as a pathogen causing sepsis and invasive disease [138]. Invasive candidiasis most commonly affects severely debilitated hosts, including the immunocompromised and those with indwelling vascular catheters, and can cause a myriad of invasive disease syndromes, including hepatosplenic candidiasis, endocarditis, endophthalmitis, and central nervous system disease [139]. Mortality from invasive candidiasis can exceed 30% [138].

The virulence of *Candida* species in sepsis stems largely from the underlying debilitated state of the host, necessitating prompt diagnosis of invasive candidiasis among at-risk patients in order to initiate empirical therapy as soon as possible (Table 11.4). Initial symptoms of invasive candidiasis are non-specific, and microbiological cultures may merely represent colonization in many cases. In general, isolation of *Candida* spp. from normally sterile body fluid in critically ill patients confirms the diagnosis [140]. Culture of respiratory tract secretions most often represents colonization and demonstration, with some exception in the severely immunocompromised. Candiduria may represent colonization, UTI, or secondary candiduria from primary candidemia. Non-culture-based methods of detection have been variably successful, with polymerase chain reaction and β-d-glucan (a cell wall component of *Candida* and other fungal species) having demonstrated the best sensitivity and specificity, depending on body site of infection and sample source [141].

Prompt source control and antifungal treatment of invasive *Candida* infections is critically important, as delays can result in significant increases in mortality risk [142]. Antifungal therapy differs based upon species-associated susceptibilities. *C. albicans* is assumed to be universally susceptible to triazoles (e.g., fluconazole), amphotericin B, and echinocandins. For other common species, particularly *C. glabrata* and *C. krusei*, fluconazole resistance is common. *C. auris* in particular can be resistant to amphotericin B, fluconazole, voriconazole, or echinocandins, necessitating broad-spectrum antifungal therapy and confirmatory susceptibility testing [143]. Suspected invasive candidiasis among ICU patients, particularly among patients with septic shock, should be treated aggressively and early; survival exceeds 80% if antifungals are started within 2 h of septic shock onset, but provider-reported practice suggests that delays in antifungal administration may exceed 30 h [144]. Finally, it is important to assess for metastatic foci of infection, particularly among patients diagnosed with candidemia, as identification of invasive candidiasis at other sites necessitates prolonged antifungal therapy.

Table 11.4 Risk factors for invasive candidiasis and/or candidemia

Patient factors	Exposure factors
Diabetes	Immunosuppressive drugs including:
Renal failure (incl. hemodialysis)	(a) Corticosteroids
Prior surgery (esp. intra-abdominal)	(b) Anti-transplant rejection drugs
Immunocompromise, including:	(c) Myeloablative chemotherapy
(a) Malignancy	Broad-spectrum antibiotics
(b) HIV	Indwelling vascular catheters
(c) Primary immunodeficiency	HSCT or SOT recipient
Premature birth (in infants only)	Prolonged ICU stay

HIV human immunodeficiency virus, *HSCT* hematologic stem cell transplant, *SOT* solid organ transplant

Conclusions

Clinicians are faced with many challenges when treating septic patients. The vast array of potential infecting organisms responsible for the development of sepsis makes the identification of targeted therapies particularly difficult. Each pathogen possesses a unique and versatile array of virulence and survival factors that can be differentially activated and expressed depending on environmental exposures and host factors, making it possible even for routine colonizing organisms to cause life-threatening disease. Understanding the role that these virulence factors, toxins, and communication mechanisms play in microorganism survival is providing valuable insight into human immune system functions and will likely prove critically important to refining the broad, syndromic diagnosis of sepsis into more discrete disease entities that will be amenable to specific and targeted therapies.

References

1. Singer M, Deutschman CS, Seymour CW, Shankar Hari M, Angus DC, Annane D, et al. The third international consensus definitions for sepsis and septic shock. J Am Med Assoc. 2016;315(8):801–10.
2. Rhodes A, Evans LE, Alhazzani W, Levy MM, Antonelli M, Ferrer R, et al. Surviving sepsis campaign: international guidelines for management of sepsis and septic shock: 2016. Intensive Care Med. 2017;43:304–77.
3. Kumar A, Paladugu B, Haery C, Kumar A, Symeoneides A, Taiberg L, et al. Timing of antibiotic administration in relation to duration of shock is a critical determinant of survival in a murine model of *E. coli* sepsis: association with serum lactate and inflammatory cytokines. J Infect Dis. 2006;193:251–8.
4. Seymour CW, Gesten F, Prescott HC, Friedrich ME, Iwashyna TJ, Phillips GS, et al. Time to treatment and mortality during mandated emergency care for sepsis. N Engl J Med. 2017;376:2235–44. https://doi.org/10.1056/NEJMoa1703058.
5. Cohen J, Vincent J-L, Adhikari FR, Machado F, Angus D, Calandra T, et al. Sepsis: a roadmap for future research. Lancet Infect Dis. 2015;15:581–614.
6. Kumar A. An alternate pathophysiologic paradigm of sepsis and septic shock: implications for optimizing antimicrobial therapy. Virulence. 2014;5(1):80–97.
7. Sullivan FL, Neckermann EF, Cannon PR. The localization and fate of bacteria in the tissues. J Immunol. 1934;26:46–67.
8. Ottenberg R. The rate and location of removal of bacteria from the blood in human disease. Arch Pathol. 1931;11:766–74.
9. Opal SM, Cross AS, Gemski PK. Antigen and its effect on serum sensitivity of rough *E. coli*. Infect Immun. 1982;37(3):956–60.
10. Miajlovic H, Smith S. Bacterial self-defence: how *Escherichia coli* evades serum killing. FEMS Microbiol Lett. 2014;354:1–9.
11. Sarma JV, Ward PA. The complement system. Cell Tissue Res. 2011;343:227–35.
12. Opal SM. Splenectomy and splenic dysfunction. In: Cohen J, Powderly W, Opal SM, editors. Infectious diseases. 4th ed. Edinburgh: Mosby, Times-Mirror International Publishers; 2016. p. 775–9.
13. Opal SM, Pop-Vicas A. Molecular mechanisms of antibiotic resistance in bacteria. In: Bennett JE, Dolin R, Blaser M, editors. Principles and practice of infectious diseases. 8th ed. Philadelphia, PA: Elsevier; 2014. p. 235–51.
14. Van der Poll T, Opal SM. The molecular pathogenesis of pneumococcal pneumonia. Lancet. 2009;374:1543–56.

15. Hacker J, Carniel E. Ecologic fitness, genomic islands and bacterial pathogenicity: a Darwinian view of evolution in microbes. EMBO Rep. 2001;2(5):371–81.
16. Finlay BB, Falkow S. Common themes in microbial pathogenicity revised. Microbiol Mol Biol Rev. 1997;61:136–69.
17. Rao AN, Barlow M, Clark LA, Boring JR, Tenover FC, McGowan JE. Class 1 integron in resistant *Escherichia coli* and *Klebsiella* spp. in US hospitals. Emerg Infect Dis. 2006;12(6):1011–4.
18. Yin W, Li H, Shen Y, Liu Z, Wang S, Shen Z, et al. Novel plasmid-mediated colistin resistance gene *mcr-3* in *Escherichia coli*. MBio. 2017;8(3):e00543-17.
19. Dellinger RP, Tomayko JF, Angus DC, Opal SM, Cupo MA, McDermott S, et al. Efficacy and safety of a phospholipid emulsion (GR270773) in gram-negative severe sepsis: results of a phase II multicenter, randomized, placebo-controlled, dose-finding clinical trial. Crit Care Med. 2009;37(11):2929–38.
20. Tidswell M, Tillis W, LaRosa SP, Lynn M, Wittek AE, Kao R, et al. Phase 2 trial of eritoran tetrasodium (E5564), a Toll-like receptor 4 antagonist, in patients with severe sepsis. Crit Care Med. 2010;38(1):72–83.
21. Wunderink RG, Laterre PF, Francois B, Perrotin D, Artigas A, Vidal LO, et al. Recombinant tissue factor pathway inhibitor in severe community-acquired pneumonia. Am J Respir Crit Care Med. 2011;183:1561–8.
22. Abraham E, Reinhart K, Opal SM, Demeyer I, Doig C, Rodriguez AL, et al. Efficacy and safety of tifacogin (recombinant tissue factor pathway inhibitor) in severe sepsis. JAMA. 2003;290(2):238–47.
23. Opal SM, Lim YP, Siryaporn E, Moldawer L, Pribble J, Palardy J, et al. Longitudinal studies of inter-alpha inhibitor proteins in severely septic patients: a potential clinical marker and mediator of severe sepsis. Crit Care Med. 2007;35(2):387–92.
24. Opal SM, Laterre PF, Francois B, LaRosa SP, Angus D, Mira JP, et al. Effect of eritoran, an antagonist of MD2-TLR4, on mortality in patients with severe sepsis. JAMA. 2013;309(11):1154–62.
25. Opal SM, Garber G, LaRosa SP, Maki D, Freebairn R, Kinasewitz G, et al. Systemic host responses in severe sepsis analyzed by causative microorganism and treatment effects of drotrecogin alfa (activated). Clin Infect Dis. 2003;37:50–8.
26. Schuster D, Metzler M, Opal S, Lowry S, Balk R, Abraham E, et al. Recombinant platelet-activating factor acetylhydrolase to prevent acute respiratory distress syndrome and mortality in severe sepsis: phase IIb, multicenter, randomized, placebo-controlled, clinical trial. Crit Care Med. 2003;31(6):1612–9.
27. Opal S, Scannon P, Vincent JL, White M, Carroll S, Palardy JE, et al. Relationship between plasma levels of lipopolysaccharide (LPS) and LPS-binding protein in patients with severe and septic shock. J Infect Dis. 1999;180:1584–9.
28. Fisher CJ, Dhainaut J-F, Opal SM, Pribble JP, Balk RA, Slotman GJ, et al. Recombinant human interleukin-1 receptor antagonist reduces the mortality of patients with sepsis syndrome as a function of disease severity: a randomized, double-blind, placebo controlled trial. JAMA. 1994;271:1836–43.
29. Warren B, Eid A, Singer P, Pillay SS, Carl P, Novak I, et al. High-dose antithrombin III in severe sepsis. JAMA. 2001;286(15):1869–78.
30. Opal SM, Laterre PF, Abraham E, Francois B, Wittebole X, Lowry S, et al. Recombinant human platelet-activating factor acetylhydrolase for treatment of severe sepsis: results of a phase III, multicenter, randomized, double-blinded, placebo-controlled, clinical trial. Crit Care Med. 2004;32(2):332–41.
31. Fisher CJ, Agosti J, Opal SM, Lowry S, Balk R, Sadoff J, et al. Treatment of septic shock with the tumor necrosis factor receptor: Fc fusion protein. N Engl J Med. 1996;334:1697–702.
32. Vincent J-L, Breasley D, Libert N, Abidi NE, O'Dwyer M, Zackarowski K, et al. Rapid diagnosis of infection in the critically ill, a multicenter study of molecular detection of bloodstream infections, pneumonia and sterile site infections. Crit Care Med. 2015;43(11):2285–93.

33. Jordana-Lluch E, Gimenez M, Quesada MD, Rivaya B, Marco C, Dominguez MJ, et al. Evaluation of the broad-range PCR/ESI-MS technology of in blood specimens for the molecular diagnosis of bloodstream infections. PLoS One. 2015;10(10):e0140865.
34. Asad S, Opal SM. Quorum sensing and the role of cell to cell communication in the pathogenesis of invasive infection. Crit Care. 2008;12(6):236–45.
35. Walters M, Sperandio V. Quorum sensing in *Escherichia coli* and *Salmonella*. Int J Med Microbiol. 2006;296(2–3):125–31.
36. Rutherford ST, Bassler BL. Bacterial quorum sensing: its role in virulence and possibilities for its control. Cold Spring Harb Perspect Med. 2012;2(11):a012427.
37. Van der Poll T, Opal SM. Host-pathogen interactions in sepsis. Lancet Infect Dis. 2008;8:32–43.
38. Mora-Rillo M, Fernandez-Romero N, Francisco N-S, Diez-Sebastian J, Romero-Gomez MP, Fernandez FA, et al. Impact of virulence genes on sepsis severity and survival in *Escherichia coli* bacteremia. Virulence. 2015;6(1):93–100. https://doi.org/10.4161/21505594.2014.991234.
39. Larsen MV, Cosentino S, Rasmussen S, Friis C, Hasman H, Marvig RL, et al. Multilocus sequence typing of total-genome-sequenced bacteria. J Clin Microbiol. 2012;50(4):1355–61.
40. Johnson J, Murray A, Kuskowski M, Schubert S, Prere M, Picard B, et al. Distribution and characteristics of clonal group A. Emerg Infect Dis. 2005;11(1):141–294.
41. Miajlovic H, MacAogain M, Collins C, Rogers T, Smith S. Characterization of *Escherichia coli* bloodstream isolates associated with mortality. J Med Microbiol. 2016;65:71–9.
42. Skjot-Rasmussen L, Ejrnaes K, Lundgren B, Hammerum AM, Frimodt-Moller N. Virulence factors and phylogenetic grouping of *Escherichia coli* isolates from patients with bacteraemia of urinary tract origin relate to sex and hospital vs. community-acquired origin. Int J Med Microbiol. 2012;302(3):129–34.
43. Cooke N, Smith S, Kelleher M, Rogers T. Major differences exist in frequencies of virulence factors and multidrug resistance between community and nosocomial *Escherichia coli* bloodstream isolates. J Clin Microbiol. 2010;48(4):1099–104.
44. Wang M, Tseng C, Chen C, Wu J, Huang J. The role of bacterial virulence and host factors in patients with *Escherichia coli* bacteria who have acute cholangitis or upper urinary tract infection. Clin Infect Dis. 2002;35(15):1161–6.
45. Johnson J, Porter S, Johnston B, Thuras P, Clock S, Crupain M, et al. Extraintestinal pathogenic and antimicrobial resistant *Escherichia coli*, including sequence type 131 (ST131), from retail chicken breasts: United States, 2013. Appl Environ Microbiol. 2017. https://doi.org/10.1128/AEM.02956-16.
46. Johnson JR, Johnston B, Clabots C, Kushowski MA, Castanheira M. *Escherichia coli* sequence type 131 as the major cause of serious multidrug resistant *E. coli* infections in the United States. Clin Infect Dis. 2010;51(3):286–94.
47. van der Mee-Marquet NL, Blanc DS, Gbaguidi-Haore H, Dos Santos Borgess S, Viboud Q, Bertrand X. Marked increase in incidence for bloodstream infections due to *Escherichia coli*, a side effect of previous antibiotic therapy in the elderly. Front Microbiol. 2015;6:646–55.
48. Anderson D, Hughes D. Antibiotic resistance and its cost: is it possible to reverse resistance? Nat Rev Microbiol. 2010;8:260–71.
49. Beceiro A, Tomas M, Bou G. Antimicrobial resistance and virulence: a successful or deleterious association in the bacterial world? Clin Microbiol Rev. 2013;26(2):185–230.
50. Geisinger E, Isberg R. Interplay between antibiotic resistance and virulence during disease promoted by multidrug-resistant bacteria. J Infect Dis. 2017;215(1):S9–S17.
51. Gomez-Simmonds A, Uhlemann A-C. Clinical implications of genomic adaptation and evolution of carbapenem-resistant *Klebsiella pneumoniae*. J Infect Dis. 2017;215(1):S18–26.
52. Holt KE, Wertheim H, Zadoks RN, Baker S, Whitehouse CA, Dance D, et al. Genomic analysis of diversity, population structure, virulence, antibiotic resistance in *Klebsiella pneumoniae*, an urgent threat to public health. Proc Natl Acad Sci U S A. 2015:E3574–81. https://doi.org/10.1073/pnas.1501049112.

53. VL Y, Hansen DS, Ko WC, Sagnimeni A, Klugman KP, von Gottberg A, et al. Virulence characteristics of Klebsiella and clinical manifestations *of K. pneumoniae* bloodstream infections. Emerg Infect Dis. 2007;13(7):986–93.
54. Logan L, Weinstein R. The epidemiology of carbapenem-resistant enterobacteriaceae: the impact and evolution of a global menace. J Infect Dis. 2017;215(1):S28–36.
55. Nassif X, Fournier J-M, Arondel J, Sansonetti PJ. Mucoid phenotype of *Klebsiella pneumoniae* is a plasmid-encoded virulence factor. Infect Immun. 1989;57(2):546–52.
56. Decré D, Verdet C, Emirian A, Le Gourrierec T, Petit J-C, Offenstadt G, et al. Emerging severe and fatal infections due to *Klebsiella pneumoniae* in two university hospitals in France. J Clin Microbiol. 2011;49(8):3012–4.
57. Fung C-P, Chang F-Y, Lee S-C, B-S H, Kuo BI-T, Liu C-Y, et al. A global emerging disease of *Klebsiella pneumoniae* liver abscess: is serotype K1 an important factor for complicated endophthalmitis? Gut. 2002;50:420–4.
58. Nadasy K, Domiati-Saad R, Tribble MA. Invasive *Klebsiella pneumoniae* syndrome in North America. Clin Infect Dis. 2007;45:e25–8.
59. Bilal S, Volz MS, Fiedler T, Podschun R, Schneider T. *Klebsiella pneumoniae*-induced liver abscesses, Germany. Emerg Infect Dis. 2014;20(11):1939–40.
60. Juan C, Pena C, Oliver A. Host and pathogen biomarkers for severe *Pseudomonas aeruginosa* infections. J Infect Dis. 2017;215(1):S44–50.
61. Bleves S, Viarre V, Salacha R, Michel Gerard PF, Filloux A, Voulhoux R. Protein secretion systems in *Pseudomonas aeruginosa*: a wealth of pathogenic weapons. Int J Med Microbiol. 2010:534–43. https://doi.org/10.1016/j.ijmm.2010.8.005.
62. Hauser A. The type III secretion system of *Pseudomonas aeruginosa*: infection by injection. Nat Rev Microbiol. 2009;7:654–65.
63. Fronzes R, Christie PJ, Waksman G. The structural biology of type IV secretion systems. Nat Rev Microbiol. 2009;7:703–14.
64. Backert S, Meyer TF. Type IV secretion systems and their effectors in bacterial pathogenesis. Curr Opin Microbiol. 2006;9:207–17.
65. Russell A, Petterson SB, Mougous JD. Type VI secretion system effectors: poisons with a purpose. Nat Rev Microbiol. 2014;12:137–48.
66. Bingle LEH, Bailey CM, Pallen MJ. Type VI secretion: a beginner's guide. Curr Opin Microbiol. 2008;11:3–8.
67. Cascales E, Cambillau C. Structural biology of type VI secretion systems. Philos Trans R Soc Lond B Biol Sci. 2012;367:1102–11.
68. Pukatzki S, McAuley SB, Miyata ST. The type VI secretion system: translocation of effectors and effector-domains. Curr Opin Microbiol. 2009;12:11–7.
69. Daleke MH, Ummels R, Bawono P, Heringa J, Vandenbrouchke-Grauls CMJE, Luirink J, et al. General secretion signal for the mycobacterial type VII secretion pathway. Proc Natl Acad Sci U S A. 2012;109(28):11342–7.
70. Simone R, Bottai D, Brosch R. ESX/type VII secretion systems and their role in host-pathogen interaction. Curr Opin Microbiol. 2009;12(1):4–10.
71. Artero A, Zaragoza R, Camarena JJ, Sancho S, González R, Nogueira JM. Prognostic factors of mortality in patients with community-acquired bloodstream infection with severe sepsis and septic shock. J Crit Care. 2010;25(2):276–81.
72. Zahar JR, Timsit JF, Garrouste-Orgeas M, Français A, Vesin A, Descorps-Declere A, et al. Outcomes in severe sepsis and patients with septic shock: pathogen species and infection sites are not associated with mortality. Crit Care Med. 2011;39(8):1886–95.
73. Puskarich MA, Trzeciak S, Shapiro NI, Arnold RC, Horton JM, Studnek JR, Kline JA, Jones AE, Emergency Medicine Shock Research Network (EMSHOCKNET). Association between timing of antibiotic administration and mortality from septic shock in patients treated with a quantitative resuscitation protocol. Crit Care Med. 2011;39(9):2066–71.
74. Malachowa N, DeLeo FR. Mobile genetic elements of *Staphylococcus aureus*. Cell Mol Life Sci. 2010;67(18):3057–71.

75. Novick RP. Staphylococcal pathogenesis and pathogenicity factors: genetics and regulation. In: Fischetti VA, Novick RP, Ferretti JJ, Portnoy DA, Rood JI, editors. Gram-positive pathogens. Washington, DC: ASM Press; 2006. p. 496–516.
76. von Eiff C, Taylor KL, Mellmann A, Fattom AI, Friedrich AW, Peters G, Becker K. Distribution of capsular and surface polysaccharide serotypes of *Staphylococcus aureus*. Diagn Microbiol Infect Dis. 2007;58:297–302.
77. Arbeit RD, Karakawa WW, Vann WF, Robbins JB. Predominance of two newly described capsular polysaccharide types among clinical isolates of *Staphylococcus aureus*. Diagn Microbiol Infect Dis. 1984;2:85–91.
78. O'Riordan K, Lee JC. *Staphylococcus aureus* capsular polysaccharides. Clin Microbiol Rev. 2004;17(1):218–34.
79. Shinefield H, Black S, Fattom A, Horwith G, Rasgon S, Ordonez J, et al. Use of a *Staphylococcus aureus* conjugate vaccine in patients receiving hemodialysis. N Engl J Med. 2002;346(7):491–6.
80. Jenkins A, Diep BA, Mai TT, Vo NH, Warrener P, Suzich J, et al. Differential expression and roles of *Staphylococcus aureus* virulence determinants during colonization and disease. MBio. 2015;6(1):e02272-14. Gilmore MS, editor
81. Crosby HA, Kwiecinski J, Horswill AR. *Staphylococcus aureus* aggregation and coagulation mechanisms, and their function in host-pathogen interactions. Adv Appl Microbiol. 2016;96:1–41.
82. Falugi F, Kim HK, Missiakas DM, Schneewind O. Role of protein A in the evasion of host adaptive immune responses *by Staphylococcus aureus*. MBio. 2013;4(5):e00575-13.
83. Vandenesch F, Lina G, Henry T. *Staphylococcus aureus* hemolysins, bicomponent leukocidins, and cytolytic peptides: a redundant arsenal of membrane-damaging virulence factors? Front Cell Infect Microbiol. 2012;2:12.
84. Guillet V, Roblin P, Werner S, Coraiola M, Menestrina G, Monteil H, et al. Crystal structure of leucotoxin S component: new insight into the Staphylococcal beta-barrel pore-forming toxins. J Biol Chem. 2004;279(39):41028–37. Epub 2004 Jul 18
85. Bukowski M, Wladyka B, Dubin G. Exfoliative toxins of Staphylococcus aureus. Toxins. 2010;2(5):1148–65.
86. Pinchuk IV, Beswick EJ, Reyes VE. Staphylococcal enterotoxins. Toxins. 2010;2(8):2177–97. https://doi.org/10.3390/toxins2082177.
87. Weigel LM, Clewell DB, Gill SR, Clark NC, McDougal LK, Flannagan SE, et al. Genetic analysis of a high-level vancomycin-resistant isolate of *Staphylococcus aureus*. Science. 2003;302(5650):1569–71.
88. Zhu W, Clark N, Patel JB. pSK41-like plasmid is necessary for Inc18-like vanA plasmid transfer from *Enterococcus faecalis to Staphylococcus aureus* in vitro. Antimicrob Agents Chemother. 2013;57(1):212–9. https://doi.org/10.1128/AAC.01587-12. Epub 2012 Oct 22
89. Hanssen AM, Ericson Sollid JU. SCCmec in staphylococci: genes on the move. FEMS Immunol Med Microbiol. 2006;46(1):8–20.
90. Geno KA, Gilbert GL, Song JY, Skovsted IC, Klugman KP, Jones C, et al. Pneumococcal capsules and their types: past, present, and future. Clin Microbiol Rev. 2015;28(3):871–99.
91. Griffin MR, Zhu Y, Moore MR, Whitney CG, Grijalva CG. U.S. hospitalizations for pneumonia after a decade of pneumococcal vaccination. N Engl J Med. 2013;369(2):155–63.
92. Keller LE, Robinson DA, McDaniel LS. Nonencapsulated *Streptococcus pneumoniae*: emergence and pathogenesis. MBio. 2016;7(2):e01792.
93. Brown AO, Mann B, Gao G, Hankins JS, Humann J, Giardina J, et al. *Streptococcus pneumoniae* translocates into the myocardium and forms unique microlesions that disrupt cardiac function. PLoS Pathog. 2014;10(9):e1004383.
94. Bandara M, Skehel JM, Kadioglu A, Collinson I, Nobbs AH, Blocker AJ, et al. The accessory Sec system (SecY2A2) in *Streptococcus pneumoniae* is involved in export of pneumolysin toxin, adhesion and biofilm formation. Microbes Infect. 2017;19(7–8):402–12. https://doi.org/10.1016/j.micinf.2017.04.003. Epub 2017 Apr 27

95. Mohan S, Hertweck C, Dudda A, et al. Tuf of *Streptococcus pneumoniae* is a surface displayed human complement regulator binding protein. Mol Immunol. 2014;62(1):249–64.
96. Rai AN, Thornton JA, Stokes J, et al. Polyamine transporter in *Streptococcus pneumoniae* is essential for evading early innate immune responses in pneumococcal pneumonia. Sci Rep. 2016;6:26964.
97. Walker MJ, Barnett TC, McArthur JD, Cole JN, Gillen CM, Henningham A, et al. Disease manifestations and pathogenic mechanisms of Group A streptococcus. Clin Microbiol Rev. 2014;27(2):264–301. https://doi.org/10.1128/CMR.00101-13.
98. Barnett TC, Scott JR. Differential recognition of surface proteins in *Streptococcus pyogenes* by two sortase gene homologs. J Bacteriol. 2002;184(8):2181–91.
99. Rezcallah MS, Hodges K, Gill DB, Atkinson JP, Wang B, Cleary PP. Engagement of CD46 and alpha5beta1 integrin by group A streptococci is required for efficient invasion of epithelial cells. Cell Microbiol. 2005;7(5):645–53.
100. Abbot EL, Smith WD, Siou GP, Chiriboga C, Smith RJ, Wilson JA, et al. Pili mediate specific adhesion of *Streptococcus pyogenes* to human tonsil and skin. Cell Microbiol. 2007;9(7):1822–33.
101. Honda-Ogawa M, Ogawa T, Terao Y, Sumitomo T, Nakata M, Ikebe K, et al. Cysteine proteinase from *Streptococcus pyogenes* enables evasion of innate immunity via degradation of complement factors. J Biol Chem. 2013;288(22):15854–64. https://doi.org/10.1074/jbc.M113.469106. Epub 2013 Apr 15
102. Collin M, Olsén A. EndoS, a novel secreted protein from *Streptococcus pyogenes* with endoglycosidase activity on human IgG. EMBO J. 2001;20(12):3046–55.
103. Egesten A, Olin AI, Linge HM, Yadav M, Mörgelin M, Karlsson A, et al. SpeB of *Streptococcus pyogenes* differentially modulates antibacterial and receptor activating properties of human chemokines. PLoS One. 2009;4(3):e4769.
104. Herwald H, Cramer H, Mörgelin M, Russell W, Sollenberg U, Norrby-Teglund A, et al. M protein, a classical bacterial virulence determinant, forms complexes with fibrinogen that induce vascular leakage. Cell. 2004;116(3):367–79.
105. Chandrahas V, Glinton K, Liang Z, Donahue DL, Ploplis VA, Castellino FJ. Direct host plasminogen binding to bacterial surface M-protein in pattern D strains of *Streptococcus pyogenes* is required for activation by its natural co-inherited SK2b protein. J Biol Chem. 2015;290(30):18833–42.
106. Sumitomo T, Nakata M, Higashino M, Jin Y, Terao Y, Fujinaga Y, Kawabata S. Streptolysin S contributes to group A streptococcal translocation across an epithelial barrier. J Biol Chem. 2011;286(4):2750–61.
107. Hryniewicz W, Pryjma J. Effect of streptolysin S on human and mouse T and B lymphocytes. Infect Immun. 1977;16(3):730–3.
108. Uchiyama S, Döhrmann S, Timmer AM, Dixit N, Ghochani M, Bhandari T, et al. Streptolysin O rapidly impairs neutrophil oxidative burst and antibacterial responses to Group A Streptococcus. Front Immunol. 2015;6:581.
109. Frick IM, Akesson P, Rasmussen M, Schmidtchen A, Björck L. SIC, a secreted protein of *Streptococcus pyogenes* that inactivates antibacterial peptides. J Biol Chem. 2003;278(19):16561–6. Epub 2003 Mar 5
110. Uchiyama S, Andreoni F, Schuepbach RA, Nizet V, Zinkernagel AS. DNase Sda1 allows invasive M1T1 Group A streptococcus to prevent TLR9-dependent recognition. PLoS Pathog. 2012;8(6):e1002736.
111. Simonsen KA, Anderson-Berry AL, Delair SF, Davies HD. Early-onset neonatal sepsis. Clin Microbiol Rev. 2014;27(1):21–47. https://doi.org/10.1128/CMR.00031-13.
112. Jackson LA, Hilsdon R, Farley MM, Harrison LH, Reingold AL, Plikaytis BD, et al. Risk factors for group B streptococcal disease in adults. Ann Intern Med. 1995;123(6):415–20.
113. Landwehr-Kenzel S, Henneke P. Interaction of *Streptococcus agalactiae* and cellular innate immunity in colonization and disease. Front Immunol. 2014;5:519.
114. Jacobsson K. A novel family of fibrinogen-binding proteins in *Streptococcus agalactiae*. Vet Microbiol. 2003;96(1):103–13.

115. Lauer P, Rinaudo CD, Soriani M, Margarit I, Maione D, Rosini R, et al. Genome analysis reveals pili in Group B streptococcus. Science. 2005;309(5731):105.
116. Konto-Ghiorghi Y, Mairey E, Mallet A, Duménil G, Caliot E, Trieu-Cuot P, et al. Dual role for pilus in adherence to epithelial cells and biofilm formation in *Streptococcus agalactiae*. PLoS Pathog. 2009;5(5):e1000422.
117. Tazi A, Disson O, Bellais S, Bouaboud A, Dmytruk N, Dramsi S, et al. The surface protein HvgA mediates group B streptococcus hypervirulence and meningeal tropism in neonates. J Exp Med. 2010;207(11):2313–22.
118. Bolduc GR, Madoff LC. The group B streptococcal alpha C protein binds alpha1beta1-integrin through a novel KTD motif that promotes internalization of GBS within human epithelial cells. Microbiology. 2007;153(Pt 12):4039–49.
119. Doran KS, Chang JC, Benoit VM, Eckmann L, Nizet V. Group B streptococcal beta-hemolysin/cytolysin promotes invasion of human lung epithelial cells and the release of interleukin-8. J Infect Dis. 2002;185(2):196–203.
120. Hensler ME, Quach D, Hsieh C-J, Doran KS, Nizet V. CAMP factor is not essential for systemic virulence of group B streptococcus. Microb Pathog. 2008;44(1):84–8.
121. Chen VL, Avci FY, Kasper DL. A maternal vaccine against group B streptococcus: past, present, and future. Vaccine. 2013;31(Suppl 4):D13–9.
122. Jarva H, Hellwage J, Jokiranta TS, Lehtinen MJ, Zipfel PF, Meri S. The group B streptococcal beta and pneumococcal Hic proteins are structurally related immune evasion molecules that bind the complement inhibitor factor H in an analogous fashion. J Immunol. 2004;172(5):3111–8.
123. Santi I, Scarselli M, Mariani M, Pezzicoli A, Masignani V, Taddei A, et al. BibA: a novel immunogenic bacterial adhesin contributing to group B streptococcus survival in human blood. Mol Microbiol. 2007;63(3):754–67.
124. Henneke P, Dramsi S, Mancuso G, Chraibi K, Pellegrini E, Theilacker C, et al. Lipoproteins are critical TLR2 activating toxins in group B streptococcal sepsis. J Immunol. 2008;180(9):6149–58.
125. Charrel-Dennis M, Latz E, Halmen KA, Trieu-Cuot P, Fitzgerald KA, Kasper DL, et al. TLR-independent type I interferon induction in response to an extracellular bacterial pathogen via intracellular recognition of its DNA. Cell Host Microbe. 2008;4(6):543–54.
126. Gupta R, Ghosh S, Monks B, DeOliveira RB, Tzeng TC, Kalantari P, et al. RNA and β-hemolysin of group B streptococcus induce interleukin-1β (IL-1β) by activating NLRP3 inflammasomes in mouse macrophages. J Biol Chem. 2014;289(20):13701–5.
127. Spaulding AR, Salgado-Pabón W, Kohler PL, Horswill AR, Leung DY, Schlievert PM. Staphylococcal and streptococcal superantigen exotoxins. Clin Microbiol Rev. 2013;26(3):422–47. https://doi.org/10.1128/CMR.00104-12.
128. McCormick JK, Yarwood JM, Schlievert PM. Toxic shock syndrome and bacterial superantigens: an update. Annu Rev Microbiol. 2001;55:77–104.
129. Li H, Llera A, Malchiodi EL, Mariuzza RA. The structural basis of T cell activation by superantigens. Annu Rev Immunol. 1999;17:435–66.
130. Dinges MM, Schlievert PM. Comparative analysis of lipopolysaccharide-induced tumor necrosis factor alpha activity in serum and lethality in mice and rabbits pretreated with the staphylococcal superantigen toxic shock syndrome toxin 1. Infect Immun. 2001;69(11): 7169–72.
131. Shands KN, Schmid GP, Dan BB, Blum D, Guidotti RJ, Hargrett NT, et al. Toxic-shock syndrome in menstruating women: association with tampon use and *Staphylococcus aureus* and clinical features in 52 cases. N Engl J Med. 1980;303(25):1436–42.
132. Davies HD, McGeer A, Schwartz B, Green K, Cann D, Simor AE, et al. Invasive group A streptococcal infections in Ontario, Canada. Ontario Group A streptococcal study group. N Engl J Med. 1996;335(8):547–54.
133. Stevens DL, Ma Y, Salmi DB, McIndoo E, Wallace RJ, Bryant AE. Impact of antibiotics on expression of virulence-associated exotoxin genes in methicillin-sensitive and methicillin-resistant *Staphylococcus aureus*. J Infect Dis. 2007;195(2):202–11.

134. Kaul R, McGeer A, Norrby-Teglund A, Kotb M, Schwartz B, O'Rourke K, et al. Intravenous immunoglobulin therapy for streptococcal toxic shock syndrome—a comparative observational study. The Canadian Streptococcal Study Group. Clin Infect Dis. 1999;28(4):800–7.
135. Inskeep TK, Stahl C, Odle J, Oakes J, Hudson L, Bost KL, et al. Oral vaccine formulations stimulate mucosal and systemic antibody responses against staphylococcal enterotoxin B in a piglet model. Clin Vaccine Immunol. 2010;17(8):1163–9.
136. Labbe AC, Pepin J, Patino C, Castonguar S, Restieri C, Laverdiere M. A single-centre 10-year experience with Candida bloodstream infections. Can J Infect Dis Med Microbiol. 2009;20:45–50.
137. Pfaller M, Neofytos D, Diekema D, Azie N, Meier-Kriesche HU, Quan SP, et al. Epidemiology and outcomes of candidemia in 3648 patients: data from the prospective antifungal therapy (PATH Alliance®) registry, 2004–2008. Diagn Microbiol Infect Dis. 2012;74(4):323–31.
138. Vallabhaneni S, Kallen A, Tsay S, Chow N, Welsh R, Kerins J, et al. Investigation of the first seven reported cases of *Candida auris*, a globally emerging invasive, multidrug-resistant fungus—United States, May 2013–August 2016. MMWR Morb Mortal Wkly Rep. 2016;65(44):1234–7.
139. Skrobik Y, Laverdiere M. Why candida sepsis should matter to ICU physicians. Crit Care Clin. 2013;29(4):853–64.
140. De Pauw B, Walsh TJ, Donnelly JP, Stevens DA, Edwards JE, Calandra T. Revised definitions of invasive fungal disease from the European Organization for Research and Treatment of Cancer/Invasive Fungal Infections Cooperative Group and the National Institute of Allergy and Infectious Diseases Mycoses Study Group (EORTC/MSG) Consensus Group. Clin Infect Dis. 2008;46:1813–21.
141. Nguyen MH, Wissel MC, Shields RK, Salomoni MA, Hao B, Press EG, et al. Performance of Candida real-time polymerase chain reaction, beta-D-glucan assay, and blood cultures in the diagnosis of invasive candidiasis. Clin Infect Dis. 2012;54:1240–8.
142. Morrell M, Fraser VJ, Kollef MH. Delaying the empiric treatment of candida bloodstream infection until positive blood culture results are obtained: a potential risk factor for hospital mortality. Antimicrob Agents Chemother. 2005;49:3640–5.
143. Kathuria S, Singh PK, Sharma C, Prakash A, Masih A, Kumar A, et al. Multidrug-resistant *Candida auris* misidentified as *Candida haemulonii*: characterization by matrix-assisted laser desorption ionization-time of flight mass spectrometry and DNA sequencing and its antifungal susceptibility profile variability by Vitek 2, CLSI broth microdilution, and Etest method. J Clin Microbiol. 2015;53(6):1823–30.
144. Kumar A, Skrobik I, Guzman J, Lapinsky S, Llaupland K, CATSS Database Research Group. The high mortality of candida septic shock is explained by excessive delays in initiation of antifungal therapy. Poster K-2174, 47th ICAAC, Chicago, IL; 2007.
145. Green E, Mecsas J. Bacterial secretion systems: an overview. Microbiol Spectr. 2016;4(1):1–32.

12 Antimicrobial Therapy

Thierry Calandra and Benoît Guery

12.1 Introduction

The management of septic patients requires a comprehensive, multidisciplinary approach based on the five fundamental pillars of sepsis medicine: early recognition of the symptoms and signs of sepsis, the use of rapid and rigorous diagnostic tools, prompt initiation of resuscitation measures and supportive care, timely administration of antimicrobial therapy, and source control. Sepsis is a time trial. Any delay in the five management steps will inexorably translate into increased morbidity and mortality. History-taking and a detailed physical examination will often provide important clues to the identification of the most likely site of infection and help to quickly assess the severity of the infectious process and the need for hemodynamic and organ support. Judicious diagnostic tests, first and foremost sampling of blood, biological fluids, and relevant tissue for microbiological studies, should be performed expeditiously and followed by the prompt administration of broad-spectrum antimicrobial agents. Imaging studies may help ruling in the most likely source of infection and decide whether source control actions are needed, such as percutaneous or surgical drainage of an abscess or debridement of infected tissue. The 2016 update of the international guidelines for the management of sepsis and septic shock of the Surviving Sepsis Campaign provides a very useful framework guiding physicians into the multifaceted elements of the management of the septic patient [1]. The aim of this chapter is to review the rationale, the basic concepts, and the modalities of antimicrobial therapy for patients with sepsis or septic shock.

T. Calandra, M.D., Ph.D. (✉) · B. Guery
Infectious Diseases Service, Department of Medicine, University Hospital and University of Lausanne, Lausanne, Switzerland
e-mail: Thierry.Calandra@chuv.ch; Benoit.Guery@chuv.ch

W. J. Wiersinga, C. W. Seymour (eds.), *Handbook of Sepsis*,
https://doi.org/10.1007/978-3-319-73506-1_12

12.2 Impact of Appropriate Antimicrobial Therapy

Numerous studies have shown that prompt administration of appropriate antimicrobial therapy improved outcome in patients with bloodstream infections (reviewed in [2, 3]). Over the last 50 years, numerous retrospective studies of patients with Gram-negative bacteremia indicated that appropriate antibiotic therapy reduced mortality when compared with inappropriate therapy, which was defined as the use of at least one agent active in vitro against the infecting pathogen [4–16]. More recently, similar findings have also been made in patients with Gram-positive bacteremia [17–19] or candidemia [20–23]. However, one should acknowledge that several studies did not found an association between the appropriateness of antibiotic therapy and patient's outcome [24–28].

A number of potential confounding factors or selection biases may account for these conflicting findings. These studies were characterized by a great deal of heterogeneity in terms of study design (retrospective vs. prospective), inclusion and exclusion criteria, sample size, comorbidities, severity of diseases (sepsis or septic shock), type of infections (community-acquired vs. nosocomial infections including hospital- or ventilator-associated pneumonias, localized vs. systemic infections), causative microorganisms (Gram-negative vs. Gram-positive, monomicrobial vs. polymicrobial infections), definitions (based on in vitro susceptibility with or without consideration of pharmacokinetic and pharmacodynamic parameters), time of assessment of appropriateness of antimicrobial therapy, type of antimicrobial therapy (empirical vs. targeted therapy), and endpoints (morbidity vs. mortality).

Methodological recommendations have been proposed to improve the quality of studies, to facilitate the comparisons of results, and to ease the generalizability of the findings [29]. Studies that have integrated these methodological recommendations have confirmed that inappropriate therapy was associated with increased mortality. For example, in a multicenter prospective study that included 801 episodes of bloodstream infections in 756 patients, inadequate empirical therapy increased mortality at day 14 and day 30 (odds ratios 2.12, 95% confidence interval, 1.34–3.34 and 1.56, 95% CI, 1.01–2.40, respectively) [30]. A systematic review and meta-analysis of 70 studies on the efficacy of appropriate antibiotic therapy for sepsis showed that patients with inappropriate therapy had higher unadjusted (univariate analysis) and adjusted (multivariate analysis) all-cause mortality (odds ratios 2.11, 95% confidence interval, 1.82–2.44 and 2.05, 95% CI, 1.69–2.49, respectively) [31]. A high level of heterogeneity was noted, and study sample size had an important influence on the observed effect of the appropriateness of therapy. Septic shock was the only confounding factor positively associated with odds ratios in a meta-regression analysis.

12.3 Empirical Therapy

Empirical therapy is defined as a probabilistic antimicrobial therapy initiated in the absence of a definitive microbiological documentation of the nature of the infection that is prior to the identification of the causative microorganism and therefore in the absence of antimicrobial susceptibility data.

Timing. The existence of statistically significant relationships between hourly delays in the administration of appropriate antibiotics and outcome of severe sepsis and septic shock has been reported in several studies [7, 8, 15, 16, 32]. A strong association was noted between a longer time until the administration of antibiotics and an increased risk-adjusted in-hospital mortality (odds ratio 1.04 per hour; 95% CI, 1.03–1.06; $P < 0.001$) in the most recent study on the impact of a 3-h bundle of sepsis care [16]. But other studies did not show similar associations [14, 26, 33]. In a meta-analysis of 11 studies that included 16,178 patients, administration of antibiotic within 3 h of emergency department triage or within 1 h of shock recognition was not associated with improved outcome [34]. As mentioned above, many studies are of low quality for a variety of reasons such as the retrospective nature of the analyses, the pooling of patient cohorts, an imprecise or lack of information regarding the appropriateness of therapy, or issues about selection of zero time points.

In the 2016 international guidelines for management of sepsis and septic shock published by the Surviving Sepsis Campaign (SSC), the recommendation is that the *"administration of IV antimicrobials be initiated as soon as possible after recognition and within one hour for both sepsis and septic shock (strong recommendation, moderate quality of evidence; grade applies to both conditions)"* [1]. This is obviously a very reasonable recommendation. However, one should also acknowledge that specific recommendations on antibiotic timing as a metric of quality of care are not supported by very robust data.

Selection of antimicrobial agents. Factors to be taken into account when choosing the initial antimicrobial regimen to be used empirically in patients with suspected infection are presented in Table 12.1. The basic principles guiding the selection of antimicrobial agents are well established. The spectrum of activity should be sufficiently broad to cover all likely pathogens with a reasonable margin of security. Given the large range of elements to be taken into account in the process of selecting an empirical antimicrobial regimen, it is difficult to make specific recommendations. The most appropriate choice may consist of one (monotherapy) or more (multidrug or combination therapy) antimicrobial agents chosen among various classes of antibiotics. These are typically extended-spectrum penicillins with or without a beta-lactamase inhibitor, third- or fourth-generation cephalosporins, carbapenems, fluoroquinolones, aminoglycosides, glycopeptides, lipopeptides, or oxazolidinones.

Table 12.1 Elements guiding the selection of antimicrobial agents in patients with sepsis

• Host factors: underlying diseases/comorbidities, immunodeficiencies (primary or acquired such as immunosuppressive therapy, neutropenia, transplantation), travels, contact with animals, prior hospitalization, immediate past medical history (recent exposure to antimicrobial agents, drug intolerance), presence of implants, or other invasive devices
• Location of the patient at the onset of infection (community or healthcare environment)
• Site of infection
• Severity of the clinical condition (sepsis, septic shock)
• Epidemiological data, local ecology (general and ward-specific)
• Colonization with resistant pathogens
• Pharmacokinetic and pharmacodynamic parameters

Facing the increase in resistance [35], carbapenems should however be considered as second-line drugs [36, 37]. Whenever possible, one should start therapy with microbicidal rather than microbiostatic antimicrobial agents. To ensure broad-spectrum empirical coverage against the most likely pathogens, it is often necessary to opt for a multidrug therapy. In theory, combinations of antibiotics provide broad-spectrum coverage, may exert additive or synergistic effects, and may reduce the risk of emergence of resistant strains [2]. Some classes of antibiotics may also exert immune modulatory effects (macrolides). Multidrug therapy is a sensible therapeutic option when multidrug-resistant pathogens (such as methicillin-resistant staphylococci [MRSA], *Pseudomonas aeruginosa,* or *Acinetobacter* species) are suspected. An increased risk of toxicity, superinfections with resistant bacteria or fungi, and higher costs are classical trade-offs of multidrug therapies. Historically, combination therapy consisted of an association of a beta-lactam with an aminoglycoside. Today empirical triple- or quadruple-agent therapy is often required to make sure that all potential pathogens are covered particularly in an environment where antimicrobial resistance is a major concern.

For empirical therapy, the 2016 guidelines of the SSC recommend *"broad-spectrum therapy with one or more antimicrobials for patients presenting with sepsis or septic shock to cover all likely pathogens (including bacterial and potentially fungal or viral coverage) (strong recommendation, moderate quality of evidence)."* In patients with septic shock, it is suggested to start *"empiric combination therapy (using at least two antibiotics of different antimicrobial classes) aimed at the most likely bacterial pathogen(s) for the initial management of septic shock (weak recommendation, low quality of evidence)"* [1].

12.4 Pharmacokinetic (PK) and Pharmacodynamic (PD) Parameters

According to the 2016 SSC guidelines, it is recommended that *"dosing strategies of antimicrobials be optimized based on accepted pharmacokinetic/pharmacodynamic principles and specific drug properties in patients with sepsis or septic shock (Best Practice Statement)"* [1]. What does that rather general statement imply concretely?

Antibiotics could be classified according to their solubility characteristics as hydrophilic or lipophilic [38]. Hydrophilic molecules like beta-lactams, aminoglycosides, or glycopeptides are affected by changes of the volumes of distribution and of renal function which occur frequently in critically ill patients. On the contrary, lipophilic molecules (fluoroquinolones and macrolides) are less influenced by the volumes of distribution but more often by renal clearance. Antibiotics could also be artificially divided in two groups, concentration-dependent or time-dependent molecules, although some molecules share properties of both groups. For concentration-dependent molecules, the maximum plasmatic concentration (Cmax) over minimum inhibitory concentration (MIC) of the pathogen is the PK/PD parameter associated with clinical success (Fig. 12.1a). For time-dependent molecules, the time over the MIC is the parameter associated with outcome (Fig. 12.1b). We will describe these

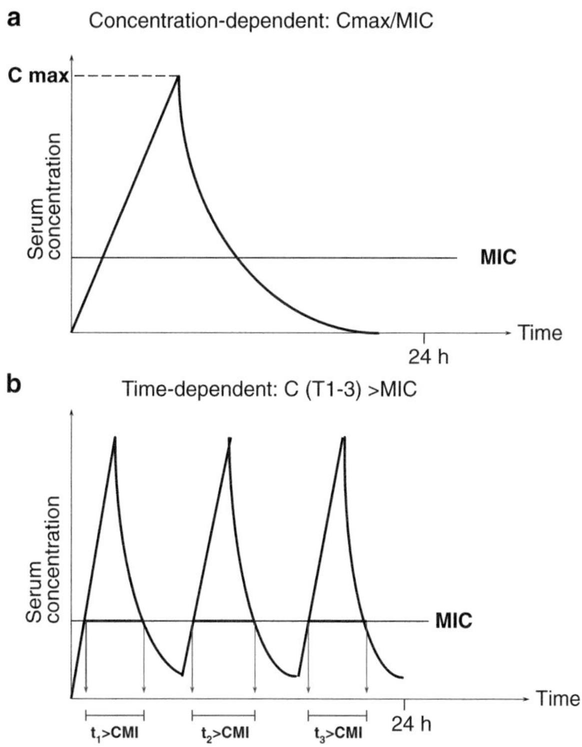

Fig. 12.1 Pharmacokinetic/pharmacodynamic parameters associated with clinical cure. (**a**) Concentration-dependent molecules, (**b**) time-dependent molecules. *Cmax* maximum plasmatic concentration, *MIC* minimum inhibitory concentration, *AUC* area under the curve

two groups underlining the role of the individual dose for concentration-dependent molecules and the rationale of continuous infusion for time-dependent molecules.

Concentration dependence and initial dosage. The best example of concentration-dependent molecules is the aminoglycosides. A seminal paper published in 1987 analyzed the clinical response to aminoglycosides in 236 patients with Gram-negative bacterial infections [39]. The authors showed a graded dose-response effect between an increasing maximal peak concentration/minimal inhibitory concentration (MIC) ratio and clinical response. A ratio greater than 8 was associated with more than 80% of clinical cure. Consistent with those data, when a Cmax/MIC equal to or greater than 10 was achieved within the first 48 h of aminoglycoside therapy, there was a 90% probability of temperature and leukocyte count resolution by day 7 in patients with nosocomial pneumonia [40]. This effect directly related to the Cmax/MIC ratio can be explained by the post-antibiotic effect. Once-daily dosing resulted in high peak concentration exposure and was associated with both an extended post-antibiotic effect and a greater bacterial killing when compared to multiple-daily dosing [41]. Initially described in vitro, this phenomenon of adaptive resistance was then confirmed in vivo in a rabbit endocarditis model [42]. Maximum adaptive resistance occurred between 8 and 16 h after amikacin exposure. After 24 h, bacteria had partially recovered their susceptibility to amikacin. It seems therefore important to use high dosage of aminoglycosides especially in critically ill patients. In patients with severe sepsis or septic shock, a first dose of 11 mg/kg of gentamicin was required to reach a peak plasma concentration equal to or greater than 30 mg/L [43]. This increase of dose is related to the modification of the volume of distribution (V_d) in septic patients. A clear relationship between aminoglycoside V_d and illness severity measured by the APACHE 2 score was also noted in a study of 42 septic patients [44]. Interestingly, in sepsis it must also be emphasized that V_d changes over time. In septic patients, gentamicin intra-patient pharmacokinetics showed that V_d decreased from 0.43 ± 0.12 L/kg to 0.29 ± 0.17 L/kg between the first and the seventh day of treatment [45]. Even with a loading dose of 25 mg/kg of amikacin (the classic dose is 15 mg/kg), a therapeutic target was achieved in only 70% of 74 patients with severe sepsis and septic shock [46]. All these data confirm that high doses of aminoglycosides should be given for 24–48 h (i.e., one or two injections) in patients with sepsis or septic shock. The goal is to be rapidly bactericidal without toxicity. The initial dose should not be decreased to obtain the highest Cmax/MIC ratio.

Fluoroquinolones belong to the group of molecules with concentration-dependent and time-dependent characteristics. In 74 acutely ill patients treated with various dosages of ciprofloxacin, the 24-h area under the concentration-time curve (AUC)/MIC ratio (AUIC) was the most important predictor of efficacy, not the Cmax/MIC ratio or the time above MIC [47]. The results also showed that an AUIC below 125 was associated with low microbiological and clinical cures (26% and 42%, respectively). Pharmacodynamic analyses of ciprofloxacin performed in 42 patients with Enterobacteriaceae bloodstream infections revealed an even higher AUIC threshold than previously suggested [48]. Clinical cure was obtained in 91.4% of the cases if the AUIC was above 250 and in only 28.6% if it was below this value. Like aminoglycosides, the dosage is critical for this group of molecules even though the V_d is less important than for aminoglycosides. Monte Carlo dosing simulations indicated that achievement of therapeutic exposures was dependent on renal function, pathogen, and MIC but that it was not related to critical illness per se [49].

Continuous infusions and time-dependent molecules. In severely ill patients, it is critical to optimize the use of antibiotics based on their PK/PD characteristics. Personalized antibiotic therapy may indeed increase the accuracy of antibiotic dosing and the effectiveness of therapy and improve patient's outcome. Intermittent dosing either as bolus injections or short infusions is the conventional mode of administration of antimicrobial agents. Yet, continuous infusions of time-dependent antibiotics like beta-lactams may increase drug exposure and antimicrobial activity and may result in a better outcome. A review of the medical literature between 2000 and 2016 supports that beta-lactam concentrations higher than five times the MIC for 100% of the time could maximize the efficacy and minimize the emergence of resistance [50].

In agreement with the previous work of several groups of investigators, a prospective, multinational, pharmacokinetic point-prevalence study on eight beta-lactam antibiotics (i.e., time-dependent antibiotics) revealed that 16% of the patients did not have free antibiotic concentrations above the MIC of the pathogen for at least 50% of the dosing interval [51]. The PK/PD endpoints of the study (i.e., antibiotic concentrations above the MIC during 50% and 100% of the dosing intervals) were associated with a positive clinical outcome in multivariate regression models.

Three randomized control trials examined the clinical influence of continuous infusions versus intermittent bolus injections of beta-lactams [52]. Continuous infusions resulted in higher plasma concentrations of piperacillin-tazobactam, meropenem, or ticarcillin-clavulanate than intermittent infusions, which exceeded the MIC of the pathogen in a much larger number of patients (82% vs. 29%, $P = 0.001$) and resulted in a better clinical response (70% vs. 43%, $P = 0.037$) in a prospective, double-blind, randomized controlled trial [52]. In a follow-up study conducted in 25 ICUs with the same antibiotics, the number of alive ICU-free days at day 28 (the primary endpoint) was similar in the continuous and intermittent treatment groups [53]. The duration of bacteremia, the number of alive organ failure-free days at day 14, the clinical cure rates 14 days post-antibiotic cessation, and the 90-day survival were also comparable in both treatment groups. In the third study conducted in patients with severe sepsis who were not on renal replacement therapy, higher clinical cure rates (56% versus 34%, $P = 0.01$) and PK/PD target attainment (day 1 97% versus 70%, $P < 0.001$; day 3 97% versus 68%, $P < 0.001$) were obtained in the continuous infusion group than in the intermittent bolus injection group [54]. A meta-analysis of these three clinical trials showed that continuous infusion of beta-lactams was associated with reduced hospital mortality (relative risk 0.74, 95% CI 0.56–1.00, $P = 0.045$) [55]. Prolonged infusions of carbapenems or piperacillin-tazobactam were also associated with lower mortality (RR 0.59, 95% CI 0.41–0.83) in a meta-analysis of 14 studies comparing extended (equal to or greater than 3 h) or continuous (24 h) versus short (20–60 min) infusions in severely ill patients [56]. In contrast, in two meta-analyses of 14 and 29 randomized controlled trials of time-dependent (beta-lactam antibiotics) or time-dependent and concentration-dependent antibiotics, continuous infusions did not improve outcome [57, 58]. Major methodological weaknesses and biases were noted, such as lack of information about the randomization process, the study blinding, the dosing of antibiotics, and a partial or selective report on data sets and outcome. No recommendation can be made regarding the use of continuous administration of antibiotics before adequately powered randomized clinical studies are performed.

Beside beta-lactams, vancomycin like fluoroquinolones also belongs to the molecules where AUIC is associated with clinical and microbiological cure. The use of intermittent or continuous administrations is still debated [59]. Only one study of methicillin-resistant *Staphylococcus aureus* infections showed that continuous infusion of vancomycin reached the targeted concentration levels faster and with a lower variability than intermittent infusions [60]. The efficacy was not different between the two groups. Like for beta-lactams, a loading dose of 35 mg/kg is required for vancomycin to rapidly achieve a targeted concentration of 20 mg/L if administered in continuous infusions in critically ill patients. To maintain target concentrations, the daily dosage was 35 mg/kg for a patient with creatinine clearance of 100 mL/min/1.73 m^2 [61].

Dosing of antimicrobials. The 2016 SSC guidelines recommend that *"dosing strategies of antimicrobials be optimized based on accepted pharmacokinetic/*

pharmacodynamic principles and specific drug properties in patients with sepsis or septic shock (best practice statement)" [1]. A large number of studies showed that PK-/PD-driven approaches for anti-infective agents are critical in intensive care unit patient and could be associated with improved clinical and microbiological cure. All these approaches rely on plasma concentration and on the MIC of the bacterial strain. There is still a debate whether measuring plasma concentration is enough when we know that only free tissue concentrations at the target site are associated with the therapeutic effect [62]. In fact, plasma concentrations often overestimate target site concentrations. Dosing antimicrobials can be motivated by several reasons: no response to treatment, evaluating toxicity (aminoglycosides and glycopeptides on renal failure risk), drug interactions (rifampicin and immunosuppressors), and targeting a plasmatic concentration (multiresistance). For example, in hemofiltration, it is often difficult to obtain the right dosage. Antibiotic levels will allow a better optimization of the therapeutic schedule [63]. Serum concentrations are important for toxicity, yet several studies have underlined, for example, with aminoglycosides and vancomycin, a major role of the patient's underlying diseases and the effect of combination of toxic drugs [64, 65].

PK/PD and resistance. If PK/PD was mostly used to optimize clinical cure, the recent increase in emergence of resistance led several authors to propose the use of PK/PD parameters to minimize the development of resistance. Most of the initial studies were performed with fluoroquinolones [66]. The notion of mutant selection window was introduced almost 20 years ago. The selection of antibiotic-resistant mutants occurs in a drug concentration ranging from the minimum inhibitory concentration (MIC) of susceptible cells to the MIC of the least susceptible single-step bacterial mutants (defining the mutant prevention concentration, MPC) [67]. The range of mutant selection window (MPC/MIC ratio) varied largely between each couple of drug/bacteria ranging from 6 to 160. This approach provides a conceptual basis to use drugs at concentrations higher than the mutant MPC or to use combination therapy to stay beyond the mutant selection window. While initially described in vitro, there also are in vivo data supporting this concept. In rabbits pneumococcal pneumonia treated with moxifloxacin, the recovery of the mutants was suppressed when the drug concentration exceeded MPC for almost half of the dosing period [68]. The mutant selection window has a large number of potential applications. One would be to optimize monotherapy and also combination therapy. This also is a critical parameter for new drugs, and it should be involved in the design and screening of new compounds [69]. However, we lack well-designed clinical studies showing an improvement on clinical cure and prognosis.

12.5 Targeted Therapy

As its name implies, targeted therapy is defined as the use of one or more antimicrobial agents active against the microorganisms identified as the causative pathogens based on antimicrobial susceptibility data.

Monotherapy versus combination therapy. Is there evidence supporting the use of more than one agent for definitive therapy in patients with sepsis, Gram-negative infections, or microbiologically documented infections caused by problematic bacteria such as *Pseudomonas aeruginosa*? In a retrospective cohort study of patients with bacterial septic shock, combination therapy defined as two antibiotics active against the isolated pathogen was associated with improved outcome [70]. Likewise, several retrospective and observational studies indicated that a survival benefit may be obtained with beta-lactam and aminoglycoside dual therapy in patients with *P. aeruginosa* bloodstream infections (reviewed in [2, 71]). However, important methodological limitations such as the use of different beta-lactam antibiotics in experimental and control treatment groups and a lack of power were noted in many studies. In a post-hoc analysis of 593 single episodes of *P. aeruginosa* bacteremia with adjustment for confounding factors, mortality at day 30 was similar in patients receiving monotherapy or combination therapy (adjusted hazard ratios for empirical or definitive therapy were 1.17, 95% CI 0.70–1.96 and 1.34, 95% CI 0.73–2.47, respectively) [72]. No survival benefit was observed in patients given combination therapy either as empirical or as definitive therapy in a meta-analysis of 19 studies (including eight RCTs) comparing beta-lactam given either alone or in combination with an aminoglycoside or a fluoroquinolone for the treatment of *P. aeruginosa* infections [73]. In the latest Cochrane review on this topic, all-cause mortality (relative risk 1.01, 95% CI 0.75–1.35) and clinical failure (relative risk 1.11, 95% CI 0.95–1.29) were similar in studies using the same beta-lactam in studies comparing beta-lactam monotherapy with a combination of beta-lactams and aminoglycosides for the treatment of patients with sepsis [71]. Similar results were obtained when analyses were limited to patients with Gram-negative infections, Gram-negative bacteremia, or *P. aeruginosa*. Monotherapy was clearly associated with a lower rate of nephrotoxicity (RR 0.30, 95% CI 0.23–0.39). In contrast to expectations, combination therapy did not prevent the development of bacterial resistance (relative risk 0.88, 95% CI 0.5–1.45). Fluoroquinolones have also been used in association with beta-lactam antibiotics providing dual therapy against Gram-negative bacteria including *P. aeruginosa* while avoiding the toxicity caused by aminoglycosides. Combination therapy with meropenem and fluoroquinolone (ciprofloxacin or moxifloxacin) was not superior to meropenem monotherapy in two multicenter studies of empirical therapy for suspected ventilator-associated pneumonia or severe sepsis [74, 75].

In summary, systematic reviews and meta-analyses of patients with Gram-negative sepsis, including *P. aeruginosa* infections, do not indicate that outcome is improved when patients are treated with dual-targeted therapy using antibiotics belonging to different antimicrobial classes. Therefore, the 2016 sepsis guidelines of the SSC suggested that *"combination therapy not be routinely used for ongoing treatment of most other serious infections, including bacteremia and sepsis without shock (weal recommendation, low quality of evidence)"* [1]. The panel also recommended *"against combination therapy for the routine treatment of neutropenic sepsis/bacteremia (strong recommendation, moderate quality of evidence)"* with a remark that *"this does not preclude the use of multidrug therapy to broaden antimicrobial therapy.*" If combination therapy is initially used for septic shock, the panel recommended *"de-escalation with discontinuation of combination therapy within the first few days in response to clinical improvement and/or evidence of infection resolution."* This recommendation applies to *"both targeted (culture-positive infections) and empiric (for culture-negative infections) combination therapy (best practice statement)."* Clearly, the persistent controversy about the place of dual-targeted therapy in the management of patients with sepsis or septic shock is unlikely to be resolved unless adequately powered randomized controlled multicenter trials are conducted.

De-escalation and duration of antimicrobial therapy. De-escalation therapy is an important component of antimicrobial stewardship programs aimed at the prevention of the development of antimicrobial resistance but also at a reduction of drug cost and adverse events. The existing evidence on the clinical and microbiological effects of de-escalation of antimicrobial therapy in patients with sepsis is rather limited. Another difficulty in the interpretation of the available literature is the lack of a standardized definition. De-escalation therapy has been defined as a reduction in the number, the spectrum, or the duration of antimicrobial therapy. In addition, numerous clinical and microbiological criteria have been used to assess the effects of de-escalation therapy. Endpoints have included the resolution of the primary infection, the occurrence of a relapse of infection, the development of superinfections, the emergence of resistant pathogens as part of the colonization flora or as an infecting microorganism, the length of ICU or hospital stay, and all-cause or attributable mortality.

A Cochrane review published in 2013 concluded that there was no direct evidence derived from published randomized clinical trial of the efficacy and safety of de-escalation therapy in patients with sepsis, severe sepsis, or septic shock [76]. Other studies have been published in the meantime. A single-center, prospective, observational study conducted in 712 ICU patients indicated that de-escalation therapy significantly reduced mortality at day 90 (OR 0.55, 95% CI 0.34–0.87, $P = 0.011$) [77]. In a multicenter, unblinded, randomized ICU study conducted in 116 patients with severe sepsis, de-escalation or continuation of empirical antibiotic therapy was associated with a comparable median length of ICU stay (9 versus 8 days, $P = 0.71$), which was the primary study endpoint [78]. But the duration of antibiotic therapy was longer (9 versus 7.5 days, $P = 0.03$), and the rate of superinfection was higher (27% versus 11%, $P = 0.03$) in the de-escalation group than in the continuation group. A small sample size, the selection process of patients, an unblinded treatment allocation, and significant imbalances between treatment groups were some of the limitations of that study [79]. A systematic review of two randomized controlled trials and 12 cohort studies on antimicrobial de-escalation in the ICU confirmed that there was a high degree of variability in the definition of de-escalation therapy. De-escalation therapy was more likely to be used in patients on broad-spectrum or appropriate antibiotics and in patients not colonized with multidrug-resistant microorganisms [80]. De-escalation therapy was associated with a lower relative risk of mortality (0.68; 95% CI 0.52–0.88). Yet, this observation should be analyzed with great caution because of a high degree of heterogeneity regarding key parameters such as the study design, the populations of patients enrolled, and the lack of adjustment for confounding variables. De-escalation therapy was also associated with a lower (OR 0.53, 95% CI 0.39–0.73) unadjusted 30-day all-cause mortality in a systematic review and meta-analysis of bloodstream infections and microbiologically documented pneumonia or sepsis [81]. However, this protective effect on outcome disappeared after adjustment (OR 0.83, 95% CI 0.56–1.16). De-escalation did not impact on the development of antimicrobial resistance, but this analysis was limited to just two studies that provided data on the emergence of resistance during therapy. It is therefore not surprising that the recommendation of the SSC guidelines could not go beyond a "best practice statement" of daily assessment for de-escalation of antimicrobial therapy in patients with sepsis and septic shock [1].

The spectrum of infections in patients with sepsis is quite large, and it explains why few studies have been able to address the question of what constitutes an appropriate duration of antimicrobial therapy in such a heterogeneous patient population. Available data are derived from studies performed in less severe patients with well-defined infections. In that context, the 2016 SSC guidelines suggested that *"an antimicrobial treatment duration of 7 to 10 days is adequate for most serious infections associated with sepsis and septic shock (weak recommendations, low quality of evidence)"* with the caveat that *"longer courses are appropriate in patients who have a slow clinical response, undrainable foci of infection, bacteremia with S. aureus, some fungal and viral infections, or immunologic deficiencies, including neutropenia. (weak recommendation, low quality of evidence)"* [1]. Conversely, shorter courses may also be appropriate in patients who improve rapidly or in whom source control was effective.

References

1. Rhodes A, Evans LE, Alhazzani W, Levy MM, Antonelli M, Ferrer R, et al. Surviving sepsis campaign: international guidelines for management of sepsis and septic shock: 2016. Intensive Care Med. 2017;43(3):304–77.
2. Bochud PY, Bonten M, Marchetti O, Calandra T. Antimicrobial therapy for patients with severe sepsis and septic shock: an evidence-based review. Crit Care Med. 2004;32(11 Suppl):S495–512.
3. Ramphal R. Importance of adequate initial antimicrobial therapy. Chemotherapy. 2005;51(4):171–6.
4. Freid MA, Vosti KL. The importance of underlying disease in patients with gram-negative bacteremia. Arch Intern Med. 1968;121(5):418–23.
5. Bryant RE, Hood AF, Hood CE, Koenig MG. Factors affecting mortality of gram-negative rod bacteremia. Arch Intern Med. 1971;127(1):120–8.
6. Kreger BE, Craven DE, McCabe WR. Gram-negative bacteremia. IV. Re-evaluation of clinical features and treatment in 612 patients. Am J Med. 1980;68(3):344–55.
7. Barie PS, Hydo LJ, Shou J, Larone DH, Eachempati SR. Influence of antibiotic therapy on mortality of critical surgical illness caused or complicated by infection. Surg Infect (Larchmt). 2005;6(1):41–54.
8. Kumar A, Roberts D, Wood KE, Light B, Parrillo JE, Sharma S, et al. Duration of hypotension before initiation of effective antimicrobial therapy is the critical determinant of survival in human septic shock. Crit Care Med. 2006;34(6):1589–96.

9. Castellanos-Ortega A, Suberviola B, Garcia-Astudillo LA, Holanda MS, Ortiz F, Llorca J, et al. Impact of the Surviving Sepsis Campaign protocols on hospital length of stay and mortality in septic shock patients: results of a three-year follow-up quasi-experimental study. Crit Care Med. 2010;38(4):1036–43.
10. El Solh AA, Akinnusi ME, Alsawalha LN, Pineda LA. Outcome of septic shock in older adults after implementation of the sepsis "bundle". J Am Geriatr Soc. 2008;56(2):272–8.
11. Ferrer R, Artigas A, Suarez D, Palencia E, Levy MM, Arenzana A, et al. Effectiveness of treatments for severe sepsis: a prospective, multicenter, observational study. Am J Respir Crit Care Med. 2009;180(9):861–6.
12. Gurnani PK, Patel GP, Crank CW, Vais D, Lateef O, Akimov S, et al. Impact of the implementation of a sepsis protocol for the management of fluid-refractory septic shock: a single-center, before-and-after study. Clin Ther. 2010;32(7):1285–93.
13. Larsen GY, Mecham N, Greenberg R. An emergency department septic shock protocol and care guideline for children initiated at triage. Pediatrics. 2011;127(6):e1585–92.
14. Puskarich MA, Trzeciak S, Shapiro NI, Arnold RC, Horton JM, Studnek JR, et al. Association between timing of antibiotic administration and mortality from septic shock in patients treated with a quantitative resuscitation protocol. Crit Care Med. 2011;39(9):2066–71.
15. Ferrer R, Martin-Loeches I, Phillips G, Osborn TM, Townsend S, Dellinger RP, et al. Empiric antibiotic treatment reduces mortality in severe sepsis and septic shock from the first hour: results from a guideline-based performance improvement program. Crit Care Med. 2014;42(8):1749–55.
16. Seymour CW, Gesten F, Prescott HC, Friedrich ME, Iwashyna TJ, Phillips GS, et al. Time to Treatment and Mortality during Mandated Emergency Care for Sepsis. N Engl J Med. 2017;376(23):2235–44.
17. Kim SH, Park WB, Lee CS, Kang CI, Bang JW, Kim HB, et al. Outcome of inappropriate empirical antibiotic therapy in patients with Staphylococcus aureus bacteraemia: analytical strategy using propensity scores. Clin Microbiol Infect. 2006;12(1):13–21.
18. Shorr AF, Micek ST, Kollef MH. Inappropriate therapy for methicillin-resistant Staphylococcus aureus: resource utilization and cost implications. Crit Care Med. 2008;36(8):2335–40.
19. Paul M, Kariv G, Goldberg E, Raskin M, Shaked H, Hazzan R, et al. Importance of appropriate empirical antibiotic therapy for methicillin-resistant Staphylococcus aureus bacteraemia. J Antimicrob Chemother. 2010;65(12):2658–65.
20. Morrell M, Fraser VJ, Kollef MH. Delaying the empiric treatment of candida bloodstream infection until positive blood culture results are obtained: a potential risk factor for hospital mortality. Antimicrob Agents Chemother. 2005;49(9):3640–5.
21. Garey KW, Rege M, Pai MP, Mingo DE, Suda KJ, Turpin RS, et al. Time to initiation of fluconazole therapy impacts mortality in patients with candidemia: a multi-institutional study. Clin Infect Dis. 2006;43(1):25–31.
22. Labelle AJ, Micek ST, Roubinian N, Kollef MH. Treatment-related risk factors for hospital mortality in Candida bloodstream infections. Crit Care Med. 2008;36(11):2967–72.
23. Zilberberg MD, Kollef MH, Arnold H, Labelle A, Micek ST, Kothari S, et al. Inappropriate empiric antifungal therapy for candidemia in the ICU and hospital resource utilization: a retrospective cohort study. BMC Infect Dis. 2010;10:150.
24. Fang CT, Shau WY, Hsueh PR, Chen YC, Wang JT, Hung CC, et al. Early empirical glycopeptide therapy for patients with methicillin-resistant Staphylococcus aureus bacteraemia: impact on the outcome. J Antimicrob Chemother. 2006;57(3):511–9.
25. Osih RB, McGregor JC, Rich SE, Moore AC, Furuno JP, Perencevich EN, et al. Impact of empiric antibiotic therapy on outcomes in patients with Pseudomonas aeruginosa bacteremia. Antimicrob Agents Chemother. 2007;51(3):839–44.
26. Corona A, Bertolini G, Lipman J, Wilson AP, Singer M. Antibiotic use and impact on outcome from bacteraemic critical illness: the BActeraemia Study in Intensive Care (BASIC). J Antimicrob Chemother. 2010;65(6):1276–85.
27. Cain SE, Kohn J, Bookstaver PB, Albrecht H, Al-Hasan MN. Stratification of the impact of inappropriate empirical antimicrobial therapy for Gram-negative bloodstream infections by predicted prognosis. Antimicrob Agents Chemother. 2015;59(1):245–50.

28. Fitzpatrick JM, Biswas JS, Edgeworth JD, Islam J, Jenkins N, Judge R, et al. Gram-negative bacteraemia; a multi-centre prospective evaluation of empiric antibiotic therapy and outcome in English acute hospitals. Clin Microbiol Infect. 2016;22(3):244–51.
29. McGregor JC, Rich SE, Harris AD, Perencevich EN, Osih R, Lodise TP Jr, et al. A systematic review of the methods used to assess the association between appropriate antibiotic therapy and mortality in bacteremic patients. Clin Infect Dis. 2007;45(3):329–37.
30. Retamar P, Portillo MM, Lopez-Prieto MD, Rodriguez-Lopez F, de Cueto M, Garcia MV, et al. Impact of inadequate empirical therapy on the mortality of patients with bloodstream infections: a propensity score-based analysis. Antimicrob Agents Chemother. 2012;56(1):472–8.
31. Paul M, Shani V, Muchtar E, Kariv G, Robenshtok E, Leibovici L. Systematic review and meta-analysis of the efficacy of appropriate empiric antibiotic therapy for sepsis. Antimicrob Agents Chemother. 2010;54(11):4851–63.
32. Gaieski DF, Mikkelsen ME, Band RA, Pines JM, Massone R, Furia FF, et al. Impact of time to antibiotics on survival in patients with severe sepsis or septic shock in whom early goal-directed therapy was initiated in the emergency department. Crit Care Med. 2010;38(4):1045–53.
33. Kaasch AJ, Rieg S, Kuetscher J, Brodt HR, Widmann T, Herrmann M, et al. Delay in the administration of appropriate antimicrobial therapy in Staphylococcus aureus bloodstream infection: a prospective multicenter hospital-based cohort study. Infection. 2013;41(5):979–85.
34. Sterling SA, Miller WR, Pryor J, Puskarich MA, Jones AE. The impact of timing of antibiotics on outcomes in severe sepsis and septic shock: a systematic review and meta-analysis. Crit Care Med. 2015;43(9):1907–15.
35. Carlet J, Rambaud C, Pulcini C, isotACldd BM-r W. WAAR (world alliance against antibiotic resistance): safeguarding antibiotics. Antimicrob Resist Infect Control. 2012;1(1):25.
36. Pakyz AL, Oinonen M, Polk RE. Relationship of carbapenem restriction in 22 university teaching hospitals to carbapenem use and carbapenem-resistant Pseudomonas aeruginosa. Antimicrob Agents Chemother. 2009;53(5):1983–6.
37. Seah XF, Ong YL, Tan SW, Krishnaswamy G, Chong CY, Tan NW, et al. Impact of an antimicrobial stewardship program on the use of carbapenems in a tertiary women's and children's hospital, Singapore. Pharmacotherapy. 2014;34(11):1141–50.
38. Roberts JA, Lipman J. Pharmacokinetic issues for antibiotics in the critically ill patient. Crit Care Med. 2009;37(3):840–51. quiz 59
39. Moore RD, Lietman PS, Smith CR. Clinical response to aminoglycoside therapy: importance of the ratio of peak concentration to minimal inhibitory concentration. J Infect Dis. 1987;155(1):93–9.
40. Kashuba AD, Nafziger AN, Drusano GL, Bertino JS Jr. Optimizing aminoglycoside therapy for nosocomial pneumonia caused by gram-negative bacteria. Antimicrob Agents Chemother. 1999;43(3):623–9.
41. Karlowsky JA, Zhanel GG, Davidson RJ, Hoban DJ. Postantibiotic effect in Pseudomonas aeruginosa following single and multiple aminoglycoside exposures in vitro. J Antimicrob Chemother. 1994;33(5):937–47.
42. Xiong YQ, Caillon J, Kergueris MF, Drugeon H, Baron D, Potel G, et al. Adaptive resistance of Pseudomonas aeruginosa induced by aminoglycosides and killing kinetics in a rabbit endocarditis model. Antimicrob Agents Chemother. 1997;41(4):823–6.
43. Allou N, Charifou Y, Augustin P, Galas T, Valance D, Corradi L, et al. A study to evaluate the first dose of gentamicin needed to achieve a peak plasma concentration of 30 mg/l in patients hospitalized for severe sepsis. Eur J Clin Microbiol Infect Dis. 2016;35(7):1187–93.
44. Marik PE. Aminoglycoside volume of distribution and illness severity in critically ill septic patients. Anaesth Intensive Care. 1993;21(2):172–3.
45. Triginer C, Izquierdo I, Fernandez R, Rello J, Torrent J, Benito S, et al. Gentamicin volume of distribution in critically ill septic patients. Intensive Care Med. 1990;16(5):303–6.
46. Taccone FS, Laterre PF, Spapen H, Dugernier T, Delattre I, Layeux B, et al. Revisiting the loading dose of amikacin for patients with severe sepsis and septic shock. Crit Care. 2010;14(2):R53.

47. Forrest A, Nix DE, Ballow CH, Goss TF, Birmingham MC, Schentag JJ. Pharmacodynamics of intravenous ciprofloxacin in seriously ill patients. Antimicrob Agents Chemother. 1993;37(5):1073–81.
48. Zelenitsky SA, Ariano RE. Support for higher ciprofloxacin AUC 24/MIC targets in treating Enterobacteriaceae bloodstream infection. J Antimicrob Chemother. 2010;65(8):1725–32.
49. Roberts JA, Cotta MO, Cojutti P, Lugano M, Della Rocca G, Pea F. Does critical illness change levofloxacin pharmacokinetics? Antimicrob Agents Chemother. 2015;60(3):1459–63.
50. Delattre IK, Taccone FS, Jacobs F, Hites M, Dugernier T, Spapen H, et al. Optimizing beta-lactams treatment in critically-ill patients using pharmacokinetics/pharmacodynamics targets: are first conventional doses effective? Expert Rev Anti Infect Ther. 2017;15(7):677–88.
51. Roberts JA, Paul SK, Akova M, Bassetti M, De Waele JJ, Dimopoulos G, et al. DALI: defining antibiotic levels in intensive care unit patients: are current beta-lactam antibiotic doses sufficient for critically ill patients? Clin Infect Dis. 2014;58(8):1072–83.
52. Dulhunty JM, Roberts JA, Davis JS, Webb SA, Bellomo R, Gomersall C, et al. Continuous infusion of beta-lactam antibiotics in severe sepsis: a multicenter double-blind, randomized controlled trial. Clin Infect Dis. 2013;56(2):236–44.
53. Dulhunty JM, Roberts JA, Davis JS, Webb SA, Bellomo R, Gomersall C, et al. A multicenter randomized trial of continuous versus intermittent beta-lactam infusion in severe sepsis. Am J Respir Crit Care Med. 2015;192(11):1298–305.
54. Abdul-Aziz MH, Sulaiman H, Mat-Nor MB, Rai V, Wong KK, Hasan MS, et al. Beta-Lactam Infusion in Severe Sepsis (BLISS): a prospective, two-centre, open-labelled randomised controlled trial of continuous versus intermittent beta-lactam infusion in critically ill patients with severe sepsis. Intensive Care Med. 2016;42(10):1535–45.
55. Roberts JA, Abdul-Aziz MH, Davis JS, Dulhunty JM, Cotta MO, Myburgh J, et al. Continuous versus intermittent beta-lactam infusion in severe sepsis. A meta-analysis of individual patient data from randomized trials. Am J Respir Crit Care Med. 2016;194(6):681–91.
56. Falagas ME, Tansarli GS, Ikawa K, Vardakas KZ. Clinical outcomes with extended or continuous versus short-term intravenous infusion of carbapenems and piperacillin/tazobactam: a systematic review and meta-analysis. Clin Infect Dis. 2013;56(2):272–82.
57. Roberts JA, Webb S, Paterson D, Ho KM, Lipman J. A systematic review on clinical benefits of continuous administration of beta-lactam antibiotics. Crit Care Med. 2009;37(6):2071–8.
58. Shiu J, Wang E, Tejani AM, Wasdell M. Continuous versus intermittent infusions of antibiotics for the treatment of severe acute infections. Cochrane Database Syst Rev. 2013;3:CD008481.
59. Rybak MJ. The pharmacokinetic and pharmacodynamic properties of vancomycin. Clin Infect Dis. 2006;42(Suppl 1):S35–9.
60. Wysocki M, Delatour F, Faurisson F, Rauss A, Pean Y, Misset B, et al. Continuous versus intermittent infusion of vancomycin in severe Staphylococcal infections: prospective multicenter randomized study. Antimicrob Agents Chemother. 2001;45(9):2460–7.
61. Roberts JA, Taccone FS, Udy AA, Vincent JL, Jacobs F, Lipman J. Vancomycin dosing in critically ill patients: robust methods for improved continuous-infusion regimens. Antimicrob Agents Chemother. 2011;55(6):2704–9.
62. Liu P, Muller M, Derendorf H. Rational dosing of antibiotics: the use of plasma concentrations versus tissue concentrations. Int J Antimicrob Agents. 2002;19(4):285–90.
63. Robatel C, Decosterd LA, Biollaz J, Eckert P, Schaller MD, Buclin T. Pharmacokinetics and dosage adaptation of meropenem during continuous venovenous hemodiafiltration in critically ill patients. J Clin Pharmacol. 2003;43(12):1329–40.
64. Jenkins A, Thomson AH, Brown NM, Semple Y, Sluman C, MacGowan A, et al. Amikacin use and therapeutic drug monitoring in adults: do dose regimens and drug exposures affect either outcome or adverse events? A systematic review. J Antimicrob Chemother. 2016;71(10):2754–9.
65. Ong LZ, Tambyah PA, Lum LH, Low ZJ, Cheng I, Murali TM, et al. Aminoglycoside-associated acute kidney injury in elderly patients with and without shock. J Antimicrob Chemother. 2016;71(11):3250–7.

66. Blondeau JM, Hansen G, Metzler K, Hedlin P. The role of PK/PD parameters to avoid selection and increase of resistance: mutant prevention concentration. J Chemother. 2004;16(Suppl 3): 1–19.
67. Zhao X, Drlica K. Restricting the selection of antibiotic-resistant mutant bacteria: measurement and potential use of the mutant selection window. J Infect Dis. 2002;185(4):561–5.
68. Etienne M, Croisier D, Charles PE, Lequeu C, Piroth L, Portier H, et al. Effect of low-level resistance on subsequent enrichment of fluoroquinolone-resistant Streptococcus pneumoniae in rabbits. J Infect Dis. 2004;190(8):1472–5.
69. Drlica K, Zhao X. Mutant selection window hypothesis updated. Clin Infect Dis. 2007;44(5):681–8.
70. Kumar A, Safdar N, Kethireddy S, Chateau D. A survival benefit of combination antibiotic therapy for serious infections associated with sepsis and septic shock is contingent only on the risk of death: a meta-analytic/meta-regression study. Crit Care Med. 2010;38(8):1651–64.
71. Paul M, Lador A, Grozinsky-Glasberg S, Leibovici L. Beta lactam antibiotic monotherapy versus beta lactam-aminoglycoside antibiotic combination therapy for sepsis. Cochrane Database Syst Rev. 2014;1:CD003344.
72. Pena C, Suarez C, Ocampo-Sosa A, Murillas J, Almirante B, Pomar V, et al. Effect of adequate single-drug vs combination antimicrobial therapy on mortality in Pseudomonas aeruginosa bloodstream infections: a post Hoc analysis of a prospective cohort. Clin Infect Dis. 2013;57(2):208–16.
73. Vardakas KZ, Tansarli GS, Bliziotis IA, Falagas ME. beta-Lactam plus aminoglycoside or fluoroquinolone combination versus beta-lactam monotherapy for Pseudomonas aeruginosa infections: a meta-analysis. Int J Antimicrob Agents. 2013;41(4):301–10.
74. Heyland DK, Dodek P, Muscedere J, Day A, Cook D, Canadian Critical Care Trials G. Randomized trial of combination versus monotherapy for the empiric treatment of suspected ventilator-associated pneumonia. Crit Care Med. 2008;36(3):737–44.
75. Brunkhorst FM, Oppert M, Marx G, Bloos F, Ludewig K, Putensen C, et al. Effect of empirical treatment with moxifloxacin and meropenem vs meropenem on sepsis-related organ dysfunction in patients with severe sepsis: a randomized trial. JAMA. 2012;307(22):2390–9.
76. Silva BN, Andriolo RB, Atallah AN, Salomao R. De-escalation of antimicrobial treatment for adults with sepsis, severe sepsis or septic shock. Cochrane Database Syst Rev. 2013;3:CD007934.
77. Garnacho-Montero J, Gutierrez-Pizarraya A, Escoresca-Ortega A, Corcia-Palomo Y, Fernandez-Delgado E, Herrera-Melero I, et al. De-escalation of empirical therapy is associated with lower mortality in patients with severe sepsis and septic shock. Intensive Care Med. 2014;40(1):32–40.
78. Leone M, Bechis C, Baumstarck K, Lefrant JY, Albanese J, Jaber S, et al. De-escalation versus continuation of empirical antimicrobial treatment in severe sepsis: a multicenter non-blinded randomized noninferiority trial. Intensive Care Med. 2014;40(10):1399–408.
79. Timsit JF, Harbarth S, Carlet J. De-escalation as a potential way of reducing antibiotic use and antimicrobial resistance in ICU. Intensive Care Med. 2014;40(10):1580–2.
80. Tabah A, Cotta MO, Garnacho-Montero J, Schouten J, Roberts JA, Lipman J, et al. A systematic review of the definitions, determinants, and clinical outcomes of antimicrobial de-escalation in the intensive care unit. Clin Infect Dis. 2016;62(8):1009–17.
81. Paul M, Dickstein Y, Raz-Pasteur A. Antibiotic de-escalation for bloodstream infections and pneumonia: systematic review and meta-analysis. Clin Microbiol Infect. 2016;22(12):960–7.

Adjunctive Immunotherapy 13

G. P. Leijte, M. Kox, and P. Pickkers

Key Points

- Overall, immunosuppressive therapy has not been found to improve sepsis outcome.
- Dampening of the immune response may be beneficial in selected sepsis patients with evidence of hyperinflammation, e.g., macrophage activation syndrome.
- Sepsis itself induces an immunosuppression, and this is increasingly recognized as an important cause for sepsis morbidity and mortality.
- Innate-immune-enhancing cytokines, GM-CSF and IFNγ have shown therapeutic promise in small clinical trials and case series.
- Adaptive-immune-enhancing molecules IL-7 and anti-PD-1/PD-L1 have shown beneficial results in preclinical studies and are under investigation in currently ongoing trials in sepsis patients.
- Adjunctive immunotherapy should be personalized by determining the immune status of the individual patient.

G. P. Leijte, M.D. · M. Kox, M.Sc. · P. Pickkers, M.D. (✉)
Department of Intensive Care Medicine, Radboud University Medical Center, Nijmegen, The Netherlands

Radboud Center for Infectious Diseases, Nijmegen, The Netherlands
e-mail: guus.leijte@radboudumc.nl; matthijs.kox@radboudumc.nl; peter.pickkers@radboudumc.nl

W. J. Wiersinga, C. W. Seymour (eds.), *Handbook of Sepsis*,
https://doi.org/10.1007/978-3-319-73506-1_13

13.1 Adjunctive Immunotherapies

Apart from antibiotics/source control and supportive measures, a sepsis-specific treatment is lacking. Nevertheless, advances in the management of sepsis and increased compliance with the Surviving Sepsis Campaign guidelines have led to major quality improvements in sepsis care. This has resulted in a significant reduction in the case fatality rate of sepsis [1]. Importantly, mortality rates still remain high, and as sepsis incidence is on the rise, the absolute sepsis mortality over the last decades has increased (Chap. 2 and [2, 3]). Hence, there is still an unmet need for adjunctive treatment for this lethal syndrome [4–8].

The search for a specific immune system-targeting therapy has dominated the scientific field for more than four decades. Over these years, our understanding of the innate and adaptive host response and immunopathology in sepsis has improved tremendously. In contrast to the former belief that sepsis patients predominantly suffer from an exaggerated pro-inflammatory response, it has now become evident that pro- and anti-inflammatory responses are mounted simultaneously and can both be harmful to the patient [5, 8–10]. Furthermore, in many septic patients, even after successful treatment of the primary infection, the host response remains dysregulated, and organ dysfunction and unwanted clinical outcome may ensue. Whether pro-inflammation or anti-inflammation is the overriding detrimental immune response differs between patients and will also evolve over time in individual patients [4]. The prominent role of the dysregulated immune response has been represented in the new definition of sepsis [11], defining sepsis as a life-threatening organ dysfunction caused by a dysregulated host response to infection. In parallel with our increased understanding of the host response in sepsis, many adjunctive immunotherapies have been developed and tested over the last decades. These therapies target specific pathological mediators or pathways that play a role in the immune response and were initially aimed at curtailing excessive inflammation but later on also focused on preventing or reversing immunosuppression. In this chapter, we will provide an overview of the most important adjunctive immunotherapies that have been studied for the treatment of sepsis and discuss future perspectives on this subject.

13.2 Immunosuppressive Strategies

From the 1970s to the turn of the century, it was commonly assumed that a pathogen-induced overzealous pro-inflammatory response resulted in organ dysfunction of the host as "collateral damage". Eventually, mortality was thought to be the consequence of this too pronounced pro-inflammatory response. As a result, therapeutic research in the sepsis field was virtually exclusively focused on dampening or preventing excessive inflammation to prevent tissue damage and to improve survival. Below, we discuss the most extensively studied immunosuppressive therapies.

13.2.1 Corticosteroids

The place of corticosteroids in the treatment of sepsis has been an important subject of debate for decades. The first trial evaluating the anti-inflammatory effects of cortisone during severe infection dates back to 1950 [12], and in the late 1970s, the use of high-dose corticosteroids in 172 septic shock patients showed an impressive reduction in mortality [13]. These findings resulted in the use of high-dose methylprednisolone or dexamethasone as standard treatment for septic shock patients. However, subsequent well-designed and larger prospective clinical trials yielded different results, as they did not reveal any treatment advantage of high-dose corticosteroids on sepsis mortality [14–16]. Strikingly, several studies even demonstrated possible harm associated with high-dose steroid treatment [17–20]. As a result, the use of high-dose corticosteroids as a treatment for septic shock was abandoned [21, 22]. Importantly, low-dose corticosteroid therapy (extensively discussed in Chap. 5) is currently mainly used in refractory septic shock patients aimed to treat relative adrenal insufficiency and not to modulate the immune response, which is therefore outside the scope of this chapter. Nevertheless, in the CORTICUS trial, low-dose hydrocortisone resulted in a higher rate of positive blood cultures following sepsis and the occurrence of secondary infections, illustrating untoward effects of suppression of the immune response even by low-dose corticosteroids [23]. An ongoing study in 3800 septic patients will hopefully resolve the longstanding controversy about the effects of hydrocortisone therapy in sepsis (Table 13.1).

13.2.2 Cytokine-Targeted Therapies

Several promising preclinical studies using antibodies targeting tumor necrosis factor (TNF)α paved the way for clinical development of agents targeting pro-inflammatory cytokines [24, 25]. However, it needs to be acknowledged that these animal studies used endotoxemia as a model for sepsis, and not a more clinically relevant model of polymicrobial sepsis such as cecal ligation and puncture, and in most studies, the cytokine-targeted treatment was administered prior to the endotoxin infusion. Such an approach is clinically not feasible in sepsis patients who arrive in the hospital with overt inflammation before treatment can be initiated. Endotoxemia is a sterile model of systemic inflammation induced by administration of the bacterial cell wall component endotoxin (also known as lipopolysaccharide [LPS]), which results in massive production of pro-inflammatory cytokines such as TNFα, in turn leading to immunopathology and multi-organ failure. Without the presence of living bacteria in the endotoxemia model, animals suffer only from the detrimental effects of the pro-inflammatory response, and it is therefore not surprising that anti-TNFα therapy showed beneficial effects. Perhaps due to these differences between the preclinical studies and clinical practice, treatment with a TNFα-neutralizing fusion protein resulted in increased mortality in septic shock patients [26]. A trial with an anti-TNFα monoclonal antibody fragment showed mild improvements in survival, but only in patients with elevated serum levels of

Table 13.1 Ongoing adjunctive immunotherapy trials in sepsis patients

Agent (study)	Proposed benefit	Study population (stratification)	Primary outcome	Anticipated completion date	Identifier
Anti-inflammatory strategies					
CytoSorb (CASAKI)	Cytokine absorption	124 severe sepsis patients (IL-6 > 1000 pg/mL)	Sepsis-induced acute kidney injury	2017	NCT02588794
Hydrocortisone (ADRENAL)	Combined hemodynamic + anti-inflammatory effects	3800 sepsis patients	90-day all-cause mortality	2017	NCT01448109
Ulinastatin	Urinary trypsin inhibitor	384 sepsis patients	28-day all-cause mortality	2018	NCT02647554
AB103 (ACCUTE)	Inhibits interaction CD28 and bacterial superantigens	290 patients with necrotizing soft tissue infections	28-day mortality	2019	NCT02469857
Thrombomodulin (ART-123)	Combined anticoagulant + anti-inflammatory effects	800 severe sepsis patients (coagulopathy: INR > 1.4)	28-day mortality	2018	NCT01598831
Immunostimulatory strategies					
Recombinant IL-7 (IRIS-7a)	Restore lymphocyte count	15 sepsis patients	>50% lymphocyte increase + mortality	2017	NCT02797431
Anti-PD-L1 Antibody	Reversing T cell exhaustion by inhibition of PD-1/PD-L1 pathway	35 severe sepsis patients	90-day all-cause mortality	2018	NCT02576457
GM-CSF (GRID trial)	Improves proliferation and function of phagocytes	488 severe sepsis (mHLA-DR < 8000 ABs/cell)	ICU acquired infections at day 28	2018	NCT02361528
Thymosin alpha 1 (TEST trial)	Augmentation of mHLA-DR	1106 sepsis patients	28-day all-cause mortality	2019	NCT02867267
BCG vaccination	Enhanced responsiveness of innate immune cells	2200 pediatric patients	Severe illness in the first 14 weeks of life	2020	NCT02606526
Anti-PD-1 Antibody	Reversing T cell exhaustion by inhibition of PD-1/PD-L1 pathway	1200 sepsis patients (lymphocytes ≤ 1.1 × 10^9 cells/L)	90-day all-cause mortality	*Start date: 2018*	–

interleukin (IL)-6 [27]. This relatively early study may have hinted to the future, as it suggests that targeted therapy based on immune status could be the way forward in immunotherapy for sepsis. A similar case could be made for IL-1-targeted treatment. Following promising preclinical and phase II clinical research, a large trial published in 1997 reports that administration of recombinant human IL-1 receptor antagonist failed to reduce 28-day mortality when compared to standard therapy [28]. Interestingly, 19 years later, a post hoc analysis of this study identified that 5.6% of the study population presented with features of macrophage activation syndrome (sepsis with concurrent hepatobiliary dysfunction/disseminated intravascular coagulation), which is representative of hyperinflammation. In this subgroup, mortality was 65% in the placebo-treated patients and 35% in the IL-1 receptor blockade patients ($p = 0.0006$) [29]. Naturally, this is a post hoc analysis, and no definitive conclusions can be drawn, but it does suggest that a specific subgroup of "hyperinflamed" sepsis patients might benefit from inhibition of the immune response.

13.2.3 Endotoxin (Signaling)-Targeted Therapy

The lipopolysaccharide cell membrane component endotoxin that is recognized by the host through Toll-like receptor 4 (TLR4) signaling is regarded as a pivotal initiator of the detrimental hyperinflammatory response in gram-negative sepsis. Therefore, several therapies targeting endotoxin or its downstream immunological effects have been evaluated over the years in several large trials [30]. The CHESS trial did not show an effect of the LPS-binding human monoclonal antibody HA-1A on 14-day mortality in patients with gram-negative septic shock [31]. A murine monoclonal antibody directed against endotoxin (E5) also failed to show improved short-term survival [32]. The most recent study on this subject, the ACCESS trial, investigated the effects of Eritoran, a synthetic lipid A antagonist that blocks binding of LPS to its receptor TLR4. In line with previous anti-endotoxin therapies, Eritoran did not reduce mortality in almost 2000 patients with severe sepsis [33].

13.2.4 Blood Purification Techniques

The removal of inflammatory mediators using blood purification techniques has also been advocated to correct the dysregulated host response in sepsis. Apart from many case series, a few randomized controlled trials have been performed during the last decade. A small study using polymyxin B hemoperfusion aimed to reduce blood endotoxin levels in abdominal sepsis patients showed more swift hemodynamic stabilization and reduced mortality [34], but the study was terminated prematurely, and endotoxin levels were not measured. In contrast to this early study, two more recent and larger randomized controlled trials did not reveal a survival benefit of polymyxin B hemoperfusion in patients with septic shock [35, 36].

13.2.5 Intravenous Immunoglobulins

A recent meta-analysis of 18 RCTs in sepsis patients showed that passive immunization using intravenous immunoglobulins (IVIGs) to improve neutralization and clearance of toxins was associated with a slight reduction in mortality [37]. However, most of the studies had notable limitations. As such, evidence supporting the use of either polyclonal standard IgG or IgM-enriched preparations is currently not available, and this therapeutic option is clinically not implemented in unselected sepsis patients.

13.3 Back to the Drawing Board: Towards Immunostimulatory Strategies

As described above, over the years, dozens of trials have convincingly demonstrated that outright inhibition of the immune response exerts no overall beneficial effects in the heterogeneous group of sepsis patients. During the last decade, observational data suggest that not an excessive pro-inflammatory response, but rather immune suppression, may be the overriding immune dysregulation in a significant proportion of sepsis patients. In addition, most patients do not die in the acute phase, but later on, suffering from uncontrolled primary or secondary (opportunistic) infections [38]. As a result of these more recent insights, sepsis research is increasingly focusing on immunostimulatory treatments aimed to restore the suppressed host response in sepsis. The suppressed immune state is characterized by impaired innate and adaptive immune responses, including impaired phagocyte function, altered *ex vivo* cytokine production, lower levels of monocyte HLA-DR (mHLA-DR) surface expression, and enhanced apoptosis and dysfunction of lymphocytes [5]. This may explain the observation that sepsis patients more likely develop secondary infections with opportunistic bacteria or fungi [38], and up to 43% of patients show positive viral polymerase chain reactions (PCRs) for multiple latent viruses in the blood, including CMV, EBV, and HSV-1, indicating reactivation of these viruses in the days to weeks following their primary bacterial infection [39]. Of note, such a phenotype is normally observed only in transplant patients that receive immunosuppressive medication [40], underlining the severity of immunosuppression in sepsis. The same study also showed that conversion from a negative to a positive virus PCR result was associated with secondary fungal and opportunistic bacterial infections and that ICU length of stay was twice as high in patients who became PCR positive versus those who remained negative [39]. Also, a seminal postmortem study revealed profound suppression of immune cell function in tissues from patients that died of sepsis versus those that died from other reasons [41]. Although this phenomenon, known as "sepsis-induced immunoparalysis", is increasingly recognized as an important immune dysfunction in septic patients [42], its clinical relevance is debated [43, 44], especially the clinical relevance of secondary infections for the patient is questionable, as a recent study demonstrated that the attributable mortality of secondary infections in sepsis may be no more than 10% [45]. Nevertheless, most agree that, at

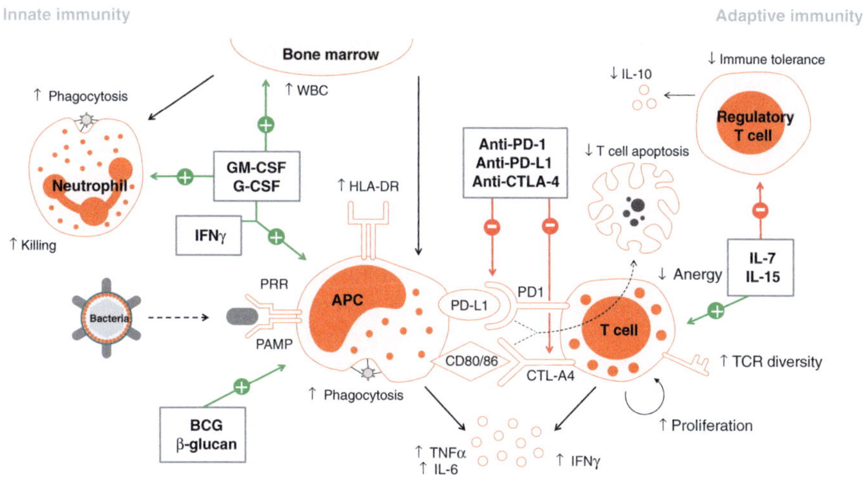

Fig. 13.1 *Immunostimulatory strategies for adjunctive immunotherapy in sepsis.* Sepsis-induced immunosuppression is characterized by impaired phagocyte function, altered cytokine production, lower levels of HLA-DR surface expression, and enhanced apoptosis and dysfunction of lymphocytes. Several immunostimulatory strategies have shown to reverse the suppressive phenotype by acting upon pathways in both the innate and adaptive immune response. *WBC* white blood count, *ROS* reactive oxygen species, *PRR* pattern recognition receptor, *PAMP* pathogen-associated molecular pattern, *HLA-DR* human leukocyte antigen-antigen D related, *APC* antigen presenting cell, *PD-L1* programmed death ligand 1, *PD1* programmed death protein 1, *CTLA-4* cytotoxic T-lymphocyte-associated protein 4, *CD* cluster of differentiation, *TCR* T cell receptor, *BCG* bacillus Calmette-Guérin, *GM-CSF* granulocyte macrophage colony-stimulating factor, *G-CSF* granulocyte colony-stimulating factor, *IFNγ* interferon γ, *TNFα* tumor necrosis factor α, *IL* interleukin

least in carefully selected immunosuppressed patients, immunostimulating therapy represents a viable and attractive treatment strategy. However, to date, the number of clinical studies that have investigated immunostimulatory therapies is very limited. Below, we review these and discuss experimental therapies that are still in preclinical development or being investigated in currently ongoing trials. An overview of the most important immunostimulatory strategies and their mode of action is illustrated in Fig. 13.1.

13.3.1 Pro-inflammatory Cytokines that Enhance Innate Immunity

Recombinant human granulocyte-macrophage colony-stimulating factor (GM-CSF) has been studied in sepsis patients as it possesses many immunostimulatory properties, e.g., it promotes survival, proliferation, and bacterial phagocytosis by neutrophils, monocytes, and macrophages [46, 47]. In one of the few biomarker-guided trials in sepsis, GM-CSF treatment (4 μg/kg/d for 8 days) was initiated in sepsis patients with evidence of severe immunosuppression (characterized by mHLA-DR

<8000 antibodies per cell for two days). GM-CSF therapy significantly increased mHLA-DR expression and improved *ex vivo* LPS-induced pro-inflammatory cytokine production, while release of the anti-inflammatory cytokine IL-10 was not influenced. These effects were associated with a more pronounced decrease in disease severity (APACHE-II), fewer days on mechanical ventilation and a trend toward shorter ICU stay [47]. With 38 patients included, the trial was underpowered to properly assess clinical endpoints. In a pediatric trial, GM-CSF treatment (in selected sepsis patients with a whole-blood *ex vivo* TNFα production of less than 200 ng/mL) restored TNFα production and reduced the incidence of secondary infections [48]. But again, the sample size (17 patients) was very small.

Granulocyte colony-stimulating factor (G-CSF) is also known for its critical role in host defense by enhancing white blood cell count, more specifically by increasing neutrophil numbers and function. In a large sepsis trial in 701 sepsis patients, G-CSF treatment (300 μg/d for 5 days or until leukocytes >$75*10^9$/L) was safe and increased white blood cell numbers, but there was no effect on 28-day mortality [49]. Summed up in a meta-analysis of randomized trials, both G-CSF and GM-CSF therapy showed an improvement of microbial clearance, however, no improvements on 28-day mortality were found in a total of 2380 patients [50].

Interferon (IFN)y is a potent activator of the innate immune system, and it was shown to reverse immunosuppression by restoring mHLA-DR expression and *in vivo* cytokine production in an experimental human model of sepsis-induced immunoparalysis [51]. Up until now, clinical data in sepsis patients is limited to case series, where it was demonstrated to reverse dysfunction of monocytes [52], increase HLA-DR expression [52–54], and improve bacterial clearance [55]. Although limited, these data do suggest that IFNγ may improve clinical outcome in sepsis-induced immunosuppression by restoring the function of innate immune cells, but an adequately powered placebo-controlled randomized clinical trial is necessary before clinical use can be advocated.

13.3.2 Adaptive Immunity-Enhancing Therapies

As immunosuppression is also characterized by apoptosis and dysfunction of lymphocytes [56], several lymphocyte-targeting cytokines are currently under investigation. IL-7 is a potent anti-apoptotic cytokine known to stimulate lymphocyte repertoire diversity as well as T cell maturation and function, which could improve lymphocyte recovery in sepsis patients [57]. Recombinant IL-7 has been shown to improve T cell defects and increase survival in murine models of sepsis [58]. Furthermore, lymphocyte function of septic patients was restored by *ex vivo* incubation with IL-7 [58, 59]. A clinical trial using IL-7 for reconstitution of immunocompetence in sepsis patients is currently ongoing (see Table 13.1). IL-15 is another promising cytokine, as it has anti-apoptotic effects on T cells and natural killer (NK) cells, activates NK cells and CD8 memory T cells, and enhances cellular cross talk [60]. In two murine models of sepsis, IL-15 administration increased plasma IFNγ levels and also the number of NK cells that produced IFNγ. IL-15 increased survival in both these polymicrobial abdominal sepsis and *P. aeruginosa* pneumonia models [60]. Human data is currently not available.

Recent work outlines important parallels between immunosuppression observed in cancer and infectious diseases, such as an increase in regulatory T cells and myeloid-derived suppressor cells, and upregulated expression of negative co-stimulatory molecules [61, 62]. Therefore, targeted therapies that have been evaluated in oncological patients are also emerging in the sepsis field. Intriguing examples are antibodies targeting inhibitory immune checkpoints in order to enhance lymphocyte immunity in sepsis. These inhibitory immune checkpoints are negative regulators of the immune response that maintain self-tolerance, thereby preventing autoimmunity and protecting tissues from immune-mediated injury [5, 8, 9]. An advantage of these immune checkpoint-targeting antibodies is that many have been studied in oncological patients, so the safety and kinetics are known, facilitating the application in sepsis patients. Indeed, there are concerns about immune-related adverse events, such as the cytokine-release syndrome [63]. The most well-known examples of immune checkpoint molecules are cytotoxic T lymphocyte-associated antigen 4 (CTLA-4) and especially the molecules of the programmed death (PD) pathway: PD-1 and its ligand PD-L1 [64, 65]. Sepsis patients exhibit increased expression of PD-1 on T cells, as well as increased PD-L1 expression on monocytes and neutrophils [66, 67]. Recent preclinical work reveals that antibodies against PD-1 or PD-L1 reverse immunosuppression and improve survival in murine models of bacterial [65, 68] and fungal sepsis [65]. Furthermore, *ex vivo* treatment of leukocytes obtained from septic patients with anti-PD-1 or anti-PD-L1 antibodies reverses lymphocyte anergy, reduces apoptosis, and decreases the release of the anti-inflammatory IL-10 [67, 69, 70]. Clinical trials investigating both anti-PD-1 and anti-PD-L1 in sepsis patients are currently ongoing or planned (Table 13.1). CTLA-4 has so far only been investigated in murine sepsis, where it was shown to decrease apoptosis [71] and improve survival [65].

13.3.3 Trained Immunity

Harnessing the non-specific immune modulatory effects of vaccines may be another strategy to improve immunity in sepsis. For instance, the vaccine against tuberculosis, bacillus Calmette-Guérin (BCG), has been shown to protect against childhood mortality, in particular neonatal sepsis, which is not related to its effect on tuberculosis [72]. Recent evidence indicates that the observed effects are due to enhancement of the innate immune response by a phenomenon called "trained immunity". Through this mechanism, BCG vaccination results in functional reprogramming of monocytes to an enhanced phenotype [73, 74]. Upon subsequent *ex vivo* stimulation with an unrelated pathogen, the trained cells show an augmented immune response, even months after the BCG administration [73, 75]. Only one study to date has evaluated the putative immune-enhancing effects of BCG on the *in vivo* immune response [76]. In this study, healthy volunteers were vaccinated with inactivated gamma-irradiated BCG, because the normal live attenuated vaccine may carry the risk of disseminated mycobacterial infection in immunosuppressed sepsis patients. Irradiated BCG did not modulate the *in vivo* response induced by intravenous endotoxin administration [76]. This is possibly the consequence of a less sustained and extensive effect of the irradiated form of BCG.

Recent work indicates that β-glucan, another molecule that induces innate immunity training, reverses endotoxin tolerance *in vitro* and *ex vivo* [77]. In view of the similarities between endotoxin tolerance and sepsis-induced immunosuppression, this finding warrants further investigation as well.

13.4 The Future for Adjunctive Immunotherapy

Most of the therapies that have been investigated in large clinical trials described in this chapter that failed to improve outcome in sepsis are characterized by a similar pattern of promising preclinical studies followed by disappointing phase II and large III trials. As such, immunotherapy, whether immunosuppressive or immunostimulatory, is bound to fail in the undifferentiated very heterogeneous sepsis patient population. In addition, mortality may not be the optimal endpoint to establish beneficial effects in these patients (future clinical trial design will be discussed in Chap. 14). For now, the lack of evidence does not support routine use of either immunosuppressive or immunostimulatory therapies in sepsis patients [50]. Nevertheless, it is conceivable that selected subgroups of patients may benefit from either form of therapy, depending on their immunologic phenotype. Therefore, it is clear that differentiation within sepsis patients is required to move this field forward, and immunophenotyping of patients may pave the way toward a more personalized approach. Immunostimulatory treatment should only be offered to those patients who suffer from a suppressed immune system, and immunosuppressive therapy could be an effective option in a carefully selected group of hyperinflamed sepsis patients.

References

1. Levy MM, Dellinger RP, Townsend SR, Linde-Zwirble WT, Marshall JC, Bion J, et al. The Surviving Sepsis Campaign: results of an international guideline-based performance improvement program targeting severe sepsis. Crit Care Med. 2010;38(2):367–74.
2. Angus DC, Linde-Zwirble WT, Lidicker J, Clermont G, Carcillo J, Pinsky MR. Epidemiology of severe sepsis in the United States: analysis of incidence, outcome, and associated costs of care. Crit Care Med. 2001;29(7):1303–10.
3. Gaieski DF, Edwards JM, Kallan MJ, Carr BG. Benchmarking the incidence and mortality of severe sepsis in the United States. Crit Care Med. 2013;41(5):1167–74.
4. Gotts JE, Matthay MA. Sepsis: pathophysiology and clinical management. BMJ. 2016;353:i1585.
5. Hotchkiss RS, Monneret G, Payen D. Sepsis-induced immunosuppression: from cellular dysfunctions to immunotherapy. Nat Rev Immunol. 2013;13(12):862–74.
6. Payen D, Monneret G, Hotchkiss R. Immunotherapy—a potential new way forward in the treatment of sepsis. Crit Care. 2013;17(1):118.
7. van der Poll T. Immunotherapy of sepsis. Lancet Infect Dis. 2001;1(3):165–74.
8. van der Poll T, van de Veerdonk FL, Scicluna BP, Netea MG. The immunopathology of sepsis and potential therapeutic targets. Nat Rev Immunol. 2017;17(7):407–20.

9. Leentjens J, Kox M, van der Hoeven JG, Netea MG, Pickkers P. Immunotherapy for the adjunctive treatment of sepsis: from immunosuppression to immunostimulation. Time for a paradigm change? Am J Respir Crit Care Med. 2013;187(12):1287–93.
10. Angus DC, van der Poll T. Severe sepsis and septic shock. N Engl J Med. 2013;369(9):840–51.
11. Singer M, Deutschman CS, Seymour CW, Shankar-Hari M, Annane D, Bauer M, et al. The third international consensus definitions for sepsis and septic shock (sepsis-3). JAMA. 2016;315(8):801–10.
12. Hahn EO, Houser HB, Rammelkamp CH Jr, Denny FW, Wannamaker LW. Effect of cortisone on acute streptococcal infections and poststreptococcal complications. J Clin Invest. 1951;30(3):274–81.
13. Schumer W. Steroids in the treatment of clinical septic shock. Ann Surg. 1976;184(3):333–41.
14. Veterans Administration Systemic Sepsis Cooperative Study Group. Effect of high-dose glucocorticoid therapy on mortality in patients with clinical signs of systemic sepsis. N Engl J Med. 1987;317(11):659–65.
15. Lefering R, Neugebauer EA. Steroid controversy in sepsis and septic shock: a meta-analysis. Crit Care Med. 1995;23(7):1294–303.
16. Sprung CL, Caralis PV, Marcial EH, Pierce M, Gelbard MA, Long WM, et al. The effects of high-dose corticosteroids in patients with septic shock. A prospective, controlled study. N Engl J Med. 1984;311(18):1137–43.
17. Wong HR, Cvijanovich NZ, Anas N, Allen GL, Thomas NJ, Bigham MT, et al. Developing a clinically feasible personalized medicine approach to pediatric septic shock. Am J Respir Crit Care Med. 2015;191(3):309–15.
18. Bone RC, Fisher CJ Jr, Clemmer TP, Slotman GJ, Metz CA, Balk RAA. controlled clinical trial of high-dose methylprednisolone in the treatment of severe sepsis and septic shock. N Engl J Med. 1987;317(11):653–8.
19. Sessler CN. Steroids for septic shock: back from the dead? (Con). Chest. 2003;123(5 Suppl):482s–9s.
20. Cronin L, Cook DJ, Carlet J, Heyland DK, King D, Lansang MA, et al. Corticosteroid treatment for sepsis: a critical appraisal and meta-analysis of the literature. Crit Care Med. 1995;23(8):1430–9.
21. Annane D, Bellissant E, Bollaert PE, Briegel J, Keh D, Kupfer Y. Corticosteroids for severe sepsis and septic shock: a systematic review and meta-analysis. BMJ. 2004;329(7464):480.
22. Gibbison B, Lopez-Lopez JA, Higgins JP, Miller T, Angelini GD, Lightman SL, et al. Corticosteroids in septic shock: a systematic review and network meta-analysis. Crit Care. 2017;21(1):78.
23. Sprung CL, Annane D, Keh D, Moreno R, Singer M, Freivogel K, et al. Hydrocortisone therapy for patients with septic shock. N Engl J Med. 2008;358(2):111–24.
24. Tracey KJ, Fong Y, Hesse DG, Manogue KR, Lee AT, Kuo GC, et al. Anti-cachectin/TNF monoclonal antibodies prevent septic shock during lethal bacteraemia. Nature. 1987;330(6149):662–4.
25. Beutler B, Milsark IW, Cerami AC. Passive immunization against cachectin/tumor necrosis factor protects mice from lethal effect of endotoxin. Science (New York, NY). 1985;229(4716):869–71.
26. Fisher CJ Jr, Agosti JM, Opal SM, Lowry SF, Balk RA, Sadoff JC, et al. Treatment of septic shock with the tumor necrosis factor receptor:Fc fusion protein. The Soluble TNF Receptor Sepsis Study Group. N Engl J Med. 1996;334(26):1697–702.
27. Panacek EA, Marshall JC, Albertson TE, Johnson DH, Johnson S, MacArthur RD, et al. Efficacy and safety of the monoclonal anti-tumor necrosis factor antibody F(ab′)2 fragment afelimomab in patients with severe sepsis and elevated interleukin-6 levels. Crit Care Med. 2004;32(11):2173–82.
28. Opal SM, Fisher CJ Jr, Dhainaut JF, Vincent JL, Brase R, Lowry SF, et al. Confirmatory interleukin-1 receptor antagonist trial in severe sepsis: a phase III, randomized, double-blind, placebo-controlled, multicenter trial. The Interleukin-1 Receptor Antagonist Sepsis Investigator Group. Crit Care Med. 1997;25(7):1115–24.

29. Shakoory B, Carcillo JA, Chatham WW, Amdur RL, Zhao H, Dinarello CA, et al. Interleukin-1 receptor blockade is associated with reduced mortality in sepsis patients with features of macrophage activation syndrome: reanalysis of a prior phase III trial. Crit Care Med. 2016; 44(2):275–81.
30. Parrillo JE. Pathogenetic mechanisms of septic shock. N Engl J Med. 1993;328(20):1471–7.
31. McCloskey RV, Straube RC, Sanders C, Smith SM, Smith CR. Treatment of septic shock with human monoclonal antibody HA-1A. A randomized, double-blind, placebo-controlled trial. CHESS Trial Study Group. Ann Intern Med. 1994;121(1):1–5.
32. Angus DC, Birmingham MC, Balk RA, Scannon PJ, Collins D, Kruse JA, et al. E5 murine monoclonal antiendotoxin antibody in gram-negative sepsis: a randomized controlled trial. E5 Study Investigators. JAMA. 2000;283(13):1723–30.
33. Opal SM, Laterre PF, Francois B, LaRosa SP, Angus DC, Mira JP, et al. Effect of eritoran, an antagonist of MD2-TLR4, on mortality in patients with severe sepsis: the ACCESS randomized trial. JAMA. 2013;309(11):1154–62.
34. Cruz DN, Antonelli M, Fumagalli R, Foltran F, Brienza N, Donati A, et al. Early use of polymyxin B hemoperfusion in abdominal septic shock: the EUPHAS randomized controlled trial. JAMA. 2009;301(23):2445–52.
35. Payen DM, Guilhot J, Launey Y, Lukaszewicz AC, Kaaki M, Veber B, et al. Early use of polymyxin B hemoperfusion in patients with septic shock due to peritonitis: a multicenter randomized control trial. Intensive Care Med. 2015;41(6):975–84.
36. Iba T, Fowler L. Is polymyxin B-immobilized fiber column ineffective for septic shock? A discussion on the press release for EUPHRATES trial. J Intensive Care. 2017;5:40.
37. Busani S, Damiani E, Cavazzuti I, Donati A, Girardis M. Intravenous immunoglobulin in septic shock: review of the mechanisms of action and meta-analysis of the clinical effectiveness. Minerva Anestesiol. 2016;82(5):559–72.
38. Otto GP, Sossdorf M, Claus RA, Rodel J, Menge K, Reinhart K, et al. The late phase of sepsis is characterized by an increased microbiological burden and death rate. Crit Care. 2011;15(4):R183.
39. Walton AH, Muenzer JT, Rasche D, Boomer JS, Sato B, Brownstein BH, et al. Reactivation of multiple viruses in patients with sepsis. PLoS One. 2014;9(2):e98819.
40. Humar A. Reactivation of viruses in solid organ transplant patients receiving cytomegalovirus prophylaxis. Transplantation. 2006;82(2 Suppl):S9–s14.
41. Boomer JS, To K, Chang KC, Takasu O, Osborne DF, Walton AH, et al. Immunosuppression in patients who die of sepsis and multiple organ failure. JAMA. 2011;306(23):2594–605.
42. Hotchkiss RS, Opal S. Immunotherapy for sepsis—a new approach against an ancient foe. N Engl J Med. 2010;363(1):87–9.
43. Cohen J, Opal S, Calandra T. Sepsis studies need new direction. Lancet Infect Dis. 2012;12(7):503–5.
44. Xiao W, Mindrinos MN, Seok J, Cuschieri J, Cuenca AG, Gao H, et al. A genomic storm in critically injured humans. J Exp Med. 2011;208(13):2581–90.
45. van Vught LA, Klein Klouwenberg PM, Spitoni C, Scicluna BP, Wiewel MA, Horn J, et al. Incidence, risk factors, and attributable mortality of secondary infections in the intensive care unit after admission for sepsis. JAMA. 2016;315(14):1469–79.
46. Nierhaus A, Montag B, Timmler N, Frings DP, Gutensohn K, Jung R, et al. Reversal of immunoparalysis by recombinant human granulocyte-macrophage colony-stimulating factor in patients with severe sepsis. Intensive Care Med. 2003;29(4):646–51.
47. Meisel C, Schefold JC, Pschowski R, Baumann T, Hetzger K, Gregor J, et al. Granulocyte-macrophage colony-stimulating factor to reverse sepsis-associated immunosuppression: a double-blind, randomized, placebo-controlled multicenter trial. Am J Respir Crit Care Med. 2009;180(7):640–8.
48. Hall MW, Knatz NL, Vetterly C, Tomarello S, Wewers MD, Volk HD, et al. Immunoparalysis and nosocomial infection in children with multiple organ dysfunction syndrome. Intensive Care Med. 2011;37(3):525–32.

49. Root RK, Lodato RF, Patrick W, Cade JF, Fotheringham N, Milwee S, et al. Multicenter, double-blind, placebo-controlled study of the use of filgrastim in patients hospitalized with pneumonia and severe sepsis. Crit Care Med. 2003;31(2):367–73.
50. Bo L, Wang F, Zhu J, Li J, Deng X. Granulocyte-colony stimulating factor (G-CSF) and granulocyte-macrophage colony stimulating factor (GM-CSF) for sepsis: a meta-analysis. Crit Care. 2011;15(1):R58.
51. Leentjens J, Kox M, Koch RM, Preijers F, Joosten LA, van der Hoeven JG, et al. Reversal of immunoparalysis in humans in vivo: a double-blind, placebo-controlled, randomized pilot study. Am J Respir Crit Care Med. 2012;186(9):838–45.
52. Docke WD, Randow F, Syrbe U, Krausch D, Asadullah K, Reinke P, et al. Monocyte deactivation in septic patients: restoration by IFN-gamma treatment. Nat Med. 1997;3(6):678–81.
53. Delsing CE, Gresnigt MS, Leentjens J, Preijers F, Frager FA, Kox M, et al. Interferon-gamma as adjunctive immunotherapy for invasive fungal infections: a case series. BMC Infect Dis. 2014;14:166.
54. Nalos M, Santner-Nanan B, Parnell G, Tang B, McLean AS, Nanan R. Immune effects of interferon gamma in persistent staphylococcal sepsis. Am J Respir Crit Care Med. 2012;185(1):110–2.
55. Jarvis JN, Meintjes G, Rebe K, Williams GN, Bicanic T, Williams A, et al. Adjunctive interferon-gamma immunotherapy for the treatment of HIV-associated cryptococcal meningitis: a randomized controlled trial. AIDS (London, England). 2012;26(9):1105–13.
56. Monneret G, Venet FA. rapidly progressing lymphocyte exhaustion after severe sepsis. Crit Care. 2012;16(4):140.
57. Venet F, Foray AP, Villars-Mechin A, Malcus C, Poitevin-Later F, Lepape A, et al. IL-7 restores lymphocyte functions in septic patients. J Immunol. 2012;189(10):5073–81.
58. Unsinger J, McGlynn M, Kasten KR, Hoekzema AS, Watanabe E, Muenzer JT, et al. IL-7 promotes T cell viability, trafficking, and functionality and improves survival in sepsis. J Immunol. 2010;184(7):3768–79.
59. Kasten KR, Prakash PS, Unsinger J, Goetzman HS, England LG, Cave CM, et al. Interleukin-7 (IL-7) treatment accelerates neutrophil recruitment through gamma delta T-cell IL-17 production in a murine model of sepsis. Infect Immun. 2010;78(11):4714–22.
60. Inoue S, Unsinger J, Davis CG, Muenzer JT, Ferguson TA, Chang K, et al. IL-15 prevents apoptosis, reverses innate and adaptive immune dysfunction, and improves survival in sepsis. J Immunol. 2010;184(3):1401–9.
61. Mellman I, Coukos G, Dranoff G. Cancer immunotherapy comes of age. Nature. 2011;480(7378):480–9.
62. Hotchkiss RS, Moldawer LL. Parallels between cancer and infectious disease. N Engl J Med. 2014;371(4):380–3.
63. Kroschinsky F, Stolzel F, von Bonin S, Beutel G, Kochanek M, Kiehl M, et al. New drugs, new toxicities: severe side effects of modern targeted and immunotherapy of cancer and their management. Crit Care. 2017;21(1):89.
64. Postow MA, Callahan MK, Wolchok JD. Immune checkpoint blockade in cancer therapy. J Clin Oncol. 2015;33(17):1974–82.
65. Chang KC, Burnham CA, Compton SM, Rasche DP, Mazuski R, Mcdonough J, et al. Blockade of the negative co-stimulatory molecules PD-1 and CTLA-4 improves survival in primary and secondary fungal sepsis. Crit Care. 2013;17(3):R85.
66. Wang JF, Li JB, Zhao YJ, Yi WJ, Bian JJ, Wan XJ, et al. Up-regulation of programmed cell death 1 ligand 1 on neutrophils may be involved in sepsis-induced immunosuppression: an animal study and a prospective case-control study. Anesthesiology. 2015;122(4):852–63.
67. Zhang Y, Li J, Lou J, Zhou Y, Bo L, Zhu J, et al. Upregulation of programmed death-1 on T cells and programmed death ligand-1 on monocytes in septic shock patients. Critical care. 2011;15(1):R70.
68. Zhang Y, Zhou Y, Lou J, Li J, Bo L, Zhu K, et al. PD-L1 blockade improves survival in experimental sepsis by inhibiting lymphocyte apoptosis and reversing monocyte dysfunction. Crit Care. 2010;14(6):R220.

69. Hotchkiss RS, Monneret G, Payen D. Immunosuppression in sepsis: a novel understanding of the disorder and a new therapeutic approach. Lancet Infect Dis. 2013;13(3):260–8.
70. Chang K, Svabek C, Vazquez-Guillamet C, Sato B, Rasche D, Wilson S, et al. Targeting the programmed cell death 1: programmed cell death ligand 1 pathway reverses T cell exhaustion in patients with sepsis. Crit Care. 2014;18(1):R3.
71. Inoue S, Bo L, Bian J, Unsinger J, Chang K, Hotchkiss RS. Dose-dependent effect of anti-CTLA-4 on survival in sepsis. Shock. 2011;36(1):38–44.
72. Breiman RF, Streatfield PK, Phelan M, Shifa N, Rashid M, Yunus M. Effect of infant immunisation on childhood mortality in rural Bangladesh: analysis of health and demographic surveillance data. Lancet. 2004;364(9452):2204–11.
73. Kleinnijenhuis J, Quintin J, Preijers F, Joosten LA, Ifrim DC, Saeed S, et al. Bacille Calmette-Guerin induces NOD2-dependent nonspecific protection from reinfection via epigenetic reprogramming of monocytes. Proc Natl Acad Sci U S A. 2012;109(43):17537–42.
74. Kleinnijenhuis J, Quintin J, Preijers F, Benn CS, Joosten LA, Jacobs C, et al. Long-lasting effects of BCG vaccination on both heterologous Th1/Th17 responses and innate trained immunity. J Innate Immun. 2014;6(2):152–8.
75. Netea MG, Quintin J, van der Meer JW. Trained immunity: a memory for innate host defense. Cell Host Microbe. 2011;9(5):355–61.
76. Hamers LA, Kox M, Arts RJ, Blok B, Leentjens J, Netea MG, et al. Gamma-irradiated bacille Calmette-Guerin vaccination does not modulate the innate immune response during experimental human endotoxemia in adult males. J Immunol Res. 2015;2015:261864.
77. Novakovic B, Habibi E, Wang SY, Arts RJ, Davar R, Megchelenbrink W, et al. beta-glucan reverses the epigenetic state of LPS-induced immunological tolerance. Cell. 2016;167(5):1354–68.e14.

Part IV

Sepsis in the Coming Decade

Novel Trial Design in Sepsis

14

Christopher W. Seymour and Derek C. Angus

Key Points

- Large, randomized clinical trials in sepsis have found few successful therapeutics in the past decade.
- Traditional randomized trials of novel therapies, both in sepsis and in other fields, typically test a single drug or intervention in a single, and often narrowly defined, patient population, randomizing patients evenly to intervention versus control.
- Newer designs in other fields have incorporated features to improve efficiency, such as the testing of multiple agents with a common control arm, the testing of a single agent within different patient subgroups, or the testing of agents within patients with different diseases but common mechanisms of action. Other features include randomization schemes that adapt over time, typically using Bayesian inference rules, to preferentially assign better performing agents within different subgroups.
- These designs may be ideal to test new precision interventions in sepsis phenotypes, although rapid patient phenotyping will be required to enable more sophisticated randomization schemes.
- Electronic health records found in many large healthcare systems are well-positioned to help deploy adaptive trials with point-of-care efficiency.

C. W. Seymour, M.D., M.Sc. (✉) · D. C. Angus, M.D., M.P.H.
Department of Critical Care Medicine, The Clinical Research, Investigation, and Systems Modeling of Acute Illness (CRISMA) Center, University of Pittsburgh School of Medicine, Pittsburgh, PA, USA
e-mail: seymourcw@upmc.edu

W. J. Wiersinga, C. W. Seymour (eds.), *Handbook of Sepsis*,
https://doi.org/10.1007/978-3-319-73506-1_14

14.1 Introduction

Sepsis is a life-threatening condition that arises when the body's response to infection injures its own tissues and organs [1]. Not all septic patients present the same [2], and there is profound variability in the signs and symptoms of overwhelming infection. A "one-size-fits-all" approach to treatment ignores this heterogeneity across patients and remains the enrollment strategy in most recent clinical trials [3]. These traditional trial designs often test a single intervention in a single cohort of patients and randomize patients in a fixed ratio. To date, few trials, if any, have delivered compelling new interventions to save lives in sepsis. Future gains, however, may come from novel trial designs that use new approaches to randomization, live perpetually in the electronic health record, and become a platform to test a suite of precision interventions among different sepsis phenotypes. In this chapter, we will review the strengths and weaknesses of traditional trials and discuss both the rationale and current experience with newer trial designs.

14.2 What Makes Sepsis a Challenge for Clinical Trials?

The pathobiology of sepsis is complex [4]. The specific response in each patient depends on the pathogen (load and virulence) and the host (genetic composition and comorbidity), with different responses at both the local and systemic levels. The host response will also evolve over time with the clinical course of the patient [5]. At a simplistic level, inflammation directed at eliminating pathogens may be responsible for "collateral" tissue damage in sepsis, whereas anti-inflammatory responses may lead to enhanced susceptibility to secondary infections that occur later in the course. These mechanisms can be characterized as an interplay between two "fitness costs": direct pathogen damage to organs and damage to organs from the host immune response [6]. The results are clinical manifestations of multiorgan system dysfunction, coagulation abnormalities, or even immune suppression [4].

As a result, no two sepsis patients are the same, and incredible complexity underlies the clinical diagnosis. The Sepsis-3 definition includes a "dysregulated host response," "causal relationship to infection," and "two or more sequential organ failure assessment score (SOFA) points" [7, 8]. A clinician must identify two criteria across more than six organ systems, which can lead to numerous combinations. These combinations also occur in patients with increasing multimorbidity, a condition of chronic comorbidity found in more 30% of ICU patients [9]. Such heterogeneity in the host, host response, and pathogen among a cohort of patients thought to be septic is a significant challenge for clinical trials, particularly those testing a therapeutic or intervention targeting a specific mechanism. In fact, across the myriad of presentations, a single drug may work in some, work variably in others, may have no effect, and potentially even be harmful in other presentations. If these factors are not measured, nor accounted for in trial design, the likelihood of uncovering new therapeutic effects is low. For example, in an in silico set of sepsis trials, if host genetic variation and pathogen features are not measured, two otherwise trials may find opposing results (e.g., net gain vs. net harm) [10].

One example of how potential treatment effects could be missed inside large sepsis clinical trials is the case of glucocorticoids in refractory septic shock. There is a meta-analysis that suggests a benefit; however, a large clinical trial—CORTICUS—showed no benefit [11]. This trial enrolled patients with clinical evidence of infection, evidence of a systemic response to infection, the onset of shock within the previous 72 h (as defined by a systolic blood pressure of <90 mmHg despite adequate fluid replacement or a need for vasopressors for at least 1 h), and hypoperfusion or organ dysfunction attributable to sepsis. CORTICUS was neutral, and likely contributing to this result was the lack of acknowledgment that patients may have a primarily inflammatory, primarily immune suppressed, or mixed phenotypes. These patient groups could be identified using biologic signatures and may have had vastly different responses to glucocorticoid replacement.

As in CORTICUS, there may be hidden groups or "phenotypes" of patients that cluster together with similar features within the broad set of inclusion criteria. From the perspective of a trialist, phenotypes are defined as a set of clinical characteristics or presenting features that group some subjects together and not others—prior to enrollment [12]. If a specific biologic mechanism is known to account for these characteristics, the groups are referred to as an endotype. In sepsis and septic shock, phenotypes and endotypes are now described in both pediatric and adult subjects, using a variety of gene expression, metabolomics, or even electronic health record data [13, 14]. An example of how electronic health record data can lead to "setting" of septic patients is shown in Fig. 14.1 using self-organizing maps. These data included only clinical, laboratory data, and vital signs for inputs, and differential colorimetric patterns reveal like and unlike patients (Fig. 14.1).

Others have used clinical trial data to derive phenotypes and then explore for treatment effects that may be differential across groups [15]. For example, in acute respiratory distress syndrome, a specific phenotype identified using inflammatory biomarkers and hypotension suggests a differential response to positive end expiratory pressure (PEEP) and fluid therapy in re-analyses of the ALVEOLI, FACTT, and ARMA trials [16, 17]. These promising findings suggest that traditional trials may be missing important treatment effects, and new strategies may be required to embrace heterogeneity and hidden phenotypes, not only in post hoc analysis but in pretrial design and simulation.

14.3 Important Features of Traditional Trials

The short-term mortality from sepsis remains near 40% in the sickest patients [18]. Traditional randomized trials have sought ways to improve these outcomes using causal inference. However, countless trials in the past two decades were neutral, with no positive treatment effects [19]. Important priorities in the design of recent trials included a balancing of covariates (e.g., baseline factors, comorbidities) across treated and untreated groups and appropriate estimation of baseline outcome rates and proposed treatment effects. A group of experts brought together by the European Drug Development Hub found [20] that despite efforts to control bias and adequately power, multiple other reasons contributed to the lack of survival improvement in sepsis trials (Table 14.1).

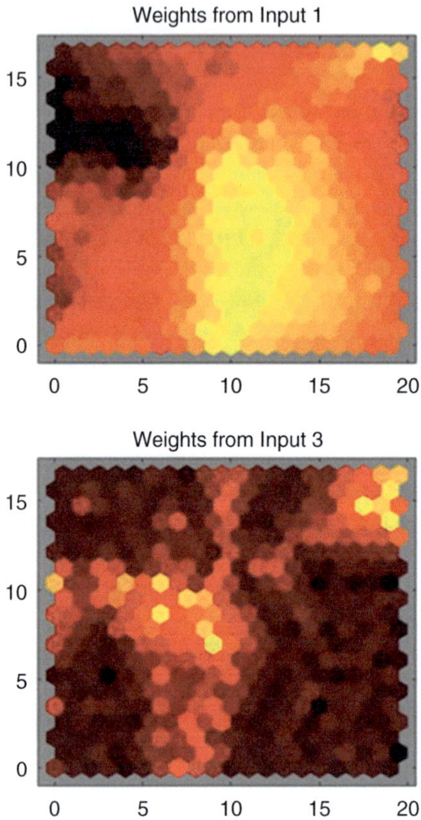

Fig. 14.1 Example of how four different clinical features can cluster septic patients in the emergency department when analyzed using self-organizing maps. Each input, numbered 1 through 4, represents a single clinical feature (e.g., heart rate, systolic blood pressure, serum lactate) on which more than 21,000 ED encounters are clustered. Color scale represents encounters that have similar values and are clustered together

Table 14.1 Reasons for lack of survival improvement in recent sepsis trials[a]

Declining baseline mortality rates in sepsis and septic shock
Suboptimal preclinical models of sepsis
Evolving knowledge of the pathophysiology of sepsis and mechanisms to target with new therapeutics
Heterogeneity in the pathobiology and source of sepsis
Low probability that a single treatment targeting a specific mechanism can influence all-cause mortality

[a]Adapted from Mebezaa et al., *J Intensive Care Med*, 2016, the European Drug Development Hub Conference, Paris, 2015

14.3.1 Narrowing or Narrowing in?

The heterogeneity of the septic population may lead to a Goldilocks phenomenon, where trialists often fail to design the trial for the "right" population. For example, in the ACCESS trial of eritoran, a toll-like receptor-4 antagonist, enrollment was restricted to septic patients with three or more SIRS criteria, one or more organ dysfunctions, and an APACHE II (Acute Physiology and Chronic Health Evaluation) score of at least 21 and not greater than 37 [21]. This is an example of "narrowing." These criteria were informed by an earlier phase 2 trial but significantly restricted the potential population of septic patients. Even though there was no significant difference in the primary endpoint of 28-day all-cause mortality with 28.1% (366/1304) in the eritoran group vs. 26.9% (177/657) in the placebo group, it is unknown if the effect of this drug in patients is lower APACHE II scores or two instead of three SIRS criteria. What is also unknown is whether the a priori narrowing of criteria resulted in a trial "narrowed in" to the population most likely to benefit. Due to the cost and infrastructure required for a future trial, these effects may never be known.

14.3.2 Enrolling Too Broad?

On the other hand, trials also may enroll patients with too broad of criteria, and the potential treatment effects may be diluted. For example, in a phase 3 trial of recombinant IL-1 receptor antagonist (anakinra), investigators randomized septic patients to receive standard supportive care versus anakinra and terminated the trial early as they were unlikely to reach the primary endpoint of reduced 28-day mortality [22]. This was the case in multiple a priori subgroups. Yet, new research in pediatric sepsis and rheumatology suggested that certain septic patients with features of macrophage activating syndrome (MAS) may have a pathophysiologic mechanism targeted by this drug [23]. This MAS phenotype was not known to investigators, effectively hidden inside their trial data. A subsequent re-analysis found a 30% absolute reduction in mortality among the group with criteria similar to MAS (i.e., disseminated intravascular coagulation and/or hepatobiliary dysfunction) compared to those without MAS [24].

Multiple other design issues also challenge traditional trials, including the choice of interventions and fixed randomization ratios. The typical approach is to take a single intervention and randomize patients to the new drug/intervention versus untreated. And yet, even if the trial is "positive," this single intervention trial may not always lead to timely practice change nor have findings replicated in subsequent trials. The resulting timeline may span multiple years, from planning to obtaining funding to validation in new sites, before findings are incorporated in clinical practice guidelines. For example, the PRISM trials (e.g., ProCESS, ARISE, and ProMISe) [25] and their meta-analysis were designed and received funding from

2005 to 2007, were published in 2015, and now contribute to international clinical practice guidelines more than 12 years later [26]. It is during this long period that background outcomes rates may change, thus impacting the power for the planned recruitment. Another issue that extends the timeline of traditional trials is a fixed 1:1 randomization ratio between intervention and control. Such equal allocation has long been the norm, believed to preserve power, internal validity, and postrandomization agnosticism by patients, caregivers, and outcome assessors as to allocation [27, 28]. It remains optimal for trials with only two arms but may lose these benefits for trials with multiple arms (>2). Also, the reliance on equal randomization may not match patient preferences, who may desire the "new" drug or an expert to decide the proper treatment. This approach also ignores potential knowledge about treatment effects that could be gleaned *during* the trial itself, perhaps assigning patients to the inferior therapy longer than necessary. As suggested by Lewis et al., the primary scientific goal of a clinical trial should not be compromised, but interim information available in a trial could be used to improve the outcomes of trial participants, especially those who enroll later in the trial [28].

14.4 Novel Trial Designs Are the Future in Sepsis

Many of the limitations of traditional trials in sepsis could theoretically be addressed using novel, efficient designs that incorporate multiple interventions and combinations of treatments in heterogeneous populations. These trials can be described using multiple terms but generally are referred to as "adaptive" trials, as key characteristics can be modified using prespecified rules in response to information accumulated during the trial itself. An extension of adaptive trials is a platform trial, which focuses not on a specific intervention or set of interventions but rather on the disease. Multiple tools are used to integrate information inside the "platform," so that multiple interventions can be evaluated simultaneously or in succession. The below sections will discuss both adaptive and platform trials in more detail with examples, as well as close relatives called umbrella or basket trials.

14.5 What Is an Adaptive Trial?

In general, an adaptive clinical trial is in which key characteristics are adjusted while enrollment in the trial is ongoing, using prospectively defined rules and in response to data collected during the trial (Fig. 14.2) [29]. This includes the randomization ratio, number of treatment groups, number and frequency of interim analyses, and even the patient subpopulation being considered. To achieve standard statistical operating characteristics, such as control of the trial's false-positive rate, the trial adaptations are entirely prespecified using extensive simulation. These simulations draw from in silico populations where the candidate treatment effect has an assigned effect, such as harm, benefit, or no effect. Then, the collective set of simulated trials that lead to correct or incorrect results according to the simulated "truth" lead to statistical estimates of error.

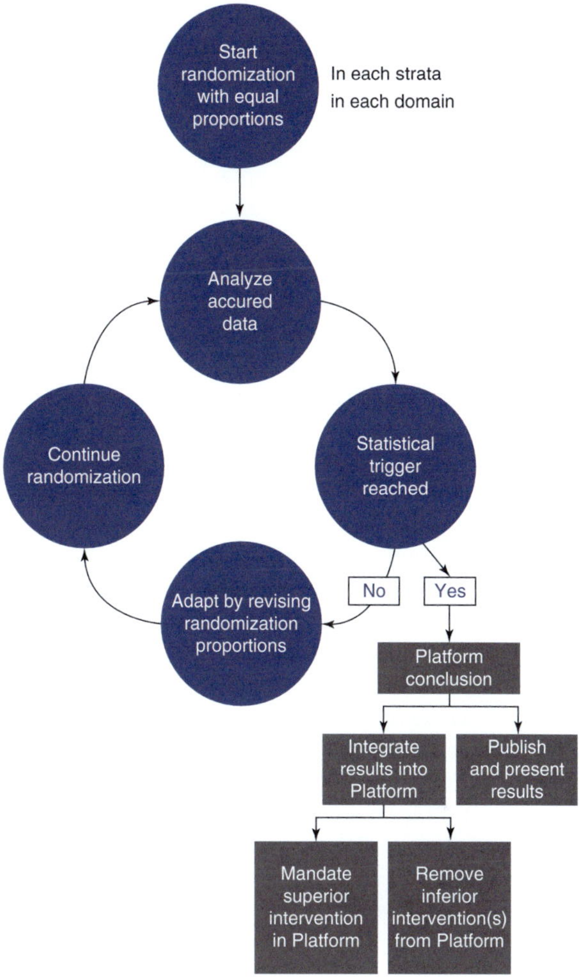

Fig. 14.2 Schematic of an adaptive platform trial. In this schematic, a trial begins with a fixed randomization ratio ("burn-in" period), and as the trial accrues data, different prespecified triggers are reached, and randomization probabilities are updated in response-adaptive randomization (dark-blue circle). When interventions are moved through the trial (gray boxes), they can be excluded for futility, graduated to confirmatory trials, or integrated into clinical practice/standard therapy as results dictate

One important adaptation is called response-adaptive randomization (RAR), where the randomization ratio used to allocate subjects across treatments can be changed during the trial so that the probability that participants who enroll later receive the treatment that is ultimately found to be performing well [30]. Response-adaptive randomization is rooted in the "play the winner" concept, a technique used in the early trial of extracorporeal membrane oxygenation (ECMO) in neonatal respiratory failure [31]. In this small randomized clinical trial, when a child who received ECMO survived, the next subject was allocated to that arm. If a child died, the study assigned the next patient to the alternate treatment—conservative care. In the 1990s, the design was criticized by many in the literature, leading to a larger validation that confirmed the survival advantage of ECMO [32]. In retrospect, this example of "play the winner" was far too small a study and is different than a design that incorporates uncertainty, where one might "probably play what is probably the winner." Two decades later, RAR builds on these concepts and seeks to maximize the risk-benefit ratio for the enrolling subject while attempting to shorten the study duration necessary for appropriately powered causal inference. In Fig. 14.3, we show an example of the relationship between power and sample size for a theoretical trial of antibiotics in sepsis, where a fixed randomization ratio is compared to a design using RAR. Important, however, is the requirement that changes to the randomization ratio are decided upon before the trial starts. The outcome of subjects must also be accumulated in a timely manner. For example, adapting randomization ratios to 1-year mortality may not be practical, and some trials may use surrogate or biomarkers for these prespecified decisions.

Another important feature of adaptive trials is the capacity to test treatments within specific groups or phenotypes, some of which may be either known before the trial or even derived during the trial itself. This approach is called "enrichment," where subjects are screened for the presence or absence of a particular marker, characteristic, or profile, and when present, treatment arms can be targeted to these specific groups. This results in a stratification of the study population. This design feature is the solution to the broad heterogeneity in sepsis discussed earlier, where an all-comer approach could miss treatment effects in specific subgroups or continue to randomize patients without the marker to receive an ineffective treatment [15].

There are different methods to enrich a study population. As described by the Food and Drug Administration [33], enrichment can fall into three broad categories. First, one can reduce heterogeneity by selecting patients within a narrower range. An example of this is the MONARCs trial of an antitumor necrosis factor monoclonal antibody, where only severe sepsis patients with elevated IL-6 were enrolled [34]. This approach could theoretically increase study power but requires certainty that (a) the biomarker actually identifies the population most likely to benefit and (b) the optimal cut-off is chosen a priori. Second, the population could be enriched for those more likely to have the study-related endpoint—called prognostic enrichment. This approach will increase the absolute event rates, but not the relative difference in outcomes. An example is the CONSENSUS trial of enalapril in high-risk subjects with congestive heart failure [35]. By enrolling only those with NYHA class IV, the investigators found a 40% reduction in mortality and hospitalization in only 253 patients. And third, enrichment could lean on biomarkers termed "drug responsive," where they identify some aspect of the patient's physiology closely linked to the putative target of the candidate treatment. This is called predictive enrichment and not only increases study efficiency but also enhances the risk-benefit ratio for the subject compared to an overall population agnostic to the marker. A recent example of the use of pathophysiologic selection is the serine/threonine-protein kinase *BRAF* mutation to identify potential responders to vemurafenib in melanoma. In early studies, patients with *BRAF* who received the drug had an improved tumor response, and in a subsequent phase 3 trial, the design enriched for only those with the *BRAF* to test vemurafenib versus standard therapy [36]. This trial was subsequently stopped at interim analyses for a 63% reduction in death with vemurafenib. All enrichment methods require the enrichment strategy (e.g., prognostic, predictive) to behave as thought, and this may not always be the case. In fact, using tools like response-adaptive randomization, the optimal threshold for biomarkers and their role as drug responsive can be "learned" during the conduct of the trial itself.

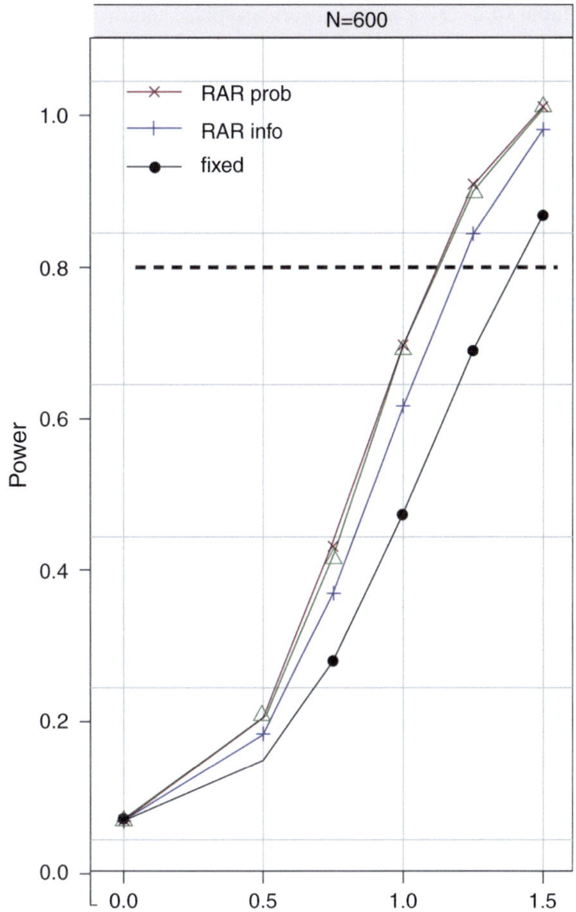

Fig. 14.3 Simulation of response-adaptive randomization in a hypothetical sepsis trial. Schematic showing the gains in trial power (y axis) of a hypothetical trial of early vs. delayed antibiotic and fluid therapy in sepsis. In this 600-subject, four-arm trial, we assume that the reduction in maximum 48-h SOFA score (x axis) is 1.0 comparing early vs. delayed treatment from a control maximum SOFA score of 4.6. We compared a "fixed" 1:1:1:1 design (black) versus two adaptive designs, which we kept standard of care (SOC) arm proportional, but varied allocation to the three treatment arms based on either the information accrued thus far (blue) or probability estimates generated from the accrued information (red). The adaptive approaches provide superior power compared to the fixed design

14.6 What Is a Platform Trial?

A platform trial is a clinical trial with a single master protocol in which multiple treatments are evaluated at the same time [28]. When combined with adaptive design, the platform can be flexible, and drop treatment arms that are not performing well, add new treatments during the course of the trial, and evaluate multiple subgroups at once. The main differences between a platform trial with an adaptive design and a traditional clinical trial are shown in Table 14.2 [28]. Platform trials also can use prespecified decision rules to determine when a candidate treatment has sufficient evidence to move from one trial phase to the next. These "graduation" decisions are based on the likelihood, knowing the treatment effects from the current trial, that the treatment/drug will be successful in a future confirmatory trial. In this way, platform trials are meant to persist beyond the evaluation of a single treatment or set of treatments and become a pipeline for academic and industry investigators to collaborate. Current platform trials, thus,

Table 14.2 Comparison between traditional clinical trial and adaptive platform trial

Feature	Traditional	Adaptive platform
Scope	Single treatment in a homogeneous population	Multiple treatments in heterogeneous population
Duration	Single question with fixed duration	Depending on candidate treatments, can extend long-term
No. of patient groups	Few	Multiple and may change during the trial
Allocation	Fixed, typically 1:1 randomization	Response-adaptive randomization
Support	Single sponsor	Collaborative funding to support long-term infrastructure

Adapted from [28]

lean on combined financial support from industry, federal, and foundation funding to maintain trial infrastructure.

A notable example of a platform trial is that designed for the Ebola virus disease (EVD) outbreak in West Africa [37]. Approved by the FDA and the US and Sierra Leone ethics committee, this platform was simulated in detail, prepared for locally at sites, but as a result of the declining epidemic in 2015, never enrolled a subject. The trial, nonetheless, is a superior example for discussion. At the time of the outbreak, no therapies for EVD existed, although many had preclinical evidence for efficacy. These drugs needed to be tested during an epidemic, when conditions are not ideal for protocol implementation, and the timeliness of results is an imperative. The resulting design allowed for each patient to be assigned a regimen, where the regimen was a single agent or combination of two agents, and agents were either primary or secondary based upon presumed efficacy. The trial would use a fixed randomization scheme, or "burn-in" phase, in which subjects were assigned 50% to primary and 50% to combination regimens. A standard of care arm was included with a minimum randomization of 20%, and adaptations were included for agents found to be superior or futile at weekly evaluations. A single statistical model governed these decisions, which was simulated in silico for various assumptions about the number and efficacy of experimental agents and their combinations, the length of the trial, and sample size. This perpetual platform proposed therapeutic evaluation, statistical analysis, and data safety monitoring committees to oversee the trial. Although never implemented, this platform included pre-prepared protocols, algorithms, simulated adaptions, and infrastructure ready for future EVD outbreaks—and the multiple agents that would require clinical trial testing. There are additional examples of platforms at different stages of development, not discussed here, which include the I-SPY2, PREPARE, and Precision Promise trials [38].

14.7 Basket and Umbrella Designs

There are other trial designs, which are similar but distinct versions of trials governed by a master protocol [39]. An "umbrella" trial is similar to a platform but tests multiple targeted therapies in a single disease in a single trial. It does not live perpetually like a platform. Examples include the BATTLE-1 trial in non-small cell lung cancer or NCI-Match trial in advanced solid tumor, lymphoma, or myeloma [40]. In contrast, a basket trial tests a single targeted therapy, but in the context of multiple disease or disease subtypes. A recent example of a basket trial is the Imatinib Target Exploration Consortium Study (B225 protocol) [41], where imatinib is compared to standard therapy across any of 40 cancers all sharing the common *bcr-abl* translocation. This basket trial has already resulted in indications for imatinib for dermatofibrosarcoma and systemic mastocytosis, among others.

14.8 Integrating Sepsis Trials in a Learning Healthcare System

As clinical trialists in sepsis consider novel designs, a key component to their success may be integration with the electronic health record and the learning healthcare system.

The electronic health record (EHR) affords many advantages when implementing newer trial designs, including point-of-care efficiency for flagging eligible patients, facilitating informed consent, and delivering randomization assignment to a clinician or study team. Once a patient is randomized, the EHR can also deliver a customized order set that includes the interventions under study that are specific to that patient. Depending on the nature of the outcomes driving randomization probabilities, the EHR can also track important endpoints such as severity of organ dysfunction, intensive care unit support, or in-hospital mortality, all of which may be routinely collected in the clinical data in real time.

An example of how this could unfold is the Diuretic Comparison Project (DCP) in the VA Office of Research and Development [42]. Comparing chlorthalidone to hydrochlorothiazide, this trial uses a point-of-care or clinically integrated design to identify, enroll, and follow subjects using the national VA electronic health records. Both cost-effective and efficient, this project is "light touch" in that there are few research coordinators and the entire trial is centrally administered across the entire USA. The DCP includes many features that could improve sepsis trials but has a fixed randomization ratio and no adaptations.

When the adaptive platform design is combined with point-of-care efficiencies inside the EHR, the trial is termed Randomized Embedded Multifactorial Adaptive Platform (REMAP) trial [43]. The REMAP trial is randomized in order to draw strong causal inferences, while a patient population is enrolled as similar as possible to those in routine clinical care in order to maximize external validity. The trial is "embedded," meaning leveraging any and all efficiency from the EHR, and the term "multifactorial" is intended to reflect the multiple treatments under evaluation. A current example is the REMAP-CAP trial, a platform trial conducted in Australia, Europe, and North America testing a suite of treatment regimens in severe, community-acquired pneumonia in the ICU [44]. The protocol includes multiple domains, such as steroids, antibiotics, and mechanical ventilation strategies, forming more than ten potential regimens. The core protocol is supplemented by region- and domain-specific appendices—which address international differences in regulatory, administrative, and clinical practice. REMAP-CAP also heavily invests in embedding. Custom order sets will be delivered at the point of care and include site-specific standard of care and concomitant therapy. Embedding will facilitate 24/7 recruitment and unload research staff from bedside screening. As REMAP-CAP continues to enroll, it may serve as an example of future, novel trials in sepsis.

Conclusions

Patient outcomes in sepsis have been slow to improve, despite a greater understanding of sepsis pathophysiology, host response, and development of new precision therapies. The design and characteristics of traditional clinical trials in sepsis may be partly to blame, and newer approaches are urgently needed. Through adaptive clinical trials that incorporate response-adaptive randomization, the scientific benefits of new treatments may be realized across the heterogeneous population of septic patients. These designs may be "patient-centered" in their intent to allocate patients to better performing treatment arms, more timely in their accrual of causal inference, and potentially less costly to funders, patients, and health systems.

References

1. Czura CJ. "Merinoff symposium 2010: sepsis"—speaking with one voice. Mol Med. 2011;17(1–2):2–3.
2. Kellum JA, Kong L, Fink MP, Weissfeld LA, Yealy DM, Pinsky MR, et al. Understanding the inflammatory cytokine response in pneumonia and sepsis: results of the Genetic and Inflammatory Markers of Sepsis (GenIMS) Study. Arch Intern Med. 2007;167(15):1655–63.
3. Huang DT, Angus DC, Barnato A, Gunn SR, Kellum JA, Stapleton DK, et al. Harmonizing international trials of early goal-directed resuscitation for severe sepsis and septic shock: methodology of ProCESS, ARISE, and ProMISe. Intensive Care Med. 2013;39(10):1760–75.
4. Angus DC, van der Poll T. Severe sepsis and septic shock. N Engl J Med. 2013;369(21):2063.
5. Boomer JS, To K, Chang KC, Takasu O, Osborne DF, Walton AH, et al. Immunosuppression in patients who die of sepsis and multiple organ failure. JAMA. 2011;306(23):2594–605.
6. Medzhitov R, Schneider DS, Soares MP. Disease tolerance as a defense strategy. Science. 2012;335(6071):936–41.
7. Singer M, Deutschman CS, Seymour CW, Shankar-Hari M, Annane D, Bauer M, et al. The third international consensus definitions for sepsis and septic shock (sepsis-3). JAMA. 2016;315(8):801–10.
8. Seymour CW, Liu VX, Iwashyna TJ, Brunkhorst FM, Rea TD, Scherag A, et al. Assessment of clinical criteria for sepsis: for the third international consensus definitions for sepsis and septic shock (sepsis-3). JAMA. 2016;315(8):762–74.
9. Christiansen CF, Christensen S, Johansen MB, Larsen KM, Tonnesen E, Sorensen HT. The impact of pre-admission morbidity level on 3-year mortality after intensive care: a Danish cohort study. Acta Anaesthesiol Scand. 2011;55(8):962–70.
10. Clermont G, Bartels J, Kumar R, Constantine G, Vodovotz Y, Chow C. In silico design of clinical trials: a method coming of age. Crit Care Med. 2004;32(10):2061–70.
11. Sprung CL, Annane D, Keh D, Moreno R, Singer M, Freivogel K, et al. Hydrocortisone therapy for patients with septic shock. N Engl J Med. 2008;358(2):111–24.

12. Seymour CW, Gomez H, Chang CH, Clermont G, Kellum JA, Kennedy J, et al. Precision medicine for all? Challenges and opportunities for a precision medicine approach to critical illness. Crit Care. 2017;21(1):257.
13. Wong HR, Sweeney TE, Hart KW, Khatri P, Lindsell CJ. Pediatric sepsis endotypes among adults with sepsis. Crit Care Med. 2017;45:e1289–91.
14. Scicluna BP, van Vught LA, Zwinderman AH, Wiewel MA, Davenport EE, Burnham KL, et al. Classification of patients with sepsis according to blood genomic endotype: a prospective cohort study. Lancet Respir Med. 2017;5(10):816–26.
15. Iwashyna TJ, Burke JF, Sussman JB, Prescott HC, Hayward RA, Angus DC. Implications of heterogeneity of treatment effect for reporting and analysis of randomized trials in critical care. Am J Respir Crit Care Med. 2015;192(9):1045–51.
16. Bos LD, Schouten LR, van Vught LA, Wiewel MA, Ong DSY, Cremer O, et al. Identification and validation of distinct biological phenotypes in patients with acute respiratory distress syndrome by cluster analysis. Thorax. 2017;72(10):876–83.
17. Famous KR, Delucchi K, Ware LB, Kangelaris KN, Liu KD, Thompson BT, et al. Acute respiratory distress syndrome subphenotypes respond differently to randomized fluid management strategy. Am J Respir Crit Care Med. 2017;195(3):331–8.
18. Rhee C, Dantes R, Epstein L, Murphy DJ, Seymour CW, Iwashyna TJ, et al. Incidence and Trends of Sepsis in US Hospitals Using Clinical vs Claims Data, 2009-2014. JAMA. 2017;318:1241–9.
19. Cohen J, Vincent JL, Adhikari NK, Machado FR, Angus DC, Calandra T, et al. Sepsis: a roadmap for future research. Lancet Infect Dis. 2015;15(5):581–614.
20. Mebazaa A, Laterre PF, Russell JA, Bergmann A, Gattinoni L, Gayat E, et al. Designing phase 3 sepsis trials: application of learned experiences from critical care trials in acute heart failure. J Intensive Care. 2016;4:24.
21. Opal SM, Laterre PF, Francois B, LaRosa SP, Angus DC, Mira JP, et al. Effect of eritoran, an antagonist of MD2-TLR4, on mortality in patients with severe sepsis: the ACCESS randomized trial. JAMA. 2013;309(11):1154–62.
22. Opal SM, Fisher CJ Jr, Dhainaut JF, Vincent JL, Brase R, Lowry SF, et al. Confirmatory interleukin-1 receptor antagonist trial in severe sepsis: a phase III, randomized, double-blind, placebo-controlled, multicenter trial. The Interleukin-1 Receptor Antagonist Sepsis Investigator Group. Crit Care Med. 1997;25(7):1115–24.
23. Carcillo JA, Halstead ES, Hall MW, Nguyen TC, Reeder R, Aneja R, et al. Three hypothetical inflammation pathobiology phenotypes and pediatric sepsis-induced multiple organ failure outcome. Pediatr Crit Care Med. 2017;18(6):513–23.
24. Shakoory B, Carcillo JA, Chatham WW, Amdur RL, Zhao H, Dinarello CA, et al. Interleukin-1 receptor blockade is associated with reduced mortality in sepsis patients with features of macrophage activation syndrome: reanalysis of a prior phase III trial. Crit Care Med. 2016;44(2):275–81.
25. The PRISM Investigators. Early, goal-directed therapy for septic shock—a patient-level meta-analysis. N Engl J Med. 2017;376:2223–34.
26. Rhodes A, Evans LE, Alhazzani W, Levy MM, Antonelli M, Ferrer R, et al. Surviving sepsis campaign: international guidelines for management of sepsis and septic shock: 2016. Intensive Care Med. 2017;43(3):304–77.
27. Lewis RJ. The pragmatic clinical trial in a learning health care system. Clin Trials. 2016;13(5):484–92.
28. Berry SM, Connor JT, Lewis RJ. The platform trial: an efficient strategy for evaluating multiple treatments. JAMA. 2015;313(16):1619–20.
29. Meurer WJ, Lewis RJ, Berry DA. Adaptive clinical trials: a partial remedy for the therapeutic misconception? JAMA. 2012;307(22):2377–8.
30. Huang X, Ning J, Li Y, Estey E, Issa JP, Berry DA. Using short-term response information to facilitate adaptive randomization for survival clinical trials. Stat Med. 2009;28(12):1680–9.

31. Bartlett RH, Roloff DW, Cornell RG, Andrews AF, Dillon PW, Zwischenberger JB. Extracorporeal circulation in neonatal respiratory failure: a prospective randomized study. Pediatrics. 1985;76(4):479–87.
32. UK Collaborative ECMO Trail Group. UK collaborative randomised trial of neonatal extracorporeal membrane oxygenation. Lancet. 1996;348(9020):75–82.
33. Administration FaD. Enrichment strategies for clinical trials to support approval of human drugs and biological products. Available at: https://www.fdagov/downloads/drugs/guidancecomplianceregulatoryinformation/guidances/ucm332181pdf. 2012.
34. Panacek EA, Marshall JC, Albertson TE, Johnson DH, Johnson S, MacArthur RD, et al. Efficacy and safety of the monoclonal anti-tumor necrosis factor antibody F(ab′)2 fragment afelimomab in patients with severe sepsis and elevated interleukin-6 levels. Crit Care Med. 2004;32(11):2173–82.
35. Group CTS. Effects of enalapril on mortality in severe congestive heart failure. Results of the Cooperative North Scandinavian Enalapril Survival Study (CONSENSUS). N Engl J Med. 1987;316(23):1429–35.
36. Chapman PB, Hauschild A, Robert C, Haanen JB, Ascierto P, Larkin J, et al. Improved survival with vemurafenib in melanoma with BRAF V600E mutation. N Engl J Med. 2011;364(26):2507–16.
37. Berry SM, Petzold EA, Dull P, Thielman NM, Cunningham CK, Corey GR, et al. A response adaptive randomization platform trial for efficient evaluation of Ebola virus treatments: a model for pandemic response. Clin Trials. 2016;13(1):22–30.
38. Berry DA. Adaptive clinical trials in oncology. Nat Rev Clin Oncol. 2012;9(4):199–207.
39. Woodcock J, LaVange LM. Master protocols to study multiple therapies, multiple diseases, or both. N Engl J Med. 2017;377(1):62–70.
40. Kim ES, Herbst RS, Wistuba II, Lee JJ, Blumenschein GR Jr, Tsao A, et al. The BATTLE trial: personalizing therapy for lung cancer. Cancer Discov. 2011;1(1):44–53.
41. Heinrich MC, Joensuu H, Demetri GD, Corless CL, Apperley J, Fletcher JA, et al. Phase II, open-label study evaluating the activity of imatinib in treating life-threatening malignancies known to be associated with imatinib-sensitive tyrosine kinases. Clin Cancer Res. 2008;14(9):2717–25.
42. NIH Collaboratory. Available from: https://www.nihcollaboratory.org/Pages/Grand-Rounds-10-07-16.aspx.
43. Angus DC. Fusing randomized trials with big data: the key to self-learning health care systems? JAMA. 2015;314(8):767–8.
44. Randomized embedded multifactorial adaptive platform trial in community acquired pneumonia. Available from: https://clinicaltrials.gov/ct2/show/NCT02735707.

15 Sepsis in Low- and Middle-Income Countries

Luciano Cesar Pontes Azevedo
and Flavia Ribeiro Machado

15.1 Introduction

Sepsis, defined as life-threatening organ dysfunction caused by a dysregulated host response to infection [1], is one of the oldest and more complex syndromes in medicine, and it remains a significant challenge to healthcare professionals worldwide. In the USA, sepsis accounts for approximately 2% of hospital admissions, half of which are treated in the intensive care unit (ICU) with annual national costs of $16.7 billion in 1995 [2]. Mortality rates worldwide can reach up to 40% for sepsis and 70% for septic shock [3]. An extrapolation of available data from high-income-countries (HIC) suggests 19.4 million sepsis cases annually with potentially 5.3 million deaths [4]. Despite these data showing a significant burden of sepsis in HICs, relevant information on its incidence, prevalence, and mortality rates is scarce, especially at the population level and for low- and middle-income countries (LMICs), which represent an important portion of the world population. The purpose of this review is to discuss the epidemiology of sepsis in LMICs, differences between LMICS and HICs, as well as possible opportunities to improve sepsis care in LMICs.

L. C. P. Azevedo, M.D., Ph.D.
Discipline of Emergency Medicine, University of São Paulo, São Paulo, Brazil

Hospital Sirio-Libanes, São Paulo, Brazil

Latin-American Sepsis Institute, R. Pedro de Toledo, 980 cj 94 São Paulo, São Paulo, Brazil

F. R. Machado, M.D., Ph.D. (✉)
Latin-American Sepsis Institute, R. Pedro de Toledo, 980 cj 94 São Paulo, São Paulo, Brazil

Discipline of Anesthesiology, Pain and Intensive Care, Federal University of São Paulo, São Paulo, Brazil
e-mail: frmachado@unifesp.br

W. J. Wiersinga, C. W. Seymour (eds.), *Handbook of Sepsis*,
https://doi.org/10.1007/978-3-319-73506-1_15

15.2 What Is an LMIC?

First, it is important to define an LMIC. The most commonly used classification is the one developed by the World Bank (www.worldbank.org). According to this stratification, economies are currently divided into four income groups: low, lower-middle, upper-middle, and high. Income is measured using gross national income (GNI) per capita, in US dollars converted from local currency. The classification is updated annually, and in 2017 the following thresholds were used: low income <1005 US$ per capita, lower middle income 1006–3955 US$ per capita, upper middle income 3956–12,235 US$ per capita, and high income >12,235 US$ per capita. It is important to understand that GNI per capita does not completely summarize a country's level of development or measure welfare. However, it has been shown to be a useful and easily available indicator that is closely correlated with other non-monetary measures of quality of life, such as life expectancy at birth, mortality rates of children, and enrollment rates in school [5].

According to this classification, a 2016–2017 list of LMICs comprised 140 countries with a population of 6248 billion inhabitants, while HICs were composed of 78 economies with a population of 1,19 billion inhabitants [5]. Thus, LMICs comprise approximately 85% of the world population, and studies estimate that more than 80% of the global mortality caused by severe infections occurs in LMICs [6], making the absence of data on the epidemiology and outcomes of sepsis even more meaningful.

It is also important to consider the significant heterogeneity within LMICs regarding access to critical care, provision of resources, and case-mix [7]. For instance, inequality and resource limitations may be extreme in some settings in Africa and parts of Southeast Asia, in contrast to some upper middle-income countries such as Thailand and some South American countries [6]. In addition, pathogens that cause sepsis are different in rural African regions compared with industrialized Asian economies, where sepsis-causative microorganisms are more similar to HICs [7].

15.3 The Burden of Sepsis in LMICs

Although LMICs include most of the world population, data on sepsis epidemiology and outcomes are very rare in these settings. Most, if not all, studies are single center or retrospective, and thus their results are not representative and are more prone to bias. Multicenter, prospective studies or those with national representativeness are more frequent in upper middle income countries such as Colombia, Brazil, and China. Population-level estimates of sepsis deaths in LMICs can be extrapolated (but probably underestimated) from deaths caused by severe infections in the global burden of disease database [8]. The extrapolation of HIC estimates of sepsis incidence to LMICs will almost certainly underestimate the number of cases in these countries because of their higher prevalence of underlying risk factors for sepsis, deficiencies in the basic healthcare system, higher rates of healthcare-associated infections [9] and antibiotic resistance [10]. The low awareness among healthcare professionals and lay people can lead to late recognition and thus the development of organ dysfunction. Conversely, other characteristics may contribute to a lower incidence of sepsis, such as a lower life expectancy. High-income countries also deliver better care to cancer, trauma, or transplanted patients, which increases the population at high risk of sepsis [11]. Therefore, prospective multinational studies showing the epidemiology of sepsis in these settings are urgently required.

Brazil is one of the LMICs with more information available on sepsis epidemiology and outcomes. The first Brazilian multicenter observational epidemiological study, BASES, included a convenience sample of five public and private ICUs and showed incidence rates for sepsis (formerly known as severe sepsis) and septic shock of 35.6 and 30 per 1000 patients-day, respectively. The mortality rate was 47.3% for sepsis and 52.2% for septic shock [12]. The next study was conducted in 2003 in 75 intensive care units (ICUs) and showed a prevalence of 17% for sepsis, with mortality rates of 34.4% and 65.3% for sepsis and septic shock, respectively [13]. Another prospective multicenter study conducted in 21 ICUs in 2004 with a primary objective to evaluate costs of sepsis care in Brazil confirmed these findings with mortality rates of 43%. Additionally, the cost of one sepsis admission was estimated to be approximately US$ 9000 per patient with no differences between public and private hospitals [14]. In the multicenter international PROGRESS study, mortality rates from sepsis in Brazil were higher (69%) than those in similar countries such as Argentina and India [15]. However, these studies were biased because all of them were based on convenient samples of ICUs. Recently, the Sepsis Prevalence Assessment Database (SPREAD) study was published, a point-prevalence sepsis cohort with outcome assessment conducted by the Latin American Sepsis Institute in 2014 in 227 Brazilian ICUs that demonstrated a prevalence of sepsis of 29% and mortality rates of 41.4% for sepsis and 58.6% for septic shock [16]. In SPREAD, a national ICU census was used to generate ICU strata by geographical region, size of the cities in which the ICUs were located, main source of income (serving general public or privately insured individuals), and ICU size. This stratification allowed a clearer picture of sepsis mortality in Brazil, as well as the study of organizational factors associated with outcome. SPREAD also provided estimations of the number of ICU-treated septic patients in Brazil per year of 420,000 cases, of whom 230,000 died in the hospital [16]. However, SPREAD did not allow the evaluation of non-ICU-treated sepsis, which may be an important issue in Brazil since restricted access to the ICU has previously been demonstrated to be associated with excess mortality in the country [17, 18]. Taniguchi et al. also estimated the burden of sepsis on a national level. These authors, using infection plus organ dysfunction as a proxy for sepsis in death certificates, identified a significant increase in the number of sepsis-associated deaths from 2002 to 2010, with age-adjusted rates of sepsis-associated mortality rising from 69.5 deaths per 100,000 to 97.8 deaths per 100,000 population from 2002 to 2010 [19].

There are also some previously published multicenter studies examining the epidemiology of sepsis in China [20]. The first study assessed ten university surgical ICUs in 2004–2005 and identified a sepsis occurrence rate of 8.68% among the total population and a mortality rate of 48.7% [21]. Another prospective, observational cohort study conducted in 22 ICUs in 2009 reported an incidence of 37.3 cases per 100 admissions for sepsis and septic shock, with a mortality rate of 33.5% [22]. More recently, a study that assessed the incidence of sepsis at the population level in a subdistrict of Beijing identified an incidence of 68 and 52 cases per 100,000 population per year for sepsis and septic shock, respectively [23]. Long-term outcomes were also assessed in Chinese septic patients. A study showed that up to 6 years after hospital discharge, sepsis survivors showed a clinically meaningful decrease in physical activity, vitality, and mental health in comparison to nonhospitalized controls [24].

In Colombia, a multicenter epidemiological study conducted in ten university hospitals demonstrated that the 28-day mortality rates due to sepsis and septic shock were 21.9% and 45.6%, respectively [25]. This is one of the few studies of LMICs to evaluate sepsis patients treated outside the ICU, which adds value as restricted ICU access is a hallmark of LMICs. The vast majority of the other studies examining the epidemiology of sepsis in LMICs used single centers or described the epidemiology of a specific type of infection and, as such, are more prone to bias and do not represent the reality of their respective countries. Sepsis mortality rates in these studies are extremely variable, ranging from 10% to 80% in some series. Detailed data derived from these studies are depicted in Table 15.1.

15.4 Major Differences Between LMICs and HIC

The outcomes of sepsis have improved in high-income countries. A recent systematic review considering only data from HICs has shown a mortality rate of 26% [4]. There are several possible explanations for these major differences between LMICs and HICs regarding sepsis outcomes. A high incidence of bacterial, parasitic, and HIV infection combined with low hygienic standards and vaccination rates, widespread malnutrition, lack of resources and ICU access, and low sepsis awareness among lay public and healthcare personnel may help to explain this disparity [41]. Although some counterbalancing factors may reduce the incidence of sepsis in LMICs, they are outweighed by other factors that contribute to a high incidence of sepsis. For example, high-income countries with longer life expectancies have a higher age-related sepsis incidence than LMICs. High complexity medical care such as chemotherapy for cancer and organ transplantation and their subsequent immunosuppression are usually more available in HICs, thus increasing the risk of sepsis [11]. Compared to HICs, sepsis in LMICs may be more commonly a disease of young and middle-aged patients with fewer comorbidities. Neonatal and maternal sepsis are also much more common in LMICs.

It is important to stress the heterogeneity of the multiple etiologies of sepsis in developing countries. While it is true that for many LMICs the most frequent sepsis-causative pathogens are the same as in HICs, in some countries, especially those located in tropical and subtropical regions, diverse pathogens such as protozoal infections, viral hemorrhagic fever, and specific diseases such as melioidosis may

Table 15.1 Studies showing sepsis outcomes in LMICs

Country	Design	Sample Size	Outcome	Reference
Brazil	Multicenter prospective ICU-treated sepsis	415	28-day mortality sepsis: 47% septic shock: 52%	[12]
Brazil	Multicenter prospective ICU-treated sepsis	521	28-day mortality sepsis: 34% septic shock: 65%	[13]
Brazil	Multicenter prospective ICU-treated sepsis	524	Hospital mortality sepsis: 43%	[14]
Brazil	Single Center prospective ICU-treated sepsis	524	28-day mortality sepsis: 50% septic shock: 73%	[26]
Brazil	Multicenter prospective ICU-treated sepsis	794	Hospital mortality sepsis: 50% septic shock: 60%	[16]
China	Multicenter prospective ICU-treated sepsis	318	Hospital mortality sepsis: 49%	[21]
China	Multicenter prospective ICU-treated sepsis	484	Hospital mortality sepsis: 34%	[22]
China	Multicenter prospective ICU-treated sepsis	479	Hospital mortality sepsis: 53%	[24]
China	Population based hospital-treated sepsis	1716	Hospital mortality sepsis: 34%	[23]
Colombia	Multicenter prospective hospital-treated sepsis	1658	Hospital mortality sepsis: 22% septic shock: 46%	[25]
Croatia	Single-center retrospective ICU-treated sepsis	214	Hospital mortality sepsis: 34% septic shock: 72%	[27]
Haiti	Single-center retrospective ER-treated sepsis	99	Hospital mortality sepsis: 24%	[28]
Iran	Single-center prospective ER-treated sepsis	145	Hospital mortality sepsis: 21%	[29]
Jamaica	Single-center ER-treated sepsis	117	Hospital mortality sepsis: 24%	[30]
Pakistan	Single-center retrospective ICU-treated sepsis	98	ICU mortality sepsis: 51%	[31]
South Africa	Single-center retrospective ER-treated surgical sepsis	675	ICU mortality sepsis: 12%	[32]
Thailand	RCT treatment of sepsis due to melioidosis	60	28-day mortality intervention: 70% placebo: 87%	[33]
Thailand	Single-center prospective ICU-treated sepsis	390	Hospital mortality sepsis: 50%	[34]

(continued)

Table 15.1 (continued)

Country	Design	Sample Size	Outcome	Reference
Thailand	Single-center prospective ICU-treated sepsis	897	ICU mortality sepsis: 11% septic shock: 47%	[35]
Turkey	Single-center retrospective hospital-treated sepsis	63	Hospital mortality sepsis: 87%	[36]
Turkey	Single-center prospective ER-treated sepsis	200	28-day mortality sepsis: 27%	[37]
Uganda	Multicenter before-after study ER-treated sepsis	671	30-day mortality before: 46% after: 33%	[38]
Uganda	Single-center prospective ER-treated sepsis	202	Hospital mortality sepsis: 32%	[39]
Uganda	Single-center prospective ward-treated sepsis	20	Hospital mortality sepsis: 10%	[40]

ICU Intensive care unit, *ER* Emergency room, *RCT* Randomized controled trial. For the sample size and mortality data, where available, only sepsis (formerly severe sepsis) and septic shock patients were considered.

also play important roles in the epidemiology of sepsis. Since sepsis research and therefore guidelines for diagnosis and treatment are mostly based on data from HICs, the generalizability of information obtained from these countries to LMICs is usually not straightforward [7]. Additionally, HIV infection in sub-Saharan Africa is very frequent and is an important risk factor for sepsis; poor primary care for HIV increases the risk of sepsis. The HIV epidemic is significantly aggravated by tuberculosis that is endemic in most parts of Africa, and both infections pose a significant burden on healthcare systems. In LMICs, sepsis has been involved in one out of four deaths in HIV/AIDS-related diagnosis, and many patients with HIV infection are not recognized until they develop sepsis [42].

Another major difference that may account for the higher mortality rates due to sepsis in LMICs is their elevated rate of healthcare-related infections. Healthcare-associated infections represent a major burden and safety issue for patients in these countries, posing even greater epidemiological relevance than in developed countries. Compared with the average prevalence of healthcare-associated infection in Europe (reported as 7.1 per 100 patients by the European Centre for Disease Prevention) and the estimated incidence in the USA (4.5 per 100 patients in 2002), the pooled prevalence of healthcare-associated infections in resource-limited settings is substantially higher, particularly in high-quality studies (15.5 per 100 patients). This difference is even higher for ICU-acquired infection (pooled density of 47.9 per 1000 patient-days in developing countries) compared with 13.6 per 1000 patient-days in the USA [43]. Developing countries have high rates of ventilator-associated pneumonia and catheter-related bloodstream infections in both adult and pediatric patients, which are mostly caused by multidrug-resistant bacteria including methicillin-resistant *Staphylococcus aureus*, extended-spectrum beta-lactamases-producing bacteria, and carbapenamase-producing Enterobacteriaceae [7]. Although antibiotic resistance is a worldwide phenomenon, the effects of antimicrobial resistance are more significant in LMICs. Essential prerequisites for infection prevention and control practices in ICU settings are human and nonhuman resources, training, and surveillance, all of which are scarce in LMICs. Understaffing is common, and lower staff–patient ratios result in more contacts between staff and multiple patients, increasing the risk of cross-infection between patients. ICUs in LMICs are commonly busy, and measures for the isolation of patients with resistant bacterial infection or colonization are seldom implemented. In addition, the availability of running water as well as adequate disinfection, sterilization, and waste disposal and environmental cleaning measures may be rare in LMICs [44]. Patients in resource-limited countries may also experience challenges identifying and treating their infections due to the absence of adequate microbiology laboratories and lack of second- and third-line antibiotics to treat resistant bacteria [45]. Most of these countries lack adequate national surveillance and infection control systems. Thus, nationally representative information is very difficult to obtain, and implementing adequate policies for restraining antimicrobial consumption is a challenge.

Resource constraints are another major problem associated with the diagnosis and treatment of sepsis in developing countries. Lack of resources may include the absence or delayed availability of laboratory tests for the diagnosis of sepsis-related organ dysfunctions, inadequate microbiological laboratories for the recovery of sepsis pathogens, and issues related to ICU bed availability and ICU main structural items. Baelani and colleagues surveyed anesthesia providers from African LMICs and from HICs during a specialty meeting to evaluate whether the current Surviving Sepsis Campaign (SSC) bundles were feasible in such resource-constrained settings. The authors reported that only 1.4% of African hospitals had the capacity to implement the SSC bundles entirely compared with 81% in the HICs [46]. In reality, this gap in resources may be much wider than described. The survey was biased toward providers who were more likely to have the fundamental structural resources required for sepsis management in their hospitals since most of them worked in private and university settings. This survey bias may be suggested by the assessment of oxygen availability, which was reported as being always available in 93.8% of those African hospitals [46]. These data are in sharp contrast to another survey conducted in 231 health centers and hospitals in 12 African countries, which reported that only 44% of facilities had uninterrupted access to oxygen [47]. In Mongolia, a survey was sent to 44 hospitals to assess the availability of resources to implement SSC bundles. At the time of the study (2009), none of the responding hospitals was able to implement the guidelines entirely, and the median percentage of implementable recommendations and suggestions combined was 52.8. Of note, 60% and 71% of the respondents reported never having available lactate and norepinephrine [48]. Similar results were reported in another survey of 66 institutions in the Congo [49]. The Brazilian SPREAD study also reported the resource availability to comply with SSC bundles, and resource constraints were an independent risk factor for mortality in the multivariable analysis [16]. From the infection control perspective, a lack of resources for the early identification of pathogens is also a major drawback in the treatment of sepsis. In Brazil, a survey was carried out to verify the adequacy of microbiology laboratories serving university hospitals or hospitals with ICUs in terms of performing routine tasks. According to the classification carried out by the authors and based on national guidelines, 85% of these laboratories did not have minimal functioning conditions. Factors associated with better quality services were as follows: serving teaching or public hospitals, serving hospitals involved in the government adverse event reporting system, and serving hospitals located in a state capital [50]. This study reveals the fragility of microbiological diagnosis in LMICs, and the results can likely be translated to the vast majority of the developing world. The lack of adequate microbiological diagnosis impedes appropriate targeting and de-escalation of antimicrobial therapy in patients with genuine bacterial sepsis and limits the ability to detect and monitor outbreaks of drug-resistant infections [44].

Inadequate access to an ICU is closely associated with resource constraints and is described as another major issue in LMICs. The spectrum of how ICUs are staffed and equipped differs vastly between countries and regions and seems to be directly correlated with their income level and healthcare spending. There is substantial variation in terms of the number of ICU beds per population in LMICs, again suggesting significant heterogeneity among these countries. The reported ICU capacity is 0.3 beds per 100,000 inhabitants in Bangladesh, 2.4 per 100,000 inhabitants in Malaysia, 2.5 per 100,000 inhabitants in Sri Lanka, and 3.9 per 100,000 inhabitants in China, while it is 11.7 per 100,000 inhabitants in Mongolia [7]. Since these countries may frequently have dissociated public and private healthcare systems, access to an ICU may also be unequal within a specific country. Considering Brazil as an example, people with health coverage only by the public system have access to 9.9 ICU beds per 100,000 inhabitants, while those with private health insurance can count on 41.4 beds per 100,000 inhabitants, exceeding even some of the richest countries in the world. The access disparity is more striking in Brazil's poorest states [51]. The unavailability of ICU beds is also related to outcomes. A study in a Brazilian university hospital demonstrated that two thirds of the patients had delayed admission to the ICU due to the lack of available beds, and this delay was significantly associated with higher mortality. The fraction of mortality risk attributable to ICU delay was 30%, and each hour of waiting was independently associated with a 1.5% increased risk of ICU death [18]. In addition, long distances and high transportation costs commonly result in delayed presentation of critically ill patients [52]. In some LMICs, the only ICUs available are located in metropolitan or urban areas, and thus travel may take several days, during which the patient's condition may deteriorate and reduce the chance of survival [53]. Inadequate care may be related to financial constraints in public and private healthcare systems in LMICs. In several countries, a substantial amount of healthcare costs must be paid by the patients or their relatives. In India, up to 75% of healthcare costs are charged to the families. This not only places a huge financial burden on patients but also substantially limits public accessibility to hospitals and, in particular, to ICUs. Unwanted consequences can be denial or refusal of ICU admission for poor patients but also premature withdrawal of life-saving interventions. In other instances, costs of care for a critically ill patient who may eventually die can exceed the limited budget of many families [7, 53].

The shortage of healthcare professionals with specific training in the care of acutely and critically ill patients is another widespread and serious challenge for the treatment of sepsis in many LMICs. These circumstances often lead to crowded ICUs, disorganization, increase in nosocomial infections, and irregularities in drug therapies. Training opportunities for critical personnel remain sparse, given the geographic inequalities in ICU distribution. Existing ICUs are often staffed by providers who are partially trained in HICs and are thus more likely to emigrate, further depleting personnel. Finally, reimbursement mechanisms for intensive care physicians are typically disorganized and relatively underfunded because the specialty is not formally recognized in many countries [54]. Studies from LMICs have already demonstrated the association of an increased nurse workload due to understaffing and the incidence of healthcare-associated infections [55], thus identifying the relationship between structural issues and adverse events.

Another important issue that may be related to the high mortality in LMICs is a low awareness of sepsis among the lay public and healthcare personnel. As a consequence of the limited knowledge of the disease and its related morbidity and mortality among the lay public, the presentation of patients to the emergency rooms (ER) is usually late. Thus, increasing public awareness about the syndrome and its warning signs may augment the perception of patients or their families of its severity and the notion that they must seek medical help as soon as sepsis symptoms develop. Most studies that have assessed sepsis awareness among the lay public were conducted in developed regions such as Europe, USA, Japan, and Singapore [56–58]. Even in these countries, perception is usually low. There is no reason to consider that these results are different in LMICs. In 2014, the Latin American Sepsis Institute carried out a sepsis poll among 2126 people in Brazil and compared awareness of sepsis with acute myocardial infarction. Only 7% of Brazilians had ever heard of sepsis, among whom only approximately 40% could adequately define the disease in a stimulated answer. Conversely, 98% of Brazilians had already heard of myocardial infarction, of whom 90% could recognize the symptoms in a stimulated answer [59]. After massive media campaigns such as World Sepsis Day, awareness among Brazilians in 2017 has increased from 7% to 14% (Azevedo et al., unpublished data). Despite this impressive improvement, much work still needs to be done to increase perception regarding the importance of sepsis, particularly in LMICs.

A reduced awareness of sepsis is also very common among healthcare providers worldwide [60]. Although a causal link has not been adequately established, it is intuitive to hypothesize that delayed diagnosis of sepsis, especially in the emergency department, may be partially caused by low suspicion of this diagnosis among the multidisciplinary team. Again, little information from LMICs is available. In Malawi, a survey performed among medical students and members of multidisciplinary teams composed mostly of relatively simple multiple-choice questions demonstrated a significant lack of knowledge regarding sepsis concepts and treatment

Table 15.2 Possible causes of high sepsis mortality in LMICs, ER, ICU, HIV

High incidence of comorbidities such as HIV and tuberculosis
Reduced awareness of sepsis among lay public and healthcare workers
Lack of formal training in ER and critical care by healthcare professionals
Inadequate access to ICU beds
Inadequate provision of critical care resources
Elevated rate of healthcare-related infections
Lack of treatment guidelines adequately validated by research in LMICs

according to SSC guidelines [61]. In a Brazilian survey, recognition of the disease continuum among emergency medicine and ICU physicians was low, especially for sepsis and severe sepsis. The percentage of physicians correctly recognizing SIRS, infection, sepsis, severe sepsis, and septic shock definitions was 78.2%, 92.6%, 27.3%, 56.7%, and 81.0%, respectively. Interestingly, most misclassifications occurred for the items sepsis and severe sepsis, thus suggesting some difficulties among these physicians in understanding the concept of organ dysfunction as important for emergency care [62]. Another important hallmark of this study is that the knowledge of sepsis was worst among physicians from public hospitals, which may partially explain (in association with structural local limitations) the increased time to sepsis diagnosis in public hospitals in Brazil reported by some studies [63, 64]. Improving awareness by the healthcare team may help to improve outcomes. In a Brazilian ER, training doctors to improve early diagnosis of sepsis resulted in significantly more diagnoses in the ER and a reduced time of referral to the ICU [65]. Several factors contribute to this "information poverty" among healthcare workers, including insufficient access to continuing medical education, the influence of traditional medical beliefs, and a critical shortage of qualified healthcare workers. In addition, lack of exposure to acute care medicine during training and limited opportunities for continuing medical education suggest that many healthcare workers have insufficient knowledge of best practices for sepsis diagnosis and treatment [66]. The possible reasons for differences in mortality between LMICs and HICs are depicted in Table 15.2.

15.5 Applications of New Sepsis Definitions for LMICS

In 2016, a task force composed of physicians from the Society of Critical Care Medicine (SCCM) and the European Society of Critical Care Medicine (ESICM) published new sepsis definitions, now called Sepsis 3. Briefly, sepsis is now considered "a life-threatening organ dysfunction caused by dysregulated host response to infection." The clinical diagnosis of organ dysfunction was suggested to be based on a variation of 2 or more points in the Sequential Organ Assessment Score (SOFA) [1]. The criteria for systemic inflammatory response syndrome (SIRS) are now not required for the definition of sepsis, but they are still useful for the diagnosis of uncomplicated infection. Since sepsis is now related to an increased disease severity with risk of death, the term "severe sepsis" has been abolished. Septic shock is now defined as "a subset of sepsis with particularly profound circulatory, cellular and metabolic abnormalities associated with a greater risk of mortality than sepsis alone." The diagnostic criteria for septic shock were referred to as "vasopressor requirement required to maintain a mean arterial pressure of >65 mmHg and a serum lactate level >2 mmol/L in the absence of hypovolemia" [67]. In addition to the above-described definitions, the task force suggested the use of a simplified SOFA score, named quick SOFA (qSOFA), as a bedside tool to rapidly identify adult patients who are more likely to die or to stay in the ICU for 3 days or more if they have infection. Therefore, qSOFA does not define sepsis and was suggested as a triage score to identify high-risk patients without the need for laboratory tests. The qSOFA score is positive if the patient has at least two of the following clinical criteria: respiratory rate of 22/min or greater, altered mentation (Glasgow Coma Scale < 15), or a systolic blood pressure of 100 mmHg or less [68].

Although the definitions have been endorsed by many medical societies worldwide, they have also generated a lot of controversy, mainly related to the increase in specificity at the expense of reducing sensitivity [69]. Major advantages of the new definition include a broader understanding of the pathophysiology of sepsis and translation of this knowledge to the definition; validation of the clinical criteria using databases instead of expert opinion as in the previous consensus; standardization of organ dysfunction criteria, which will facilitate the inclusion of similar patients in clinical studies; removal of SIRS variables as diagnostic criteria for sepsis because they are not sensitive or specific enough for sepsis [70, 71]; and simplification of the nomenclature since severe sepsis shall not be used anymore.

Conversely, there are important drawbacks of the new definitions, especially for LMICs. First, the authors themselves recommend retrospective and prospective validation of the new definitions (more specifically the clinical criteria) in developing countries [1]. The databases that were used to validate the new criteria originated from HICs, and as stated previously, the case-mix and outcomes of septic patients in the developing world are different from HICs. In addition, another main concern generated by the new definitions is the reduced sensitivity for the detection of cases that might have an unfavorable course, mainly in LMICs. The new concepts limit the criteria for organ dysfunction and tend to select a more severely ill population [72]. This phenomenon may have advantages for HICs, where patients are usually recognized early, but it is a concern in settings such as busy understaffed ERs or wards from LMICs, where delayed recognition is very common. Another problem with the new definitions is the use of the SOFA score, since the score is not well known out of the critical care community. Thus, the application of SOFA by other healthcare professionals who also treat sepsis is not straightforward. Using SOFA in quality improvement programs to detect sepsis is unfeasible and might delay diagnosis and the initiation of antibiotics [69]. Additionally, the exclusion of lactate as a marker of organ dysfunction in septic patients without hypotension is another issue. This approach undermines the relevance of lactate as a disease severity marker that should be collected in all sepsis-suspected patients irrespective of blood pressure levels. This phenomenon might compromise the early detection of patients with sepsis and cryptic shock who have high mortality rates despite normal blood pressure [73]. Thus, in quality improvement initiatives, the new broad Sepsis 3 definition of sepsis should be used, meaning that any life-threating organ dysfunction must be considered as sepsis, including fluid-reversible hypotension, an altered level of consciousness (GCS13–14), and hyperlactatemia, although none of them isolated reach a variation of 2 points in the SOFA score. This result is in alignment with the Surviving Sepsis Campaign definitions of organ dysfunction. The new definition of septic shock, which includes lactate levels, may also limit the diagnosis of this condition in scenarios in which lactate is not available, a common issue in many low-income countries [46, 48, 49]. If the definition is not homogeneous among countries, it may hinder the comparison of septic shock mortality rates as patients under vasopressors would be erroneously considered to have sepsis, resulting in biased epidemiologic studies in these scenarios. The final major issue concerning the definitions is the use of qSOFA beyond the purpose for which it was validated. qSOFA was validated as a severity score but was suggested to be used as a triage test, and it was not validated for this purpose [1]. The statistical model used to select the cutoff of 2 points aimed to predict morbidity and mortality and not to be used as a screening tool for early sepsis diagnosis. In addition, the proposal to use this score for screening might lead to the misinterpretation that patients without two qSOFA points are not severely ill, potentially delaying adequate patient treatment and allocation, especially in LMICs.

Very few studies have assessed the validation of sepsis definitions in LMICs. In Brazil, a study conducted in a university hospital ICU showed that sepsis-3 definitions, as expected, could more precisely select patients at high risk of death than the previous definitions. Again as expected, the accuracy of the new definitions increased with disease severity, which is not necessarily in the best interest of LMICs. Interestingly, patients with infection and no organ dysfunction assessed by SOFA, but with lactate concentrations above 4 mmol/L, have similar mortality rates to patients with sepsis according to the new definition. These data suggest the importance of measuring lactate in all patients with severe infection/sepsis to identify a group with high mortality, irrespective of their arterial pressure [74]. Although confirming its ability to predict mortality and morbidity, many studies in HICs have now clearly confirmed the low sensitivity of qSOFA [75–79], which means that its use as a screening tool would result in a high percentage of patients being missed. The only prospective study in ER patients that demonstrated a reasonable sensitivity of qSOFA collected the score variables during the entire ER stay and not prior to the sepsis diagnosis, which does not adequately mimics a screening tool [80].

Very few data from LMICs regarding qSOFA evaluation are currently available. In a Greek study of 65 departments, the sensitivity of qSOFA to predict death was 60.8% for patients outside the ICU. The sensitivity of qSOFA for organ dysfunction outside the ICU was 48.7%, thus demonstrating that this tool may be inadequate for triage [81]. In Gabon, a prospective collected sample of 329 SIRS(+)-infected patients in a resource-constrained hospital showed a good sensitivity of 87% (95%

CI 60–98%) and specificity of 75% (95% CI 70–80%), with an AUROC of 0.83. In addition to the small sample size, an odd finding of this study was the mortality rate of 4.5%, which was very low for infected patients in LMICs, thus suggesting that their results may not be generalizable [82]. In patients with pneumonia in an ER in China, qSOFA had a sensitivity of 12% and specificity of 97% to predict mortality, and patients with qSOFA of zero and 1 had mortality rates of 16.3% and 24.4%, respectively. These mortality rates are much higher than the ones reported for sepsis patients with similar qSOFA scores in the Sepsis 3 validation cohort, thus suggesting that adequate application of qSOFA to LMICs may pend further validation studies [83]. The preliminary prospectively collected data from the Latin American Sepsis Institute showed that among 1890 septic patients from 55 institutions, 58.7% were qSOFA-negative with a mortality rate of 17.6%. The mortality rate of qSOFA-negative patients in public hospitals was 40%. However, as a severity score, qSOFA showed good performance with an ROC curve of 0.74±0.01 (95% CI: 0.72–0.75) [84]. Considering the current evidence, qSOFA is not recommended as a screening tool in LMICs, although it is still useful to identify, among patients who had already been detected using other available screening tools, those who are at an increased risk of death.

15.6 Quality Improvement Initiatives for Sepsis in LMICs

Essentially, most opportunities to evolve sepsis care in LMICs are related to improvements in the several limitations in structure and critical care provision described previously in this chapter.

Few studies have assessed adherence to sepsis guidelines, and quality improvement initiatives were reported from LMICs. In an Asian study conducted in 2009 involving LMICs and HICs, Phua et al. demonstrated that overall compliance with SSC guidelines was very poor, and LMICs were less likely to be compliant with the bundles. Hospital mortality rate was 47% for low-income countries and 50% for middle-income countries, whereas it was 38% for HICs. Undergoing treatment in an HIC as well as in an ICU with an accredited fellowship program was a factor associated with reduced mortality [85]. In another study in Asia, the impact of quality improvement initiatives for sepsis management was assessed in five countries, among which China and India were the LMICs. In that study, educational activities in the ER and ICU increased compliance with the bundle from 13.3% to 54.5% over the six quartiles of implementation. Compliance with the bundle was associated with reduction in mortality, but this effect was lost after correction for confounding variables [86]. In China, three cohort studies, two conducted in patients with sepsis and the other in patients with severe pneumonia, demonstrated overall low compliance with the bundles, but those patients who were compliant had a lower hospital mortality [87–89]. In a prospective cohort of septic patients with *S. aureus* bacteremia in a single hospital in Thailand, the authors identified a mortality rate of 53% and highly variable adherence to SSC guidelines [90]. In one before-after study in Thailand, the authors identified very low adherence to the guidelines (0%) in the pre-intervention phase associated with a significant mortality rate (40%). These numbers significantly improved to 37% adherence and 18% mortality following adoption of the sepsis 6-hour bundle in the ER [91]. In Uganda, a before-after study was conducted in which dedicated study medical officers treated sepsis patients with protocols in two hospitals. These authors identified a significant increase in the number of patients who received antibiotics during the first hour of sepsis and a significant reduction in mortality even after correction for potential confounders [38].

In Brazil, some single-center studies carried out in private institutions (which are usually more comparable to HICs) demonstrated that quality improvement initiatives such as the implementation of treatment protocols are associated with reductions in mortality [92–94]. In addition, two multicenter reports were from the Latin American Sepsis Institute quality improvement initiative. The first pre and post-intervention was conducted in ten private hospitals in São Paulo and demonstrated an increase in bundle compliance from 13% to 62% during the intervention, with a significant reduction in mortality rates from 55% at baseline to 26%. In addition to the reduction of mortality, the intervention was also cost saving, with a reduction of 11,000 dollars in total cost per patient from baseline to the last 3 months of the intervention [95]. Using the LASI database with 21,000 patients from 2005 to 2014 comprising both public and private hospitals, we recently demonstrated that compliance to the bundles and reduced mortality were largely dependent on the main source of hospital income. For instance, a comparison of the first period with the last period of intervention showed that compliance with the 6-hour bundle increased from 13.5% to 58.2% in private institutions, with a much lower increment from 7.4% to 15.7% in public hospitals. Mortality rates significantly decreased throughout the program in private institutions, from 47.6% to 27.2% in the eighth period [96]. However, in public hospitals, mortality significantly diminished only in the first two periods. The quality improvement initiative was also associated with a reduction in the time to sepsis diagnosis, in addition to a reduction in the severity of illness, suggesting an improvement in sepsis awareness [96]. In public settings, the time to sepsis diagnosis, although improved, was still very long after several periods of intervention. Possible reasons to explain these differences between public and private settings include the case-mix (increased disease severity in public hospitals), resource constraints, understaffing and high turnover of healthcare workers, and difficulties in access to the ICU.

All these studies have shown that most of the sepsis bundles proposed by the Surviving Sepsis guidelines can be fully implemented or adapted for application in middle-income countries, as the required resources are usually available. Some of the recommended interventions, however, require tools and monitoring capabilities that are inaccessible for many district and regional hospitals in middle-income countries and in the majority of settings in low-income countries. Additionally, blind adoption of established interventions in high-income settings may prove to be ineffective in lower-income scenarios. Examples are the use of fluid bolus resuscitation in children with infection and impaired perfusion in Africa (mostly malaria), which was associated with increased short-term mortality irrespective of the solution administered (saline or albumin) [97]. In Zambia, the adoption of an adapted

EGDT guideline in a single-center study resulted in increased mortality in the group of patients with hypoxemic respiratory failure and early termination of the trial [98]. In Haiti, the use of a World Health Organization-adapted protocol for early sepsis treatment that focused mostly on fluids and antibiotics failed to improve mortality, time to fluids, or time to antimicrobials [99]. Taken together, these results underscore the need to generate specific guidelines focused on the context of resource constraints of LMICs and to enhance research to identify the appropriate answers to the questions that are relevant to those who work in these settings. Building an adequate research capacity is one key step toward achieving these goals.

Conclusion

Very few data exist regarding the epidemiology of sepsis in LMICs, but the limited evidence suggests that this disease poses a significant burden to these countries because it is a major cause of short-term mortality and a high-cost condition. Developing countries face significant issues regarding sepsis care, as demonstrated by low awareness of the disease among the lay public and healthcare team, a lack of preventive measures for infections, a high prevalence of nosocomial infections, and inadequate ICU access and structure. Little research has also been conducted in sepsis management in LMICs, and most sepsis guidelines are developed for HICs with recommendations that are not feasible for adoption in many parts of the developing world. Hence, it is imperative to address sepsis burden in LMICs through research, increased awareness, capacity building, and the introduction of practical clinical guidelines that are reproducible in these settings.

References

1. Singer M, Deutschman CS, Seymour CW, Shankar-Hari M, Annane D, Bauer M, et al. The third international consensus definitions for sepsis and septic shock (sepsis-3). JAMA. 2016;315(8):801–10. https://doi.org/10.1001/jama.2016.0287.
2. Angus DC, Linde-Zwirble WT, Lidicker J, Clermont G, Carcillo J, Pinsky MR. Epidemiology of severe sepsis in the United States: analysis of incidence, outcome, and associated costs of care. Crit Care Med. 2001;29(7):1303–10.
3. Jawad I, Luksic I, Rafnsson SB. Assessing available information on the burden of sepsis: global estimates of incidence, prevalence and mortality. J Glob Health. 2012;2(1):010404. https://doi.org/10.7189/jogh.02.010404.
4. Fleischmann C, Scherag A, Adhikari NK, Hartog CS, Tsaganos T, Schlattmann P, et al. Assessment of global incidence and mortality of hospital-treated sepsis—current estimates and limitations. Am J Respir Crit Care Med. 2016;193:259–72. https://doi.org/10.1164/rccm.201504-0781OC.
5. World-Bank. Countries by income (2017). Accessed 27 July 2017.
6. Cheng AC, West TE, Limmathurotsakul D, Peacock SJ. Strategies to reduce mortality from bacterial sepsis in adults in developing countries. PLoS Med. 2008;5(8):e175. https://doi.org/10.1371/journal.pmed.0050175.
7. Schultz MJ, Dunser MW, Dondorp AM, Adhikari NK, Iyer S, Kwizera A, et al. Current challenges in the management of sepsis in ICUs in resource-poor settings and suggestions for the future. Intensive Care Med. 2017;43(5):612–24. https://doi.org/10.1007/s00134-017-4750-z.

8. Adhikari NK, Fowler RA, Bhagwanjee S, Rubenfeld GD. Critical care and the global burden of critical illness in adults. Lancet. 2010;376(9749):1339–46. https://doi.org/10.1016/S0140-6736(10)60446-1.
9. Rosenthal VD, Maki DG, Mehta Y, Leblebicioglu H, Memish ZA, Al-Mousa HH, et al. International Nosocomial Infection Control Consortium (INICC) report, data summary of 43 countries for 2007–2012. Device-associated module. Am J Infect Control. 2014;42(9):942–56. https://doi.org/10.1016/j.ajic.2014.05.029.
10. Guzman-Blanco M, Labarca JA, Villegas MV, Gotuzzo E, Latin America Working Group on Bacterial Resistance. Extended spectrum beta-lactamase producers among nosocomial Enterobacteriaceae in Latin America. Braz J Infect Dis. 2014;18(4):421–33. https://doi.org/10.1016/j.bjid.2013.10.005.
11. Cohen J, Vincent JL, Adhikari NK, Machado FR, Angus DC, Calandra T, et al. Sepsis: a roadmap for future research. Lancet Infect Dis. 2015;15(5):581–614. https://doi.org/10.1016/S1473-3099(15)70112-X.
12. Silva E, Pedro Mde A, Sogayar AC, Mohovic T, Silva CL, Janiszewski M, et al. Brazilian sepsis epidemiological study (BASES study). Crit Care. 2004;8(4):R251–60. https://doi.org/10.1186/cc2892.
13. Sales Junior JA, David CM, Hatum R, Souza PC, Japiassu A, Pinheiro CT, et al. An epidemiological study of sepsis in Intensive Care Units: sepsis Brazil study. Revista Brasileira de terapia intensiva. 2006;18(1):9–17.
14. Sogayar AM, Machado FR, Rea-Neto A, Dornas A, Grion CM, Lobo SM, et al. A multicentre, prospective study to evaluate costs of septic patients in Brazilian intensive care units. Pharmacoeconomics. 2008;26(5):425–34.
15. Beale R, Reinhart K, Brunkhorst FM, Dobb G, Levy M, Martin G, et al. Promoting Global Research Excellence in Severe Sepsis (PROGRESS): lessons from an international sepsis registry. Infection. 2009;37(3):222–32. https://doi.org/10.1007/s15010-008-8203-z.
16. Machado FR, Cavalcanti AB, Bozza FA, Ferreira EM, Carrara FS, Souza JL, Caixeta N, Salomao R, Angus DC, Azevedo LC. The epidemiology of sepsis in Brazilian intensive care units: the Sepsis PREvalence Assessment Database (SPREAD), an observational study. Lancet Infect Dis. 2017;17(11):1180–9.
17. Bozza FA, Salluh JI. An urban perspective on sepsis in developing countries. Lancet Infect Dis. 2010;10(5):290–1. https://doi.org/10.1016/S1473-3099(10)70074-8.
18. Cardoso LT, Grion CM, Matsuo T, Anami EH, Kauss IA, Seko L, et al. Impact of delayed admission to intensive care units on mortality of critically ill patients: a cohort study. Crit Care. 2011;15(1):R28. https://doi.org/10.1186/cc9975.
19. Taniguchi LU, Bierrenbach AL, Toscano CM, Schettino GP, Azevedo LC. Sepsis-related deaths in Brazil: an analysis of the national mortality registry from 2002 to 2010. Crit Care. 2014;18(6):608. https://doi.org/10.1186/s13054-014-0608-8.
20. Liao X, Du B, Lu M, Wu M, Kang Y. Current epidemiology of sepsis in mainland China. Ann Transl Med. 2016;4(17):324. https://doi.org/10.21037/atm.2016.08.51.
21. Cheng B, Xie G, Yao S, Wu X, Guo Q, Gu M, et al. Epidemiology of severe sepsis in critically ill surgical patients in ten university hospitals in China. Crit Care Med. 2007;35(11):2538–46. https://doi.org/10.1097/01.CCM.0000284492.30800.00.
22. Zhou J, Qian C, Zhao M, Yu X, Kang Y, Ma X, et al. Epidemiology and outcome of severe sepsis and septic shock in intensive care units in mainland China. PLoS One. 2014;9(9):e107181. https://doi.org/10.1371/journal.pone.0107181.
23. Zhou J, Tian H, Du X, Xi X, An Y, Duan M, et al. Population-based epidemiology of sepsis in a subdistrict of Beijing. Crit Care Med. 2017;45(7):1168–76. https://doi.org/10.1097/CCM.0000000000002414.
24. Zhang K, Mao X, Fang Q, Jin Y, Cheng B, Xie G, et al. Impaired long-term quality of life in survivors of severe sepsis : Chinese multicenter study over 6 years. Anaesthesist. 2013;62(12):995–1002. https://doi.org/10.1007/s00101-013-2257-8.
25. Rodriguez F, Barrera L, De La Rosa G, Dennis R, Duenas C, Granados M, et al. The epidemiology of sepsis in Colombia: a prospective multicenter cohort study in ten university hospitals. Crit Care Med. 2011;39(7):1675–82. https://doi.org/10.1097/CCM.0b013e318218a35e.

26. Kauss IA, Grion CM, Cardoso LT, Anami EH, Nunes LB, Ferreira GL, et al. The epidemiology of sepsis in a Brazilian teaching hospital. Braz J Infect Dis. 2010;14(3):264–70.
27. Degoricija V, Sharma M, Legac A, Gradiser M, Sefer S, Vucicevic Z. Survival analysis of 314 episodes of sepsis in medical intensive care unit in university hospital: impact of intensive care unit performance and antimicrobial therapy. Croat Med J. 2006;47(3):385–97.
28. Papali A, Verceles AC, Augustin ME, Colas LN, Jean-Francois CH, Patel DM, et al. Sepsis in Haiti: prevalence, treatment, and outcomes in a Port-au-Prince referral hospital. J Crit Care. 2017;38:35–40. https://doi.org/10.1016/j.jcrc.2016.09.031.
29. Jalili M, Barzegari H, Pourtabatabaei N, Honarmand AR, Boreiri M, Mehrvarz A, et al. Effect of door-to-antibiotic time on mortality of patients with sepsis in emergency department: a prospective cohort study. Acta Med Iran. 2013;51(7):454–60.
30. Edwards R, Hutson R, Johnson J, Sherwin R, Gordon-Strachan G, Frankson M, et al. Severe sepsis in the emergency department—an observational cohort study from the university hospital of the West Indies. West Indian Med J. 2013;62(3):224–9.
31. Asghar A, Hashmi M, Rashid S, Khan FH. Incidence, outcome and risk factors for sepsis—a two year retrospective study at surgical intensive care unit of a teaching hospital in Pakistan. J Ayub Med Coll Abbottabad. 2016;28(1):79–83.
32. Green S, Kong VY, Clarke DL, Sartorius B, Odendaal J, Bruce JL, et al. The spectrum and outcome of surgical sepsis in Pietermaritzburg, South Africa. S Afr Med J. 2017;107(2):134–6. https://doi.org/10.7196/SAMJ.2017.v107i2.11339.
33. Cheng AC, Limmathurotsakul D, Chierakul W, Getchalarat N, Wuthiekanun V, Stephens DP, et al. A randomized controlled trial of granulocyte colony-stimulating factor for the treatment of severe sepsis due to melioidosis in Thailand. Clin Infect Dis. 2007;45(3):308–14. https://doi.org/10.1086/519261.
34. Khwannimit B, Bhurayanontachai R. The epidemiology of, and risk factors for, mortality from severe sepsis and septic shock in a tertiary-care university hospital setting. Epidemiol Infect. 2009;137(9):1333–41. https://doi.org/10.1017/S0950268809002027.
35. Khwannimit B, Bhurayanontachai R. The direct costs of intensive care management and risk factors for financial burden of patients with severe sepsis and septic shock. J Crit Care. 2015;30(5):929–34. https://doi.org/10.1016/j.jcrc.2015.05.011.
36. Tanriover MD, Guven GS, Sen D, Unal S, Uzun O. Epidemiology and outcome of sepsis in a tertiary-care hospital in a developing country. Epidemiol Infect. 2006;134(2):315–22. https://doi.org/10.1017/S0950268805004978.
37. Gunes Ozaydin M, Guneysel O, Saridogan F, Ozaydin V. Are scoring systems sufficient for predicting mortality due to sepsis in the emergency department? Turk J Emerg Med. 2017;17(1):25–8. https://doi.org/10.1016/j.tjem.2016.09.004.
38. Jacob ST, Banura P, Baeten JM, Moore CC, Meya D, Nakiyingi L, et al. The impact of early monitored management on survival in hospitalized adult Ugandan patients with severe sepsis: a prospective intervention study*. Crit Care Med. 2012;40(7):2050–8. https://doi.org/10.1097/CCM.0b013e31824e65d7.
39. Amir A, Saulters KJ, Olum S, Pitts K, Parsons A, Churchill C, et al. Outcomes of patients with severe sepsis after the first 6 hours of resuscitation at a regional referral hospital in Uganda. J Crit Care. 2016;33:78–83. https://doi.org/10.1016/j.jcrc.2016.01.023.
40. Rudd KE, Tutaryebwa LK, West TE. Presentation, management, and outcomes of sepsis in adults and children admitted to a rural Ugandan hospital: a prospective observational cohort study. PLoS One. 2017;12(2):e0171422. https://doi.org/10.1371/journal.pone.0171422.
41. Dunser MW, Festic E, Dondorp A, Kissoon N, Ganbat T, Kwizera A, et al. Recommendations for sepsis management in resource-limited settings. Intensive Care Med. 2012;38(4):557–74. https://doi.org/10.1007/s00134-012-2468-5.
42. Rello J, Leblebicioglu H, members of ESGCIP. Sepsis and septic shock in low-income and middle-income countries: need for a different paradigm. Int J Infect Dis. 2016;48:120–2. https://doi.org/10.1016/j.ijid.2016.04.017.
43. Allegranzi B, Bagheri Nejad S, Combescure C, Graafmans W, Attar H, Donaldson L, et al. Burden of endemic health-care-associated infection in developing countries: systematic review and meta-analysis. Lancet. 2011;377(9761):228–41. https://doi.org/10.1016/S0140-6736(10)61458-4.

44. Dondorp AM, Limmathurotsakul D, Ashley EA. What's wrong in the control of antimicrobial resistance in critically ill patients from low- and middle-income countries? Intensive Care Med. 2017. https://doi.org/10.1007/s00134-017-4795-z.
45. Bebell LM, Muiru AN. Antibiotic use and emerging resistance: how can resource-limited countries turn the tide? Glob Heart. 2014;9(3):347–58. https://doi.org/10.1016/j.gheart.2014.08.009.
46. Baelani I, Jochberger S, Laimer T, Otieno D, Kabutu J, Wilson I, et al. Availability of critical care resources to treat patients with severe sepsis or septic shock in Africa: a self-reported, continent-wide survey of anaesthesia providers. Crit Care. 2011;15(1):R10. https://doi.org/10.1186/cc9410.
47. Belle J, Cohen H, Shindo N, Lim M, Velazquez-Berumen A, Ndihokubwayo JB, et al. Influenza preparedness in low-resource settings: a look at oxygen delivery in 12 African countries. J Infect Dev Ctries. 2010;4(7):419–24.
48. Bataar O, Lundeg G, Tsenddorj G, Jochberger S, Grander W, Baelani I, et al. Nationwide survey on resource availability for implementing current sepsis guidelines in Mongolia. Bull World Health Organ. 2010;88(11):839–46. https://doi.org/10.2471/BLT.10.077073.
49. Baelani I, Jochberger S, Laimer T, Rex C, Baker T, Wilson IH, et al. Identifying resource needs for sepsis care and guideline implementation in the Democratic Republic of the Congo: a cluster survey of 66 hospitals in four eastern provinces. Middle East J Anaesthesiol. 2012;21(4):559–75.
50. Costa LB, Cardoso MR, Ferreira CG, Levy CE, Borba HM, Sallas J, et al. National prevalence survey in Brazil to evaluate the quality of microbiology laboratories: the importance of defining priorities to allocate limited resources. Rev Panam Salud Publica. 2013;33(1):73–8.
51. Machado FR. All in a Day's Work—Equity vs. Equality at a Public ICU in Brazil. N Engl J Med. 2016;375(25):2420–1. https://doi.org/10.1056/NEJMp1610059.
52. Firth P, Ttendo S. Intensive care in low-income countries—a critical need. N Engl J Med. 2012;367(21):1974–6. https://doi.org/10.1056/NEJMp1204957.
53. Dunser MW, Baelani I, Ganbold L. A review and analysis of intensive care medicine in the least developed countries. Crit Care Med. 2006;34(4):1234–42. https://doi.org/10.1097/01.CCM.0000208360.70835.87.
54. Murthy S, Adhikari NK. Global health care of the critically ill in low-resource settings. Ann Am Thorac Soc. 2013;10(5):509–13. https://doi.org/10.1513/AnnalsATS.201307-246OT.
55. Daud-Gallotti RM, Costa SF, Guimaraes T, Padilha KG, Inoue EN, Vasconcelos TN, et al. Nursing workload as a risk factor for healthcare associated infections in ICU: a prospective study. PLoS One. 2012;7(12):e52342. https://doi.org/10.1371/journal.pone.0052342.
56. Shime N, Shinohara T, Shigemi K, Parker M. Knowledge and perception about sepsis: a survey in Japan. Anaesth Intensive Care. 2012;40(4):737–8.
57. Rubulotta FM, Ramsay G, Parker MM, Dellinger RP, Levy MM, Poeze M, et al. An international survey: public awareness and perception of sepsis. Crit Care Med. 2009;37(1):167–70.
58. Phua J, Lim HF, Tay CK, Aung NW. Public awareness of sepsis and stroke in Singapore: a population-based survey. Ann Acad Med Singapore. 2013;42(6):269–77.
59. Azevedo LC, Carrara F, Machado FR, Lubarino J, Salomao R, Costa-Filho RC. Conhecimento do público leigo sobre sepse no Brasil: uma comparação com infarto agudo do miocárdio (in portuguese). Revista Brasileira de terapia intensiva. 2014;S1:S7–S43.
60. Poeze M, Ramsay G, Gerlach H, Rubulotta F, Levy M. An international sepsis survey: a study of doctors' knowledge and perception about sepsis. Crit Care. 2004;8(6):R409–13. https://doi.org/10.1186/cc2959.
61. Marshall-Brown P, Namboya F, Pollach G. Evaluating sepsis training for medical students and nonphysicians in Malawi. J Clin Anesth. 2016;34:352–7. https://doi.org/10.1016/j.jclinane.2016.05.013.
62. Assuncao M, Akamine N, Cardoso GS, Mello PV, Teles JM, Nunes AL, et al. Survey on physicians' knowledge of sepsis: do they recognize it promptly? J Crit Care. 2010;25(4):545–52. https://doi.org/10.1016/j.jcrc.2010.03.012.

63. Freitas FG, Salomao R, Tereran N, Mazza BF, Assuncao M, Jackiu M, et al. The impact of duration of organ dysfunction on the outcome of patients with severe sepsis and septic shock. Clinics. 2008;63(4):483–8.
64. Conde KA, Silva E, Silva CO, Ferreira E, Freitas FG, Castro I, et al. Differences in sepsis treatment and outcomes between public and private hospitals in Brazil: a multicenter observational study. PLoS One. 2013;8(6):e64790. https://doi.org/10.1371/journal.pone.0064790.
65. Rezende E, Silva JM Jr, Isola AM, Campos EV, Amendola CP, Almeida SL. Epidemiology of severe sepsis in the emergency department and difficulties in the initial assistance. Clinics. 2008;63(4):457–64.
66. Papali A, McCurdy MT, Calvello EJ. A "three delays" model for severe sepsis in resource-limited countries. J Crit Care. 2015;30(4):861 e9–14. https://doi.org/10.1016/j.jcrc.2015.04.003.
67. Shankar-Hari M, Phillips GS, Levy ML, Seymour CW, Liu VX, Deutschman CS, et al. Developing a new definition and assessing new clinical criteria for septic shock: for the third international consensus definitions for sepsis and septic shock (sepsis-3). JAMA. 2016;315(8):775–87. https://doi.org/10.1001/jama.2016.0289.
68. Seymour CW, Liu VX, Iwashyna TJ, Brunkhorst FM, Rea TD, Scherag A, et al. Assessment of clinical criteria for sepsis: for the third international consensus definitions for sepsis and septic shock (sepsis-3). JAMA. 2016;315(8):762–74. https://doi.org/10.1001/jama.2016.0288.
69. Machado FR, Assuncao MS, Cavalcanti AB, Japiassu AM, Azevedo LC, Oliveira MC. Getting a consensus: advantages and disadvantages of Sepsis 3 in the context of middle-income settings. Revista Brasileira de terapia intensiva. 2016;28(4):361–5. https://doi.org/10.5935/0103-507X.20160068.
70. Kaukonen KM, Bailey M, Pilcher D, Cooper DJ, Bellomo R. Systemic inflammatory response syndrome criteria in defining severe sepsis. N Engl J Med. 2015;372(17):1629–38. https://doi.org/10.1056/NEJMoa1415236.
71. Churpek MM, Zadravecz FJ, Winslow C, Howell MD, Edelson DP. Incidence and prognostic value of the systemic inflammatory response syndrome and organ dysfunctions in ward patients. Am J Respir Crit Care Med. 2015;192(8):958–64. https://doi.org/10.1164/rccm.201502-0275OC.
72. Simpson SQ. New sepsis criteria: a change we should not make. Chest. 2016;149(5):1117–8. https://doi.org/10.1016/j.chest.2016.02.653.
73. Ranzani OT, Monteiro MB, Ferreira EM, Santos SR, Machado FR, Noritomi DT, et al. Reclassifying the spectrum of septic patients using lactate: severe sepsis, cryptic shock, vasoplegic shock and dysoxic shock. Revista Brasileira de terapia intensiva. 2013;25(4):270–8. https://doi.org/10.5935/0103-507X.20130047.
74. Besen BA, Romano TG, Nassar AP Jr, Taniguchi LU, Azevedo LC, Mendes PV, et al. Sepsis-3 definitions predict ICU mortality in a low-middle-income country. Ann Intensive Care. 2016;6(1):107. https://doi.org/10.1186/s13613-016-0204-y.
75. Churpek MM, Snyder A, Han X, Sokol S, Pettit N, Howell MD, et al. Quick Sepsis-related Organ Failure Assessment, Systemic Inflammatory Response Syndrome, and Early Warning Scores for Detecting Clinical Deterioration in Infected Patients outside the Intensive Care Unit. Am J Respir Crit Care Med. 2017;195(7):906–11. https://doi.org/10.1164/rccm.201604-0854OC.
76. Finkelsztein EJ, Jones DS, Ma KC, Pabon MA, Delgado T, Nakahira K, et al. Comparison of qSOFA and SIRS for predicting adverse outcomes of patients with suspicion of sepsis outside the intensive care unit. Crit Care. 2017;21(1):73. https://doi.org/10.1186/s13054-017-1658-5.
77. Singer AJ, Ng J, Thode HC Jr, Spiegel R, Weingart S. Quick SOFA scores predict mortality in adult emergency department patients with and without suspected infection. Ann Emerg Med. 2017;69(4):475–9. https://doi.org/10.1016/j.annemergmed.2016.10.007.
78. Henning DJ, Puskarich MA, Self WH, Howell MD, Donnino MW, Yealy DM, et al. An emergency department validation of the SEP-3 sepsis and septic shock definitions and comparison with 1992 consensus definitions. Ann Emerg Med. 2017;70:544–52. https://doi.org/10.1016/j.annemergmed.2017.01.008.
79. Askim A, Moser F, Gustad LT, Stene H, Gundersen M, Asvold BO, et al. Poor performance of quick-SOFA (qSOFA) score in predicting severe sepsis and mortality—a prospective study of

patients admitted with infection to the emergency department. Scand J Trauma Resusc Emerg Med. 2017;25(1):56. https://doi.org/10.1186/s13049-017-0399-4.
80. Freund Y, Lemachatti N, Krastinova E, Van Laer M, Claessens YE, Avondo A, et al. Prognostic accuracy of sepsis-3 criteria for in-hospital mortality among patients with suspected infection presenting to the emergency department. JAMA. 2017;317(3):301–8. https://doi.org/10.1001/jama.2016.20329.
81. Giamarellos-Bourboulis EJ, Tsaganos T, Tsangaris I, Lada M, Routsi C, Sinapidis D, et al. Validation of the new Sepsis-3 definitions: proposal for improvement in early risk identification. Clin Microbiol Infect. 2017;23(2):104–9. https://doi.org/10.1016/j.cmi.2016.11.003.
82. Huson MA, Kalkman R, Grobusch MP, van der Poll T. Predictive value of the qSOFA score in patients with suspected infection in a resource limited setting in Gabon. Travel Med Infect Dis. 2017;15:76–7. https://doi.org/10.1016/j.tmaid.2016.10.014.
83. Chen YX, Wang JY, Guo SB. Use of CRB-65 and quick sepsis-related organ failure assessment to predict site of care and mortality in pneumonia patients in the emergency department: a retrospective study. Crit Care. 2016;20(1):167. https://doi.org/10.1186/s13054-016-1351-0.
84. Machado FR, Westphal GA, Cavalcanti AB, Souza JL, Bossa A, Monteiro MB, Bafi AT, Azevedo LCP. Is qSOFA an adequate tool to identify sepsis? A Brazilian multicenter study. Revista Brasileira de terapia intensiva. 2016;(Suppl. 1):S4.
85. Phua J, Koh Y, Du B, Tang YQ, Divatia JV, Tan CC, et al. Management of severe sepsis in patients admitted to Asian intensive care units: prospective cohort study. BMJ. 2011;342:d3245. https://doi.org/10.1136/bmj.d3245.
86. Na S, Kuan WS, Mahadevan M, Li CH, Shrikhande P, Ray S, et al. Implementation of early goal-directed therapy and the surviving sepsis campaign resuscitation bundle in Asia. Int J Qual Health Care. 2012;24(5):452–62. https://doi.org/10.1093/intqhc/mzs045.
87. Li ZQ, Xi XM, Luo X, Li J, Jiang L. Implementing surviving sepsis campaign bundles in China: a prospective cohort study. Chin Med J (Engl). 2013;126(10):1819–25.
88. Guo Q, Li HY, Li YM, Nong LB, YD X, He GQ, et al. Compliance with severe sepsis bundles and its effect on patient outcomes of severe community-acquired pneumonia in a limited resources country. Arch Med Sci. 2014;10(5):970–8. https://doi.org/10.5114/aoms.2014.46216.
89. Wang Z, Xiong Y, Schorr C, Dellinger RP. Impact of sepsis bundle strategy on outcomes of patients suffering from severe sepsis and septic shock in china. J Emerg Med. 2013;44(4):735–41. https://doi.org/10.1016/j.jemermed.2012.07.084.
90. Mahavanakul W, Nickerson EK, Srisomang P, Teparrukkul P, Lorvinitnun P, Wongyingsinn M, et al. Feasibility of modified surviving sepsis campaign guidelines in a resource-restricted setting based on a cohort study of severe S. aureus sepsis [corrected]. PLoS One. 2012;7(2):e29858. https://doi.org/10.1371/journal.pone.0029858.
91. Apibunyopas Y. Mortality rate among patients with septic shock after implementation of 6-hour sepsis protocol in the emergency department of Thammasat University Hospital. J Med Assoc Thai. 2014;97(Suppl 8):S182–93.
92. Shiramizo SC, Marra AR, Durao MS, Paes AT, Edmond MB, Pavao dos Santos OF. Decreasing mortality in severe sepsis and septic shock patients by implementing a sepsis bundle in a hospital setting. PLoS One. 2011;6(11):e26790. https://doi.org/10.1371/journal.pone.0026790.
93. Westphal GA, Koenig A, Caldeira Filho M, Feijo J, de Oliveira LT, Nunes F, et al. Reduced mortality after the implementation of a protocol for the early detection of severe sepsis. J Crit Care. 2011;26(1):76–81. https://doi.org/10.1016/j.jcrc.2010.08.001.
94. Assuncao MS, Teich V, Shiramizo SC, Araujo DV, Carrera RM, Serpa Neto A, et al. The cost-effectiveness ratio of a managed protocol for severe sepsis. J Crit Care. 2014;29(4):692 e1–6. https://doi.org/10.1016/j.jcrc.2014.03.008.
95. Noritomi DT, Ranzani OT, Monteiro MB, Ferreira EM, Santos SR, Leibel F, et al. Implementation of a multifaceted sepsis education program in an emerging country setting: clinical outcomes and cost-effectiveness in a long-term follow-up study. Intensive Care Med. 2014;40(2):182–91. https://doi.org/10.1007/s00134-013-3131-5.
96. Machado FR, Ferreira EM, Sousa JL, Silva C, Schippers P, Pereira A, et al. Quality improvement initiatives in sepsis in an emerging country: does the institution's main source of income

influence the results? an analysis of 21,103 patients. Crit Care Med. 2017;45(10):1650–9. https://doi.org/10.1097/CCM.0000000000002585.

97. Maitland K, Kiguli S, Opoka RO, Engoru C, Olupot-Olupot P, Akech SO, et al. Mortality after fluid bolus in African children with severe infection. N Engl J Med. 2011;364(26):2483–95. https://doi.org/10.1056/NEJMoa1101549.
98. Andrews B, Muchemwa L, Kelly P, Lakhi S, Heimburger DC, Bernard GR. Simplified severe sepsis protocol: a randomized controlled trial of modified early goal-directed therapy in Zambia. Crit Care Med. 2014;42(11):2315–24. https://doi.org/10.1097/CCM.0000000000000541.
99. Papali A, Eoin West T, Verceles AC, Augustin ME, Nathalie Colas L, Jean-Francois CH, et al. Treatment outcomes after implementation of an adapted WHO protocol for severe sepsis and septic shock in Haiti. J Crit Care. 2017;41:222–8. https://doi.org/10.1016/j.jcrc.2017.05.024.

Sepsis: The Road Ahead

16

Jianfeng Xie and Craig M. Coopersmith

Key Points

- Remarkable progress has been made in understanding the pathophysiology of sepsis.
- New insights into sepsis have not been associated with new treatments for sepsis.
- The road ahead will include improved recognition of sepsis.
- The road ahead will include improved compliance with evidence-based management of sepsis.
- The road ahead will lead to an increased understanding of the global burden of sepsis.
- The road ahead will have increased screening and better methods for identifying sepsis.
- The road ahead will lead to include precision medicine approaches for entry into clinical trials as well as new trial designs for sepsis.
- The road ahead will lead to improvements in the diagnosis of both infection and sepsis.
- The road ahead will lead to a more robust understanding of both organ dysfunction and the dysregulated host response in sepsis.
- Although numerous pathways of discovery will be undertaken, especially promising routes include modulating both the microbiome and the immune system.

J. Xie, M.D.
Department of Critical Care Medicine, Zhongda Hospital, School of Medicine, Southeast University, Nanjing, China
e-mail: jianfeng.xie@emory.edu

C. M. Coopersmith, M.D. (✉)
Department of Surgery and Emory Critical Care Center, Emory University School of Medicine, Atlanta, GA, USA
e-mail: cmcoop3@emory.edu

W. J. Wiersinga, C. W. Seymour (eds.), *Handbook of Sepsis*,
https://doi.org/10.1007/978-3-319-73506-1_16

The term sepsis was first introduced by Hippocrates nearly 2500 years ago to describe the process of decay of organic matter [1]. However, little progress in understanding or treating sepsis occurred until the past 40–50 years. Remarkable progress has been made in understanding the pathophysiology of sepsis during the last few decades, with new insights occurring at an accelerating pace. These insights, however, have not been met with new therapies for sepsis since the only widely accepted treatments for sepsis are rapid antibiotic and fluid administration [2], combined with general supportive care.

This has led to an interesting paradox. More and more patients are getting septic. In the United States, there was an increase of 192% of sepsis as a diagnosis leading to hospital stay between 2005 and 2014 [3]. Whereas in 2005 sepsis was not listed among the top ten principal diagnoses for inpatient stays, in 2014 sepsis was ranked third, behind only pregnancy and newborns/neonates. At the same time, despite an absence of new treatments, the case fatality is decreasing [4–6], presumably related, at least in part, to earlier and increased recognition as well as improved management.

While the road ahead for sepsis will assuredly not be linear, it is nearly a guarantee that patient-centric outcomes will improve over time. The reasons for our optimism lie in two complementary paths—(1) improved recognition and management of sepsis using existing clinical knowledge that has incomplete penetration with practitioners and (2) discovery of new knowledge and translation of both new and existing preclinical insights to the bedside.

16.1 Improving Recognition of Sepsis

There is no question that timely recognition and management of sepsis saves lives. However, for years sepsis was a syndrome which was poorly recognized by many medical professionals and barely recognized (if at all) as even existing by the lay public. Unfortunately, delayed or absent recognition leads to delayed (or worse, no) treatment of sepsis. Fortunately, awareness of sepsis has risen markedly over the last 15 years, with a rapid increase in the slope of both public and professional recognition of sepsis. The reason behind this is multifactorial and will likely set the path for sepsis recognition in the future.

On a professional level, the Surviving Sepsis Campaign has dramatically raised awareness of sepsis in the inpatient setting. The Surviving Sepsis Campaign guidelines, which have been published every 4 years since 2004 [2, 7–9] combined with the campaign's bundles, have been incorporated into healthcare systems throughout the world. The future will lead to an expansion of the campaign's activities with pediatric sepsis guidelines, studies of sepsis in resource-limited nations, studies of sepsis on the hospital wards, and a research arm to determine priorities for future sepsis research. The road ahead will have a much wider audience in healthcare providers across (a) the world, (b) spectrum of resources available, (c) entire spectrum of age, and (d) entire spectrum of healthcare (i.e., not just in the emergency department and ICU but in the outpatient setting, hospital wards, rehabilitation facilities, etc.).

However, the reach of professional societies—while broad—is not unlimited and has dominantly been aimed at healthcare providers. Numerous foundations—many unfortunately borne out of personal tragedy—have been successful in raising the public profile of sepsis, both with the general public and regulatory agencies and legislators who can affect broad-based change in sepsis. These have resulted in a high-profile campaign by the Centers for Disease Control and Prevention aimed toward engaging and educating both providers and the public about sepsis [10]. Similarly, the World Health Organization recently approved a resolution on improving the prevention, diagnosis, and management of sepsis [11].

Further, the concept of sepsis survivorship is in its infancy, and most patients who survive sepsis do not think of themselves as sepsis survivors. Similarly, most of their families and friends do not think of their loved one as a survivor nor do their healthcare providers. This contrasts greatly with other diseases like cancer, where there is a long-standing tradition of patients (and families and providers) thinking of themselves as survivors, years after treatment. There are literally thousands of support groups for cancer. In contrast, currently there are only sporadic pockets of support groups for sepsis, including the recently formed THRIVE initiative from the Society of Critical Care Medicine which seeks to improve patient and family support after critical illness [12].

It is important to note that many sepsis advocacy groups are grassroots organizations and are quite new. The increase in the public profile of sepsis over the last few years has been extraordinary, but there continues to be a marked disconnect between the human suffering and financial costs of sepsis with public recognition of the disease and the massive burden it imposes on society. The future will likely lead to increasingly large organizations working on behalf of sepsis in multiple domains (awareness, regulatory, research, etc.) in a manner not possible with smaller groups. At the same time, it is likely that a positive feedback effect will occur, leading to increasing numbers of advocacy groups, increasing recognition of sepsis survivorship—and thus survivor groups—and a general uptick in public awareness of sepsis.

16.2 Improved Compliance with Evidence-Based Sepsis Guidelines and Bundles

A recent 7.5 year study of nearly 30,000 sepsis patients in over 200 hospitals from the Surviving Sepsis Campaign database demonstrated that for every quarter a hospital participated in the campaign, mortality decreased 0.7% per quarter [5].While association cannot prove causation, this is consistent with a broad-based literature demonstrating that participation in quality improvement initiatives in sepsis is associated with improved outcomes. This study also demonstrated a striking difference in mortality depending on bundle compliance, with 38.6% of patients dying in hospitals with low compliance bundle, compared to 29.0% in hospital with high bundle compliance. While this is very exciting on the surface, a quick look at what constitutes high bundle compliance demonstrates a remarkable opportunity for improvement since performing all elements within the bundle was performed less than 40% of the time in the "high" compliance group. Similarly, compliance is poor in low- and middle-income countries [13, 14] with bundle compliance occurring less than 8% in a study of 150 ICUs in 16 Asian countries. It is difficult to justify how performing all elements of sepsis bundles less than 50% of the time is a desired outcome. Comparing sepsis to other high-acuity, high-intensity conditions, mortality on a per-case basis is significantly higher for sepsis than for myocardial infarction, trauma, or cerebrovascular accident. However, it is difficult to imagine less than half of patients with these life-threatening conditions being treated in a timely fashion. For instance, 93% of patients with ST-segment elevation myocardial infarction in the United States are treated with percutaneous coronary intervention within the recommended 90 min of arrival to the emergency department, with an average door to balloon time of 59 min [15].

The road ahead will assuredly close this chasm between what the literature supports and what is provided at the bedside. The reason for these changes will be multifactorial. Part of this will likely happen organically. Culture change takes years to occur, and as more studies come out on sepsis and public and medical recognition of sepsis increases, attitudes about sepsis truly being an emergency requiring all elements of care to be provided swiftly and accurately will almost certainly increase.

At the same time, these changes may occur more slowly than many would consider acceptable. Based upon this, mandates on sepsis care have begun to be implemented. Starting in 2013, New York State began requiring hospitals to follow protocols for the early identification and treatment of sepsis. A high profile study of 49,331 septic patients from 149 hospitals examined after this mandate demonstrated an 82.5% compliance with sepsis bundles [16]. Whether regulatory mandates for sepsis care are beneficial has been debated with some investigators arguing for caution or more precision before implementing them [17, 18]. Nonetheless, we believe that the road ahead will be met with increased regulations and mandates related to sepsis throughout the world. There are a number of reasons we believe that sepsis management will be the target of increasing regulatory mandates. First, septic shock has a mortality of greater than 40% [19]. The poor bundle compliance in hospitals left to manage sepsis on their own as compared to the markedly higher bundle compliance in hospitals mandated to have a sepsis protocol will almost certainly lead to strong public pressure to have increased regulation. Further, sepsis is the single most expensive hospital condition to treat [20], and it is likely that the results from New York State will engender further efforts from policymakers who could easily see a correlation between earlier and better care and decreased costs.

16.3 Understanding the Global Burden of Sepsis

The best estimate of the global burden of sepsis is that there are 31.5 cases of sepsis and 19.4 million cases of severe sepsis potentially causing 5.3 million deaths annually [21]. These estimates are based upon a total of 27 studies from high-income countries without any population incidence levels in low- and middle-income countries. However confidence in these statistics is relatively low considering that 87% of the world's population lives in low- and middle-income countries and the fact that sepsis is treated as a "garbage code" in the Global Burden of Disease statistics, where most deaths from sepsis are classified as being caused by the underlying infection, rather than from sepsis [11].

Even in higher-income countries, it is still unclear how many people have sepsis and how many people die from the disease. For instance, in the United States, most recent estimates state that between 894,000 and 3.1 million people develop sepsis with between 230,000 and 370,000 dying from the disease each year, depending on which of four different techniques were used to identify septic patients [22]. This differs markedly from an estimate of 146,000–159,000 deaths from using death certificate data generated by a Centers for Disease Control and Prevention database [23] in the United States and even more markedly from an estimate of under 39,000 deaths from "septicemia" from the National Vital Statistics in the same country in 2014 [24].

Thus the current situation leaves both healthcare professionals and the general public without a clear understanding of how many people get septic and how many people die from the disease. The road ahead will assuredly help to clarify this situation. The effort to do so will likely be multifactorial and will depend upon issues ranging from which population is studied to which definition of sepsis is used. As outlined above, as public awareness of sepsis rises worldwide, it will likely be unacceptable to have essentially no understanding of the burden of sepsis in low- and middle-income countries, which will likely lead to efforts to quantify this. Similarly, in higher-income countries, a greater degree of accuracy will likely be demanded, which will result in more refined estimates.

There are multiple methods in which the burden of sepsis can be calculated. These include (but are not limited to) administrative claims data for ICD-9 or ICD-10 code for infection, for organ dysfunction, or for a severe sepsis code or via death certificates [22, 23, 25–28]. Each technique has its own advantages and disadvantages, which is related to a broader discussion as to the intended use of sepsis diagnostic criteria. An intellectual framework by Seymour et al. identified five different purposes of sepsis diagnostic criteria—clinical care, clinical research, basic research, surveillance and epidemiology, and quality improvement and audit [29, 30]. It is likely that the road ahead will offer a richer and more diverse array of sepsis diagnostic criteria, depending on the indication examined. This will have the advantage of giving deeper and more robust information depending on the question asked, but may unfortunately lead to confusion, where multiple definitions and criteria for sepsis exist [31–34].

16.4 Sepsis Definitions, Clinical Criteria, and Screening Criteria

The definition of sepsis has evolved greatly from the time of Hippocrates. The well-known 1991 definitions included the spectrum of sepsis, severe sepsis, and septic shock in the setting of the systemic inflammatory response syndrome with suspected infection with organ dysfunction and hypotension refractory to fluid resuscitation for the latter two entities [32]. A revised version in 2001 further defined organ dysfunction but did not fundamentally change the definition [35]. While the definition served the medical community well for a quarter of a century, it was subjected to numerous criticisms. Many of these centered on the very nonspecific systemic inflammatory response syndrome, since almost half of all patients develop this in the hospital without being septic and 1/8 of patients die with sepsis without having this [36–38]. Further, the definitions were not a traditional definition, which per the dictionary expresses the essential nature of something or describes what something is. Much like the essence of a myocardial if not an elevated troponin (which is instead a bedside test used as part of clinical diagnosis), the essence of sepsis is unlikely to be an elevated heart rate and temperature in the setting of suspected infection.

Based upon these, the Sepsis 3 definitions were published in 2016 [33]. There has been significant confusion between the clinical criteria used to diagnose sepsis (much like troponin in myocardial infarction) and screening criteria used to potentially identify septic patients who will have a prolonged ICU stay or die and the actual definition. The definition of sepsis is life-threatening organ dysfunction caused by a dysregulated host response to infection. This is an intellectual construct that is the best method we have today of understanding what sepsis is. This is distinct from the clinical criteria used for identifying sepsis—a sequential organ failure assessment (SOFA) score ≥ 2 in the setting of suspected infection [33]. It is also distinct from a screening test that can be done (most successfully outside the ICU)—qSOFA—which examines respiratory rate, blood pressure, and mental status [39]. The clinical criteria and qSOFA have the subject of significant academic debate [40–43]. In contrast, the actual definition of sepsis has received near uniform praise as an intellectual construct.

In charting the road forward, it is best to separate the clinical criteria and screening criteria from the definition as the former are perhaps more tangible and certainly have a more narrow scope than the latter. The SOFA score was first described in 1996 to describe organ dysfunction and failure in sepsis [44]. It has reliably been used in critical care, and delta SOFA (rather than fixed-day SOFA) has been shown to be reliably and consistently associated with mortality in randomized controlled trials [45]. While SOFA has been—and continues to be—of tremendous utility, it also incorporates elements not typically used in sepsis management such as "renal dose" dopamine. In addition, with the advent of big data and complex systems analysis, it is likely that further refinements in either the SOFA score or a different scoring system for sepsis will likely be more accurate in the future. Since the publication of Sepsis 3, there has been a concerted effort to validate qSOFA as a screening tool both outside and inside the ICU and in different socioeconomic environments [46–51]. It is likely that the future will bring numerous studies demonstrating where and when qSOFA has utility for bedside providers and that subsequent analyses will lead to more accurate predictive criteria.

16.5 Precision Medicine and Trial Design

Implicit in most trials to date is the assumption that all sepsis patients are the same (or similar) and that there is a common host response. All along as a patient has the diagnosis of sepsis, they have been enrolled in clinical trials—independent of the initiating microorganism, the patient's underlying genetics or comorbidities, the patient's host response, the severity of disease, etc. In some ways, this strategy of enrolling all comers is analogous to enrolling patients with cancer (regardless of the cell type or stage) into a clinical trial.

It is nearly a given, however, that all septic patients are not the same, and strategies that might be effective in one patient population would be ineffective or harmful in a different patient population of septic patients. There is significant preclinical literature demonstrating that the identical intervention can have significant differences in efficacy depending on a variety of host variables [52–57]. Further, there is emerging data that endotypes exist in which patients have a different and disparate response to sepsis [58–60]. Further, while IL-1 receptor antagonist fails to improve 28-day survival in septic patients, a reanalysis of this same phase 3 trial demonstrated significantly reduced mortality in a subgroup patients with macrophage activation syndrome [61]. In the future, a multipronged engine aimed at precision has been proposed including (a) optimizing patient stratification and identifying potential targets; (b) running in silico trials, confirming targets, and examining and refining mechanisms in both cells and rodents; and (c) evaluating large mammal, which then loops back on optimizing patient stratification [62]. The road ahead will assuredly look more similar to oncology where patients are enrolled in clinical trials based upon molecular signatures and/or "omics" (genomics, transcriptomics, proteomics, or metabolomics) criteria as well as related criteria.

The gold standard study to date in sepsis has generally been considered to the randomized controlled trial using mortality as an endpoint. However, it is likely sepsis trials in the future will look quite different. Randomized trials are inefficient in that they only examine two groups. In contrast, adaptive trial design can increase trial efficiency by discarding ineffective doses or drugs or by increasing arms with a higher likelihood of success [63]. Trial designs can use either predictive enrichment with patients based on likelihood of treatment response independent of disease severity or prognostic enrichment with a patient population at high risk of outcome event (or both) [64]. Further, while short to intermediate mortality is obviously an important outcome in sepsis, it is not the only potential outcome of interest, especially with increased understanding of the burden of sepsis long after patients leave the ICU. There are multiple other patient-centric outcomes that will likely be examined in the road ahead including those within the ICU (ventilator days, pressor days, length of stay), within the hospital (length of stay), and beyond the ICU since septic patients have been shown to have long-term functional disabilities [65], cognitive decline, [66, 67] and healthcare usage [68, 69].

16.6 Sepsis 3 and the Road Ahead for Diagnosing Sepsis

The new definition of sepsis contains four distinct components—(a) life-threatening, (b) organ dysfunction, (c) dysregulated host response, and (d) suspected infection. The definition of life-threatening is subjective, but the details of how to predict this are generally covered above. Infection is generally suspected by nonspecific findings such as altered temperature and white blood cell count and less commonly by organ dysfunction without a clear etiology. This leaves a large opportunity for the future in that in many ways, the manner in which infection is either suspected or diagnosed has not changed in decades, resulting in the very real limitation of lack of specificity for suspecting infection and lack of both accuracy and timeliness in diagnosing infection. For example, blood cultures are positive in approximately one third of septic patients [70], and half of septic patients are culture negative [71]. Further, those that are culture positive require a time frame of days for full sensitivities to result after samples are manually streaked on an agar plate. This has significant implications for antibiotic stewardship and also can cause delays in therapy—associated with increased mortality—if initial broad-spectrum antibiotics are not effective against the pathogen that is ultimately cultured. While Sepsis 3 intentionally did not comment on the definition of infection [33], the road forward will almost certainly result in both more accurate diagnosis of infection and the capacity to diagnose infection in a much shorter time frame than is commonly done at the bedside. Although an overview of advances in diagnostic microbiology is outside the scope of this chapter, it is important to note that numerous rapid microbial pathogen tests using modern technology are being developed and tested in patients which can identify pathogens more accurately and rapidly than current techniques [72–78].

Complementary to more rapid and effective diagnosis of infection is more rapid and effective diagnosis of sepsis. Since earlier therapy of sepsis has been associated with improved outcomes, it stands to reason that if sepsis can be diagnosed (and hence treated) before signs and symptoms are obvious to the healthcare team, many of the more morbid complications of sepsis can potentially be attenuated or even prevented. Analysis of "big data" for patterns within easily accessible data that are not obvious to the bedside practitioner is a field that is in its infancy but holds tremendous promise. A few recent studies have demonstrated that it is feasible to predict sepsis prior to clinical manifestations occurring. For instance, using routinely available physiologic and laboratory data from ICU patients, a targeted real-time early warning score identified patients before the onset of septic shock with an area under the curve ROC of 0.83. Further, with a specificity of 0.67, this score achieved a sensitivity of 0.85 and identified patients a median of 28.2 h before onset, of which two thirds were identified before any sepsis-related organ dysfunction [79]. Similarly, a machine learning approach using multivariable combinations of easily obtained data was superior to other sepsis screening tools both in detecting sepsis at onset and 1–4 h preceding sepsis onset, even when 60% of input data was missing [80]. In addition, a point-of-care microfluidic biochip for quantification of CD64 expression on only 10 microliters of whole blood when combined with measurements from the electronic medical record showed utility for improved sepsis diagnosis [81]. The road ahead will almost certainly incorporate "big data" and complex systems into predictive algorithms that will transform the way sepsis is identified.

16.7 Sepsis 3 and the Road Ahead for Organ Dysfunction and Host Response

Blood pressure, mental status, platelet count, and creatinine are commonly assessed at the bedside as surrogates of cardiovascular, brain, hematologic, and renal function. While there is obvious utility to examining gross organ dysfunction, it is likely that we are missing insights on a cellular or subcellular level that might be critical in understanding or treating sepsis. For instance, it is likely that intracellular bioenergetics, cell death (apoptosis, necrosis, pyroptosis, autophagy), barrier function, and functional status of cells (activated, naive, memory, exhausted, etc.) play a role in determining organ function or dysfunction. The tools for measuring each of these currently exist in animal models, and some are being used experimentally in patients. The transition of understanding and measurement of organ dysfunction to a more cellular and subcellular level will likely occur in the intermediate to long-term future as deeper understanding of these (and many other) processes reach maturity and real-time assays allow their measurement at the bedside. Similarly, measuring a dysregulated host response (as opposed to an adaptive regulated host response) is currently impossible at the bedside. A tremendous number of possibilities exist for monitoring and modulating both organ function and the host response to infection that are outside the scope of this chapter; however, we will briefly highlight two especially promising areas of research that will guide the road ahead in sepsis.

One promising road for modulation is the microbiome. The microbiome is the ecological community of microorganisms that reside in the whole body. The most intensively studied branch is the gut microbiome which consists of 40 trillion microbes, as many cells as we have in our bodies [82]. Within 6 h of the onset of sepsis [83], the microbiome is converted into the "pathobiome" [84, 85] which is highlighted by (a) a loss of microbial diversity, (b) dominance of pathogenic microorganisms, and (c) alterations in bacteria present to become more virulent [86, 87]. In addition, ICU treatment or conditions (antibiotics, vasoactive drugs, fasting or altered nutrition) can also disrupt the microbiome. Together, these induce extremely low microbial diversity which is associated with worse outcomes in sepsis patients [84–86]. Numerous studies have been done altering the microbiome in the ICU—with strategies ranging from probiotics to fecal microbial transplant to selective decontamination of the digestive system [88–95]. Each of these has been demonstrated to improve patient-centric outcomes such as ventilator-associated pneumonia, diarrhea, and mortality. However, our understanding of the microbiome is still very much in the nascent stage. The road ahead will allow us to understand our inner microbial community on a cellular and subcellular level and how to potentially modulate this community in a precision manner to improve outcomes in a more targeted, mechanistic method.

Another promising treatment is immunomodulation. Historically, many trials have attempted to decrease the pro-inflammatory response in sepsis. While this approach has often been successful in preclinical trials of inbred mice when the precise time of onset of sepsis is known, they have generally been unsuccessful in septic patients [96]. However, recent data suggests that immune cells are exhausted in sepsis, with increased levels of multiple co-inhibitory markers such as PD-1, CTLA-4, BLA, and 2B4 in both animal studies and septic patients [97–103]. This can lead to secondary infection in the immunosuppressive stage of sepsis, which is a common cause of late death in sepsis [104, 105]. Notably, co-inhibitor blockade is associated with improved survival in multiple preclinical models of sepsis. While clinical trials examining co-inhibitory blockade in septic patients are just beginning to enroll patients, immune augmentation represents an attractive strategy in the future for sepsis. Further, a better understanding of a patient's immune status (pro-inflammatory, anti-inflammatory, exhausted, immunosuppressed, etc.) on an ongoing basis will likely allow for targeted immunotherapy.

Reference

1. Marshall JC. Sepsis: rethinking the approach to clinical research. J Leukoc Biol. 2008;83(3):471–82.
2. Rhodes A, Evans LE, Alhazzani W, et al. Surviving sepsis campaign: international guidelines for management of sepsis and septic shock: 2016. Crit Care Med. 2017;45(3):486–552.
3. McDermott KW, Elixhauser A, Sun R. Trends in Hospital Inpatient Stays in the United States, 2005–2014. Healthcare cost and utilization project (HCUP) 2017;Available from: https://www.hcup-us.ahrq.gov/reports/statbriefs/sb225-Inpatient-US-Stays-Trends.jsp.
4. Kaukonen KM, Bailey M, Suzuki S, et al. Mortality related to severe sepsis and septic shock among critically ill patients in Australia and New Zealand, 2000–2012. JAMA. 2014;311(13):1308–16.
5. Levy MM, Rhodes A, Phillips GS, et al. Surviving sepsis campaign: association between performance metrics and outcomes in a 7.5-year study. Crit Care Med. 2015;43(1):3–12.
6. Seymour CW, Rea TD, Kahn JM, et al. Severe sepsis in pre-hospital emergency care: analysis of incidence, care, and outcome. Am J Respir Crit Care Med. 2012;186(12):1264–71.
7. Dellinger RP, Carlet JM, Masur H, et al. Surviving sepsis campaign guidelines for management of severe sepsis and septic shock. Crit Care Med. 2004;32(3):858–73.
8. Dellinger RP, Levy MM, Carlet JM, et al. Surviving Sepsis Campaign: international guidelines for management of severe sepsis and septic shock: 2008. Crit Care Med. 2008;36(1):296–327.
9. Dellinger RP, Levy MM, Rhodes A, et al. Surviving sepsis campaign: international guidelines for management of severe sepsis and septic shock: 2012. Crit Care Med. 2013;41(2):580–637.
10. Making health care safer—think sepsis. Time matters. https://www.cdcgov/vitalsigns/sepsis/2017. Accessed 1 Aug 2017.
11. Reinhart K, Daniels R, Kissoon N, et al. Recognizing sepsis as a global health priority—a WHO resolution. N Engl J Med. 2017;377:414–7.
12. THRIVE. Society of Critical Care Medicine 2017. Available from: http://www.myicucare.org/thrive/Pages/default.aspx. Accessed 1 Aug 2017.
13. Phua J, Koh Y, Du B, et al. Management of severe sepsis in patients admitted to Asian intensive care units: prospective cohort study. BMJ. 2011;342:d3245.
14. Levy MM, Artigas A, Phillips GS, et al. Outcomes of the surviving sepsis campaign in intensive care units in the USA and Europe: a prospective cohort study. Lancet Infect Dis. 2012;12(12):919–24.

15. Masoudi FA, Ponirakis A, de Lemos JA, et al. Executive summary: trends in U.S. cardiovascular care: 2016 report From 4 ACC national cardiovascular data registries. J Am Coll Cardiol. 2017;69(11):1424–6.
16. Seymour CW, Gesten F, Prescott HC, et al. Time to treatment and mortality during mandated emergency care for sepsis. N Engl J Med. 2017;376(23):2235–44.
17. Rhee C, Gohil S, Klompas M. Regulatory mandates for sepsis care—reasons for caution. N Engl J Med. 2014;370(18):1673–6.
18. Klompas M, Rhee C. The CMS sepsis mandate: right disease, wrong measure. Ann Intern Med. 2016;165(7):517–8.
19. Shankar-Hari M, Phillips GS, Levy ML, et al. Developing a new definition and assessing new clinical criteria for septic shock: for the third international consensus definitions for sepsis and septic shock (sepsis-3). JAMA. 2016;315(8):775–87.
20. Torio CM, Andrews RM. National inpatient hospital costs: the most expensive conditions by payer, 2011. Statistical Brief #160. 2006 February.
21. Fleischmann C, Scherag A, Adhikari NK, et al. Assessment of global incidence and mortality of hospital-treated sepsis. Current estimates and limitations. Am J Respir Crit Care Med. 2016;193(3):259–72.
22. Gaieski DF, Edwards JM, Kallan MJ, et al. Benchmarking the incidence and mortality of severe sepsis in the United States. Crit Care Med. 2013;41(5):1167–74.
23. Epstein L, Dantes R, Magill S, et al. Varying estimates of sepsis mortality using death certificates and administrative codes—United States, 1999–2014. MMWR Morb Mortal Wkly Rep. 2016;65(13):342–5.
24. Kochanek KD, Murphy SL, Xu J, et al. Deaths: final data for 2014. Natl Vital Stat Rep. 2016;65(4):1–122.
25. Angus DC, Linde-Zwirble WT, Lidicker J, et al. Epidemiology of severe sepsis in the United States: analysis of incidence, outcome, and associated costs of care. Crit Care Med. 2001;29(7):1303–10.
26. Martin GS, Mannino DM, Eaton S, et al. The epidemiology of sepsis in the United States from 1979 through 2000. N Engl J Med. 2003;348(16):1546–54.
27. Dombrovskiy VY, Martin AA, Sunderram J, et al. Rapid increase in hospitalization and mortality rates for severe sepsis in the United States: a trend analysis from 1993 to 2003. Crit Care Med. 2007;35(5):1244–50.
28. Wang HE, Shapiro NI, Angus DC, et al. National estimates of severe sepsis in United States emergency departments. Crit Care Med. 2007;35(8):1928–36.
29. Seymour CW, Coopersmith CM, Deutschman CS, et al. Application of a framework to assess the usefulness of alternative sepsis criteria. Crit Care Med. 2016;44(3):e122–30.
30. Angus DC, Seymour CW, Coopersmith CM, et al. A framework for the development and interpretation of different sepsis definitions and clinical criteria. Crit Care Med. 2016;44(3):e113–21.
31. Rhee C, Kadri S, Huang SS, et al. Objective sepsis surveillance using electronic clinical data. Infect Control Hosp Epidemiol. 2016;37(2):163–71.
32. Bone RC, Balk RA, Cerra FB, et al. Definitions for sepsis and organ failure and guidelines for the use of innovative therapies in sepsis. The ACCP/SCCM Consensus Conference Committee. American College of Chest Physicians/Society of Critical Care Medicine. Chest. 1992;101(6):1644–55.
33. Singer M, Deutschman CS, Seymour CW, et al. The third international consensus definitions for sepsis and septic shock (sepsis-3). JAMA. 2016;315(8):801–10.
34. Frohlich S, Murphy N, Doolan A, et al. Acute respiratory distress syndrome: underrecognition by clinicians. J Crit Care. 2013;28(5):663–8.
35. Levy MM, Fink MP, Marshall JC, et al. 2001 SCCM/ESICM/ACCP/ATS/SIS international sepsis definitions conference. Crit Care Med. 2003;31(4):1250–6.
36. Churpek MM, Zadravecz FJ, Winslow C, et al. Incidence and prognostic value of the systemic inflammatory response syndrome and organ dysfunctions in ward patients. Am J Respir Crit Care Med. 2015;192(8):958–64.

37. Kaukonen KM, Bailey M, Pilcher D, et al. Systemic inflammatory response syndrome criteria in defining severe sepsis. N Engl J Med. 2015;372(17):1629–38.
38. Vincent JL. Dear SIRS, I'm sorry to say that I don't like you. Crit Care Med. 1997;25(2):372–4.
39. Seymour CW, Liu VX, Iwashyna TJ, et al. Assessment of clinical criteria for sepsis: for the third international consensus definitions for sepsis and septic shock (sepsis-3). JAMA. 2016;315(8):762–74.
40. Sprung CL, Schein RM, Balk RA. The new sepsis consensus definitions: the good, the bad and the ugly. Intensive Care Med. 2016;42(12):2024–6.
41. Simpson SQ. New sepsis criteria: a change we should not make. Chest. 2016;149(5):1117–8.
42. Bhattacharjee P, Edelson DP, Churpek MM. Identifying patients with sepsis on the hospital wards. Chest. 2017;151(4):898–907.
43. Abraham E. New definitions for sepsis and septic shock: continuing evolution but with much still to be done. JAMA. 2016;315(8):757–9.
44. Vincent JL, Moreno R, Takala J, et al. The SOFA (Sepsis-related Organ Failure Assessment) score to describe organ dysfunction/failure. On behalf of the Working Group on Sepsis-Related Problems of the European Society of Intensive Care Medicine. Intensive Care Med. 1996;22(7):707–10.
45. de Grooth HJ, Geenen IL, Girbes AR, et al. SOFA and mortality endpoints in randomized controlled trials: a systematic review and meta-regression analysis. Crit Care. 2017;21(1):38.
46. Raith EP, Udy AA, Bailey M, et al. Prognostic accuracy of the SOFA score, SIRS criteria, and qSOFA score for in-hospital mortality among adults with suspected infection admitted to the intensive care unit. JAMA. 2017;317(3):290–300.
47. Freund Y, Lemachatti N, Krastinova E, et al. Prognostic accuracy of sepsis-3 criteria for in-hospital mortality among patients with suspected infection presenting to the emergency department. JAMA. 2017;317(3):301–8.
48. Churpek MM, Snyder A, Han X, et al. Quick sepsis-related organ failure assessment, systemic inflammatory response syndrome, and early warning scores for detecting clinical deterioration in infected patients outside the intensive care unit. Am J Respir Crit Care Med. 2017;195(7):906–11.
49. Forward E, Konecny P, Burston J, et al. Predictive validity of the qSOFA criteria for sepsis in non-ICU inpatients. Intensive Care Med. 2017;43(6):945–6.
50. Finkelsztein EJ, Jones DS, Ma KC, et al. Comparison of qSOFA and SIRS for predicting adverse outcomes of patients with suspicion of sepsis outside the intensive care unit. Crit Care. 2017;21(1):73.
51. Donnelly JP, Safford MM, Shapiro NI, et al. Application of the third international consensus definitions for sepsis (sepsis-3) classification: a retrospective population-based cohort study. Lancet Infect Dis. 2017;17(6):661–70.
52. Liang Z, Xie Y, Dominguez JA, et al. Intestine-specific deletion of microsomal triglyceride transfer protein increases mortality in aged mice. PLoS One. 2014;9(7):e101828.
53. Dominguez JA, Xie Y, Dunne WM, et al. Intestine-specific Mttp deletion decreases mortality and prevents sepsis-induced intestinal injury in a murine model of Pseudomonas aeruginosa pneumonia. PLoS One. 2012;7(11):e49159.
54. Csoka B, Nemeth ZH, Mukhopadhyay P, et al. CB2 cannabinoid receptors contribute to bacterial invasion and mortality in polymicrobial sepsis. PLoS One. 2009;4(7):e6409.
55. Tschop J, Kasten KR, Nogueiras R, et al. The cannabinoid receptor 2 is critical for the host response to sepsis. J Immunol. 2009;183(1):499–505.
56. Rios-Santos F, Benjamim CF, Zavery D, et al. A critical role of leukotriene B4 in neutrophil migration to infectious focus in cecal ligation and puncture sepsis. Shock. 2003;19(1):61–5.
57. Eichacker PQ, Parent C, Kalil A, et al. Risk and the efficacy of antiinflammatory agents: retrospective and confirmatory studies of sepsis. Am J Respir Crit Care Med. 2002;166(9):1197–205.
58. Grunwell JR, Weiss SL, Cvijanovich NZ, et al. Differential expression of the Nrf2-linked genes in pediatric septic shock. Crit Care. 2015;19:327.

59. Wong HR, Cvijanovich NZ, Anas N, et al. Developing a clinically feasible personalized medicine approach to pediatric septic shock. Am J Respir Crit Care Med. 2015;191(3):309–15.
60. Wong HR, Cvijanovich NZ, Anas N, et al. Prospective testing and redesign of a temporal biomarker based risk model for patients with septic shock: implications for septic shock biology. EBioMedicine. 2015;2(12):2087–93.
61. Shakoory B, Carcillo JA, Chatham WW, et al. Interleukin-1 receptor blockade is associated with reduced mortality in sepsis patients with features of macrophage activation syndrome: reanalysis of a prior phase III trial. Crit Care Med. 2016;44(2):275–81.
62. Buchman TG, Billiar TR, Elster E, et al. Precision medicine for critical illness and injury. Crit Care Med. 2016;44(9):1635–8.
63. Perner A, Gordon AC, Angus DC, et al. The intensive care medicine research agenda on septic shock. Intensive Care Med. 2017;43:1294–305.
64. Shankar-Hari M, Rubenfeld GD. The use of enrichment to reduce statistically indeterminate or negative trials in critical care. Anaesthesia. 2017;72(5):560–5.
65. Yende S, Austin S, Rhodes A, et al. Long-term quality of life among survivors of severe sepsis: analyses of two international trials. Crit Care Med. 2016;44(8):1461–7.
66. Annane D, Sharshar T. Cognitive decline after sepsis. Lancet Respir Med. 2015;3(1):61–9.
67. Heming N, Mazeraud A, Verdonk F, et al. Neuroanatomy of sepsis-associated encephalopathy. Crit Care. 2017;21(1):65.
68. Goodwin AJ, Rice DA, Simpson KN, et al. Frequency, cost, and risk factors of readmissions among severe sepsis survivors. Crit Care Med. 2015;43(4):738–46.
69. Prescott HC, Langa KM, Liu V, et al. Increased 1-year healthcare use in survivors of severe sepsis. Am J Respir Crit Care Med. 2014;190(1):62–9.
70. Bochud PY, Bonten M, Marchetti O, et al. Antimicrobial therapy for patients with severe sepsis and septic shock: an evidence-based review. Crit Care Med. 2004;32(11 Suppl):S495–512.
71. Gupta S, Sakhuja A, Kumar G, et al. Culture-negative severe sepsis: nationwide trends and outcomes. Chest. 2016;150(6):1251–9.
72. Vincent JL, Brealey D, Libert N, et al. Rapid diagnosis of infection in the critically Ill, a multicenter study of molecular detection in bloodstream infections, pneumonia, and sterile site infections. Crit Care Med. 2015;43(11):2283–91.
73. Clerc O, Prod'hom G, Vogne C, et al. Impact of matrix-assisted laser desorption ionization time-of-flight mass spectrometry on the clinical management of patients with Gram-negative bacteremia: a prospective observational study. Clin Infect Dis. 2013;56(8):1101–7.
74. Clerc O, Prod'hom G, Senn L, et al. Matrix-assisted laser desorption ionization time-of-flight mass spectrometry and PCR-based rapid diagnosis of Staphylococcus aureus bacteraemia. Clin Microbiol Infect. 2014;20(4):355–60.
75. Huang AM, Newton D, Kunapuli A, et al. Impact of rapid organism identification via matrix-assisted laser desorption/ionization time-of-flight combined with antimicrobial stewardship team intervention in adult patients with bacteremia and candidemia. Clin Infect Dis. 2013;57(9):1237–45.
76. Cambau E, Durand-Zaleski I, Bretagne S, et al. Performance and economic evaluation of the molecular detection of pathogens for patients with severe infections: the EVAMICA open-label, cluster-randomised, interventional crossover trial. Intensive Care Med. 2017;43(11):1616–25.
77. Buehler SS, Madison B, Snyder SR, et al. Effectiveness of practices to increase timeliness of providing targeted therapy for inpatients with bloodstream infections: a laboratory medicine best practices systematic review and meta-analysis. Clin Microbiol Rev. 2016;29(1):59–103.
78. Timbrook TT, Morton JB, McConeghy KW, et al. The effect of molecular rapid diagnostic testing on clinical outcomes in bloodstream infections: a systematic review and meta-analysis. Clin Infect Dis. 2017;64(1):15–23.
79. Henry KE, Hager DN, Pronovost PJ, et al. A targeted real-time early warning score (TREWScore) for septic shock. Sci Transl Med. 2015;7(299):299ra122.

80. Desautels T, Calvert J, Hoffman J, et al. Prediction of sepsis in the intensive care unit with minimal electronic health record data: a machine learning approach. JMIR Med Inform. 2016;4(3):e28.
81. Hassan U, Ghonge T, Reddy B Jr, et al. A point-of-care microfluidic biochip for quantification of CD64 expression from whole blood for sepsis stratification. Nat Commun. 2017;8:15949.
82. Sender R, Fuchs S, Milo R. Are we really vastly outnumbered? Revisiting the ratio of bacterial to host cells in humans. Cell. 2016;164(3):337–40.
83. Hayakawa M, Asahara T, Henzan N, et al. Dramatic changes of the gut flora immediately after severe and sudden insults. Dig Dis Sci. 2011;56(8):2361–5.
84. Krezalek MA, Defazio J, Zaborina O, et al. The shift of an intestinal "microbiome" to a "pathobiome" governs the course and outcome of sepsis following surgical injury. Shock. 2016;45(5):475–82.
85. Alverdy JC, Krezalek MA. Collapse of the microbiome, emergence of the pathobiome, and the immunopathology of sepsis. Crit Care Med. 2017;45(2):337–47.
86. McDonald D, Ackermann G, Khailova L, et al. Extreme dysbiosis of the microbiome in critical illness. mSphere. 2016;1(4):e00199-16.
87. Lankelma JM, van Vught LA, Belzer C, et al. Critically ill patients demonstrate large interpersonal variation in intestinal microbiota dysregulation: a pilot study. Intensive Care Med. 2017;43:59–68.
88. Price R, Maclennan G, Glen J. Selective digestive or oropharyngeal decontamination and topical oropharyngeal chlorhexidine for prevention of death in general intensive care: systematic review and network meta-analysis. BMJ. 2014;348:g2197.
89. Manzanares W, Lemieux M, Langlois PL, et al. Probiotic and synbiotic therapy in critical illness: a systematic review and meta-analysis. Crit Care. 2016;19:262.
90. Li Q, Wang C, Tang C, et al. Successful treatment of severe sepsis and diarrhea after vagotomy utilizing fecal microbiota transplantation: a case report. Crit Care. 2015;19:37.
91. Wei Y, Yang J, Wang J, et al. Successful treatment with fecal microbiota transplantation in patients with multiple organ dysfunction syndrome and diarrhea following severe sepsis. Crit Care. 2016;20(1):332.
92. Fay KT, Ford ML, Coopersmith CM. The intestinal microenvironment in sepsis. Biochim Biophys Acta. 2017;1863:2574–83.
93. Klingensmith NJ, Coopersmith CM. The gut as the motor of multiple organ dysfunction in critical illness. Crit Care Clin. 2016;32(2):203–12.
94. Meng M, Klingensmith NJ, Coopersmith CM. New insights into the gut as the driver of critical illness and organ failure. Curr Opin Crit Care. 2017;23(2):143–8.
95. Lyons JD, Coopersmith CM. Pathophysiology of the gut and the microbiome in the host response. Pediatr Crit Care Med, 2017. 18(3_suppl Suppl 1):S46–9.
96. Stortz JA, Raymond SL, Mira JC, et al. Murine models of sepsis and trauma: can we bridge the gap? ILAR J. 2017;58:1–16.
97. Boomer JS, Shuherk-Shaffer J, Hotchkiss RS, et al. A prospective analysis of lymphocyte phenotype and function over the course of acute sepsis. Crit Care. 2012;16(3):R112.
98. Brahmamdam P, Inoue S, Unsinger J, et al. Delayed administration of anti-PD-1 antibody reverses immune dysfunction and improves survival during sepsis. J Leukoc Biol. 2010;88(2):233–40.
99. Chang K, Svabek C, Vazquez-Guillamet C, et al. Targeting the programmed cell death 1: programmed cell death ligand 1 pathway reverses T cell exhaustion in patients with sepsis. Crit Care. 2014;18(1):R3.
100. Chang KC, Burnham CA, Compton SM, et al. Blockade of the negative co-stimulatory molecules PD-1 and CTLA-4 improves survival in primary and secondary fungal sepsis. Crit Care. 2013;17(3):R85.
101. Shubin NJ, Chung CS, Heffernan DS, et al. BTLA expression contributes to septic morbidity and mortality by inducing innate inflammatory cell dysfunction. J Leukoc Biol. 2012;92(3):593–603.

102. Shubin NJ, Monaghan SF, Heffernan DS, et al. B and T lymphocyte attenuator expression on CD4+ T-cells associates with sepsis and subsequent infections in ICU patients. Crit Care. 2013;17(6):R276.
103. Chen CW, Mittal R, Klingensmith NJ, et al. Cutting edge: 2B4-mediated coinhibition of CD4+ T cells underlies mortality in experimental sepsis. J Immunol. 2017;199:1961–6.
104. Delano MJ, Ward PA. Sepsis-induced immune dysfunction: can immune therapies reduce mortality? J Clin Invest. 2016;126(1):23–31.
105. van Vught LA, Klein Klouwenberg PM, Spitoni C, et al. Incidence, risk factors, and attributable mortality of secondary infections in the intensive care unit after admission for sepsis. JAMA. 2016;315(14):1469–79.

MIX
Papier aus verantwortungsvollen Quellen
Paper from responsible sources
FSC® C105338

If you have any concerns about our products,
you can contact us on
ProductSafety@springernature.com

In case Publisher is established outside the EU,
the EU authorized representative is:
Springer Nature Customer Service Center GmbH
Europaplatz 3, 69115 Heidelberg, Germany

Printed by Libri Plureos GmbH
in Hamburg, Germany